Methods and Techniques in Chinese Medicine

Methods and Techniques in Chinese Medicine

Edited by **Penelope Williams**

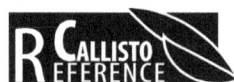

R CALLISTO REFERENCE

New York

Published by Callisto Reference,
106 Park Avenue, Suite 200,
New York, NY 10016, USA
www.callistoreference.com

Methods and Techniques in Chinese Medicine
Edited by Penelope Williams

International Standard Book Number: 978-1-63239-738-6 (Hardback)

Contents

Preface

This book has been a concerted effort by a group of academicians, researchers and scientists, who have contributed their research works for the realization of the book. This book has materialized in the wake of emerging advancements and innovations in this field. Therefore, the need of the hour was to compile all the required researches and disseminate the knowledge to a broad spectrum of people comprising of students, researchers and specialists of the field.

This book traces the progress in the field of chinese medicine and highlights some of its key concepts and applications. It elucidates the theories and innovative techniques around prospective developments with respect to this field. Chinese medicine refers to the system of treatment which uses the traditional methods like acupuncture, massage, exercise, herbal medicine, etc. It is based on the special terms of 'qi' known as life force or energy and uses this concept to treat mind, body and spirit. This text includes topics of utmost significance, which are bound to provide incredible insights to the readers about the interesting concepts in the field of chinese medicine. It aims to present researches that have transformed this discipline and has aided its advancement. Those with an interest in this area would find this book beneficial.

At the end of the preface, I would like to thank the authors for their brilliant chapters and the publisher for guiding us all-through the making of the book till its final stage. Also, I would like to thank my family for providing the support and encouragement throughout my academic career and research projects.

Editor

Long-Term Treatment with an Herbal Formula MCC Ameliorates Obesity-Associated Metabolic Dysfunction in High Fat Diet-Induced Obese Mice: A Comparative Study among MCC and Various Combinations of Its Constituents

Pou Kuan Leong[1], Hoi Yan Leung[1], Hoi Shan Wong[1], Ji Hang Chen[1], Wing Man Chan[1], Chung Wah Ma[2], Yi Ting Yang[2], Kam Ming Ko[1*]

[1]Division of Life Science, Hong Kong University of Science and Technology, Hong Kong, China
[2]Infinitus (China) Company Ltd., Guangzhou, China
Email: *bcrko@ust.hk

Abstract

Obesity has been found to be associated with increased incidence of various metabolic disorders. Anti-obesity interventions are therefore urgently needed. An earlier study has demonstrated that treatment with an herbal formula MCC, which comprises the fruit of *Momordica charantia* (MC), the pericarpium of *Citri reticulate* (CR) and L-carnitine (CA), reduced the weight gain in high fat diet (HFD)-fed mice. In the present study, we investigated the effect of long-term treatment with MCC (6 g/kg/day × 40 doses) and various combinations of its constituents in HFD-fed female ICR mice. Body weight change was monitored during the course of the experiment. Total and differential adiposity, plasma lipid contents, metabolic enzyme activities and mitochondrial coupling efficiency in skeletal muscle were measured. Glucose homeostasis was also assessed. Results showed that HFD increased the body weight, total and differential adiposity, and plasma lipid contents as well as impaired metabolic status in skeletal muscle and glucose homeostasis. MCC and all combinations of its constituents reduced the weight gain in HFD-fed mice, which was accompanied with an improvement on glucose homeostasis. While MC, CA and CR independently suppressed the HFD-induced weight gain in mice, MC seems to be the most effective in weight reduction, all of which correlated with the induction of mitochondrial uncoupling in skeletal muscle. Only CA and

CR, but not MC, significantly reduced the total adiposity and visceral adiposity as well as plasma cholesterol level. However, the two component combinations, MC + CR and MC + CA, decreased the degree of visceral adiposity and plasma cholesterol level, respectively. MCC treatment at 1.5 g/kg (but not a higher dose of 6 g/kg) suppressed visceral adiposity and induced mitochondrial uncoupling in skeletal muscle in HFD-fed mice. The finding suggests that MCC may offer a promising prospect for ameliorating the diet-induced obesity and metabolic disorders in humans.

Keywords

High Fat Diet; Obesity; Weight Control; Momordica Charantia; Citri Reticulata; L-Carnitine

1. Introduction

The worldwide epidemic of obesity has been found to be associated with increased incidence of cardiovascular diseases, type 2 diabetes as well as the metabolic syndrome, leading to severe economic burden on healthcare system in modern society. Body mass index (BMI), which indicates the ratio of body weight to height, is a conventional metrics for assessing the health risk arising from obesity. Recent studies have demonstrated an inverse relationship of obesity and mortality in cardiovascular diseases and diabetes, suggesting that BMI may be not a reliable benchmark of healthy individual [1]. Alternatively, the mass of visceral fat pad, which is the fat pad of intra-abdominal cavity, is causally related to metabolic diseases, presumably by virtue of its secretion of pro-inflammatory adipokines [2]. In addition to visceral fat mass, a high ratio of low-density lipoprotein cholesterol (LDL-C) to high-density lipoprotein cholesterol (HDL-C) in combination with hypertriglyceridemia correlates well with a high risk of coronary heart disease [3]. In this regard, anti-obesity interventions, which aimed at controlling not only body weight but also plasma lipids as well as visceral fat mass, are urgently needed.

Regular physical exercise combined with low calorie diet is a commonly used intervention for the treatment of obesity. However, only a small portion of obese individuals with intervention on lifestyle can maintain a prolonged and sustained weight control [4]. Therapeutic interventions, including the use of pancreatic lipase inhibitor and stimulator of central noradrenaline release, are alternative approach to treating obesity. Despite their efficacy of weight reduction, adverse effects, such as steatorrhoea and liver injury, were observed in some obese individuals [5]. Recently, Tseng *et al.* have proposed a novel target of obesity therapy by increasing cellular bioenergetics [6]. As such, the dissipation of proton gradient across the mitochondrial inner membrane (*i.e.* mitochondrial uncoupling) can cause an inefficient generation of cellular ATP, with a resultant increase in energy expenditure. In this connection, the induction of mitochondrial uncoupling, particularly in skeletal muscle, offers a potential treatment of obesity [7].

In an effort to develop safe interventions for obesity, herbal medicine, which has a long history of use in weight reduction, has attracted a lot of interest. An herbal formula MCC, which is comprised of the fruit of *Momordica charantia* (MC, also called bitter melon), the pericarpium of *Citri reticulata* (CR) and L-carnitine (CA), was found to reduce the weight gain, visceral fat mass and hyperlipidemia in high fat diet (HFD)-induced obese mice [8]. However, the role of the three constituents of MCC formula in producing the pharmacological action remains to be investigated.

In the present study, we endeavored to define the role of the three constituents of MCC formula by comparing the weight reduction effect of MCC and various combinations of its constituents (*i.e.*, 1- and 2-component combinations), using a mouse model of HFD-induced obesity. The body weight gain was monitored during the course of 8-week experiment. To examine the degree of adiposity and plasma lipid levels, the mass of gonadal fat, mesenteric fat and subcutaneous fat as well as various plasma lipid contents [triglyceride (TG), LDL-C and HDL-C] were measured after the 8-week HFD feeding. To investigate the glucose homeostasis of HFD-fed mice, plasma glucose levels after 24-h fasting as well as glucose intolerance and insulin sensitivity index in oral glucose tolerance test (OGTT) were measured. To assess the metabolic status of skeletal muscle, activities of myocellular phosphofructokinase (PFK), β-hydroxyacyl-Co A dehydrogenase (β-HAD), carnitine palmitoyl CoA transferase (CPT) and citrate synthase (CS), as well as state 3 and state 4 respiratory rates of isolated mitochondria of skeletal muscle were assayed. The mitochondrial coupling efficiency was then estimated by computing the ratio of state 3 to state 4 mitochondrial respiratory rate.

2. Materials and Methods

2.1. Chemicals

PicoLab® Rodent diet 20 (normal diet) was purchased from LabDiet® (City, State, USA). The "Original" High Fat Diet (Diet-induced Obesity Formula D12492, 60% energy from fat) purchased from Research Diets, Inc. (New Brunswick, NJ, USA). TG and cholesterol assay kits were purchased from Wako Pure Chemical Industries, Ltd (Okasa, Japan). HDL-C test kit was purchased from Wako Diagnostics (Richmond, VA, USA). Glucose assay reagent was obtained from Sigma Chemical Co. (St. Louis, MO, USA). ELISA kit for measuring mouse insulin was purchased from Crystal Chem Inc. (Downers Grove, USA). The water extracts of MC and CR as well as CA were manufactured and supplied by Infinitus (China) Company Ltd., Guangzhou, China. The MCC formula is comprised of MC, CR and CA with the mass ratio of MC:CR:CA being 1:3.5:10. All other chemicals were of analytical grade.

2.2. Animal Care

Female ICR mice (8 - 10 weeks old, 20 - 25 g) were maintained under a 12-hour dark/light cycle at about 22°C, and allowed food and water *ad libitum* in the Animal and Plant Care Facilities at the Hong Kong University of Science and Technology (HKUST). All experimental protocols were approved by the University Committee on Research Practice at HKUST

2.3. Animal Treatment

In a preliminary study, MCC treatment was found to reduce the high fat diet-induced weight gain in both male and female ICR mice, with similar changes in the tested biochemical parameters. In the present study, only female ICR mice were used, which were randomly assigned to 10 groups, with 10 - 15 mice in each group: 1) Normal diet (ND, 13% energy from fat, PicoLab) control; 2) High fat diet (HFD, 60% energy from fat, Test Diet) control; 3) HFD, MC 0.17 g/kg; 4) HFD, CR, 0.6 g/kg; 5) HFD, CA, 1.71 g/kg; 6) HFD, MC + CR, 0.17 + 0.6 g/kg; 7) HFD, MC + CA, 0.17 + 1.71 g/kg; 8) HFD, CR + CA, 0.6 + 1.71 g/kg; 9) HFD, MCC, 1.5 g/kg; 10) HFD, MCC, 6.0 g/kg; 11) Emodin, 40 mg/kg. Doses of various combinations were equivalent to 6.0 g/kg of MCC. Mice were administered intragastrically at the indicated dose 5 days per week for 8 weeks. Control mice received water (vehicle) only. Twenty-four hours after the last dosing, blood samples were drawn from overnight fasted, phenobarbital-anesthetized mice by cardiac excision using syringes rinsed with 0.5% heparin in saline (w/v), and the mice were then sacrificed by cervical dislocation. Samples of gastrocnemius muscle and fat pads (gonadal, mesenteric and subcutaneous fat) were excised, and they were subjected to further analysis.

2.4. Preparation of Samples

Plasma samples were obtained by centrifuging whole blood samples at 1500 × g for 10 minutes at 4°C. Plasma samples were then subjected to biochemical analysis.

Minced gastrocnemius muscle tissues were digested by collagenase solution [0.075% (w/v) in buffer] at 4°C for 20 min. After removing the collagenase solution by centrifugation, the digested tissues were mixed with 20 mL of ice-cold homogenizing buffer (100 mM KCl, 50 mM MOPS, 10 mM EGTA, pH 7.2) and subjected to homogenization with a Teflon-glass homogenizer at 4000 rpm for 25 - 30 complete strokes. Then the homogenates were centrifuged at 600 × g for 10 min at 4°C. The resultant supernatant was nucleus-free fraction. For measurements of β-HAD, CS and CPT activities, nucleus-free fraction was diluted with 0.2% Triton X-100 (w/v, in K_2HPO_4 buffer) [8].

Mitochondrial pellets were prepared from nucleus-free fractions of muscle homogenates by centrifugation at 9200 × g at 4°C for 30 min. The mitochondrial pellets were then resuspended in a buffer containing 250 mM sucrose, 50 mM Tris, pH 7.5 and constituted the mitochondrial fractions [8].

2.5. Measurement of Body Weight and Fat Pad Weight

Body weight of mice was measured once a week during the 8-week course of experiment. Gonadal, mesenteric, and subcutaneous fat pads were weighed. The ratio of a particular fat pad weight to body weight was estimated and expressed as fat pad index [8].

2.6. Biochemical Analysis

Plasma glucose levels were measured using an assay kit basing on coupled hexokinase-catalyzed and glucose-6-phosphate dehydrogenase-catalyzed reactions, with a resultant NAD reduction. Absorbance changes at 340 nm were monitored spectrophotometrically by Victor[3] Multi-label Counter (Perkin Elmer, Turku, Finland). Plasma levels of TG, HDL-C, and TC levels were measured using assay kits. LDL-C level was estimated by Friedewald's formula: $LDL = TC - (HDC - C + TG/5)$ [9]. Plasma insulin level was measured using an ELISA kit. PFK, β-HAD, CS and CPT activities in skeletal muscle were measured using enzymatic methods, as described as Leong $et\ al.$ and Colberg $et\ al.$ [8] [10].

2.7. Oral Glucose Tolerance Test

After 8 weeks of experiment, oral glucose tolerance test (OGTT) was performed. Six hour post-fasting, blood samples were collected as initial levels of plasma glucose and insulin ($i.e.$ time = 0). Then, glucose (2 g/kg) was orally administered to the mice. Blood samples were collected at 15, 30, 60 and 120 min post-dosing of glucose. Plasma glucose and insulin levels were measured. Glucose intolerance was estimated by computing the area under the curve (AUC) plotting plasma glucose level against time and expressed in arbitrary unit. Insulin sensitivity index (ISI) was estimated by following equation:

$$1000 / \left\{ \text{Square root of} \left[(FPG \times FPI) \right] \times (\text{Mean OGTT glucose}) \times (\text{mean OGTT insulin}) \right\},$$

where FPG = fasting plasma glucose; FPI = fasting plasma insulin [10].

2.8. Measurement of Mitochondrial Respiration

Mitochondrial respiratory was measured polarographically by a Clark-type oxygen electrode (Hansatech Instruments Ltd., Norfolk, UK) at 30°C. Mitochondrial fraction (~0.5 mg protein/mL) was incubated in a buffer containing 30 mM KCl, 6 mM MgCl$_2$, 75 mM sucrose, 1 mM EDTA, 20 mM KH$_2$PO$_4$ and 0.1% (w/v) fatty acid-free BSA, pH 7.0. Substrate solution containing 10 mM glutamate and 2.5 mM malate was added, and after a stable state 2 respiration had been established, state 3 respiration (coupling) was initiated by the addition of ADP (final concentration 0.6 mM). When all of the added ADP was used up for ATP generation, oligomycin (ATP synthase inhibitor) was added to induce the state 4 respiration (uncoupling). The respiratory control ratio (RCR) was estimated by calculating the ratio of state 3 to state 4 respirations [11].

2.9. Statistical Analysis

The time dependent changes in the body weight during the course of 8 week experiment was analyzed by mixed Analysis of Variance (mixed ANOVA). Other data were analyzed by one-way Analysis of Variance (ANOVA). Post-hoc multiple comparisons were performed using Least Significant Difference (LSD). P values < 0.05 were regarded as statistically significant.

3. Results

3.1. Effects of MCC and Various Combinations of Its Constituents on Body Weight Gain in HFD-Fed Mice

ND slightly but not significantly increased the body weight during the course of 8-week experiment in mice. HFD accelerated the body weight increase during the course of experiment in mice, with the degree of stimulation being 24%, when compared with that of ND (**Figure 1**). MCC and all combinations of its constituents were found to inhibit the HFD-induced body weight gain (**Table 1**). While MC (0.17 g/kg) completely abrogated the HFD-induced body weight gain, MC + CR (0.17 and 0.6 g/kg) caused the largest degree of suppression (91.6%) among the 2-component combinations (**Table 1**). The 3-component combination MCC (6.0 g/kg) also suppressed the HFD-induced body weight gain, with the extent of inhibition being 76% (**Figure 1** and **Table 1**).

3.2. Effects of MCC and Various Combinations of Its Constituents on Various Fat Pad Indices in HFD-Fed Mice

The HFD-induced body weight gain was associated with an increase in total fat pad index (162%), as well as

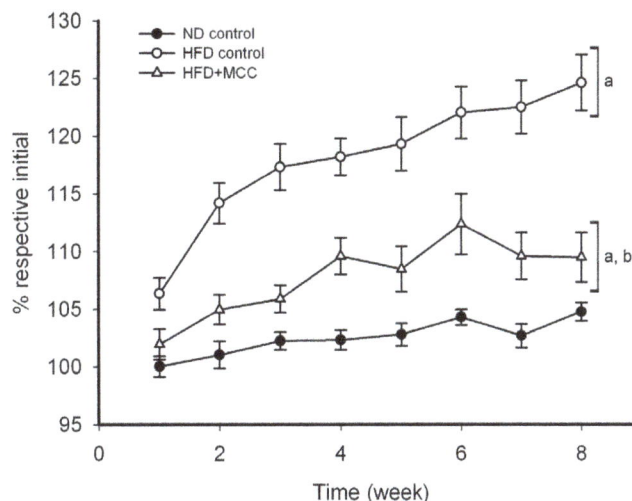

Figure 1. Effect of MCC on body weight gain during the course of 8-week experiment in HFD-fed mice. Mice were allowed food [ND (13% energy from fat) or HFD (60% energy from fat)] and water *ad libitum*, during the course of 8-week experiment. In the drug treatment groups, mice were intragastrically administered with MCC (6 g/kg/day) 5 days per week for 8 weeks (*i.e.* 40 doses), while control mice received water (vehicle) only. Body weights of mice were monitored by measuring the body weight of mice every week during the 8-week period. Data were expressed as % initial, by normalizing with initial body weight (*i.e.* time = week 0) of the respective mouse. Value given are means ± SEM, with n = 10 - 15. The initial values of body weight of each group were given as follows: 1) ND control = 33.1 ± 0.5 g; 2) HFD control = 33.2 ± 1.0 g; 3) HFD + 6 g/kg MCC = 36.1 ± 0.7 g. [a]Significantly different from time-matched ND-fed control; [b]significantly different from time-matched HFD-fed control.

Table 1. Effects of MCC and various combinations of its constituents on body weight in HFD-fed mice.

Treatment	Body weight (% control)	% Suppression of weight gain
ND		
Control	104.8 ± 0.8	
HFD		
Control	124.6 ± 2.4[a]	
MC	103.5 ± 2.9[b]	106.3
CR	108.6 ± 2.4[b]	80.6
CA	112.2 ± 2.2[b]	62.4
MC + CR	106.4 ± 2.8[b]	91.6
MC + CA	106.7 ± 3.1[b]	90.5
CR + CA	109.3 ± 2.6[b]	77.0
MCC	109.5 ± 2.1[b]	76.2

[a]Significantly different from ND-fed control; [b]significantly different from HFD-fed control.

differential increases in gonadal fat pad (184%), mesenteric fat pad (93%) and subcutaneous fat pad (162%) indices, when compared with the ND control (**Table 2**). Among the single-component treatments, MC and CR suppressed the HFD-induced increases in total fat pad index (39% and 36%, respectively) as well as gonadal fat pad index (47% and 38%), whereas CA reduced the gonadal fat pad index (46%) and mesenteric fat pad index

(103%) in HFD-fed mice (**Table 2**). CR further suppressed the subcutaneous fat by 23%. Among the 2-component treatments, MC + CR and MC + CA decreased the total fat pad index (41% and 74%, respectively) and gonadal fat pad index (57% and 87%) in HFD-fed mice. In addition, MC + CA also suppressed increases in fat pad indices of total fat pad (64%) and subcutaneous fat pad (50%) of HFD-fed mice. CR + CA reduced the subcutaneous fat index (27%) in HFD-fed mice (**Table 2**). MCC (6.0 g/kg) did not produce detectable changes the total and differential fat pad indices.

3.3. Effects of MCC and Various Combinations of Its Constituents on Plasma Lipid Levels in HFD-Fed Mice

The HFD-induced increases in total and differential fat pad indices were paralleled by increases in plasma levels of TG and TC and (36% and 79%, respectively), as well as the ratio of LDL-C to HDL-C (27%) in HFD-fed mice (**Figure 2**). MCC (6.0 g/kg) and various combinations of its constituents differentially modulated the plasma lipid level in HFD-fed mice (**Figure 2**). The HFD-induced elevation in plasma TG level was decreased by MCC and all tested combinations (except CA), with complete suppression produced by MC + CA, CR + CA and MCC. MCC and all tested combinations reduced the plasma TC level in HFD-fed mice, with the extent of suppression afforded by CR + CA (77%) being most prominent, followed by MCC (71%). The HFD-induced increase in LDL-C/HDL-C ratio was suppressed by MCC and all tested combinations (except MC and MC + CA), with the complete inhibition produced by MCC.

3.4. Effects of MCC and Various Combinations of Its Constituents on Glucose Homeostasis in HFD-Fed Mice

In addition to increases in plasma lipid levels, HFD also impaired the glucose homeostasis, as indicated by increases in fasting plasma glucose level (28%) and oral glucose intolerance (25%) as well as the decrease in insulin sensitivity (65%) (**Figures 3(A)-(C)**). MCC and all tested combinations caused reversal changes on fasting plasma glucose level, oral glucose intolerance and insulin sensitivity in HFD-fed mice. Treatment with CR, MC + CR or CA + CR caused complete normalization of fasting plasma glucose level in HFD-fed mice (**Figure 3(A)**). In the oral glucose tolerance test, MC, MC + CR, MC + CA, CR + CA and MCC completely reversed the glucose intolerance, while CA, MC + CR, MC + CA and MCC completely restored the insulin sensitivity in HFD-fed mice.

3.5. Effects of MCC and Various Combinations of Its Constituents on Various Metabolic Enzyme Activities of Skeletal Muscle in HFD-Fed Mice

The HFD-induced impairment of glucose homeostasis was associated with the reduced PFK activity (20%) of

Table 2. Effects of MCC and various combinations of its constituents on various fat pad indices in HFD-fed mice.

Treatment	Total		Differential	
	Fat pad index	Subcutaneous fat pad index	Gonadal fat pad index	Mesenteric fat pad index
ND				
Control	0.044 ± 0.004	0.017 ± 0.001	0.021 ± 0.002	0.0064 ± 0.0005
HFD				
Control	0.115 ± 0.010^a	0.043 ± 0.004^a	0.059 ± 0.006^a	0.0124 ± 0.0009^a
MC	0.082 ± 0.11^b	0.033 ± 0.005	0.038 ± 0.005^b	0.0112 ± 0.0014
CR	0.079 ± 0.09^b	0.032 ± 0.004^b	0.037 ± 0.005^b	0.0104 ± 0.0012
CA	0.087 ± 0.008	0.039 ± 0.004	0.039 ± 0.004^b	0.0087 ± 0.0009^b
MC+CR	0.092 ± 0.014	0.043 ± 0.008	0.038 ± 0.006^b	0.0103 ± 0.0011
MC+CA	0.073 ± 0.017^b	0.031 ± 0.007^b	0.033 ± 0.010^b	0.0084 ± 0.0014^b
CR+CA	0.097 ± 0.020	0.029 ± 0.006^b	0.057 ± 0.013	0.0102 ± 0.0015
MCC	0.101 ± 0.008	0.035 ± 0.003	0.056 ± 0.005	0.0109 ± 0.0008

[a]Significantly different from ND-fed control; [b]significantly different from HFD-fed control.

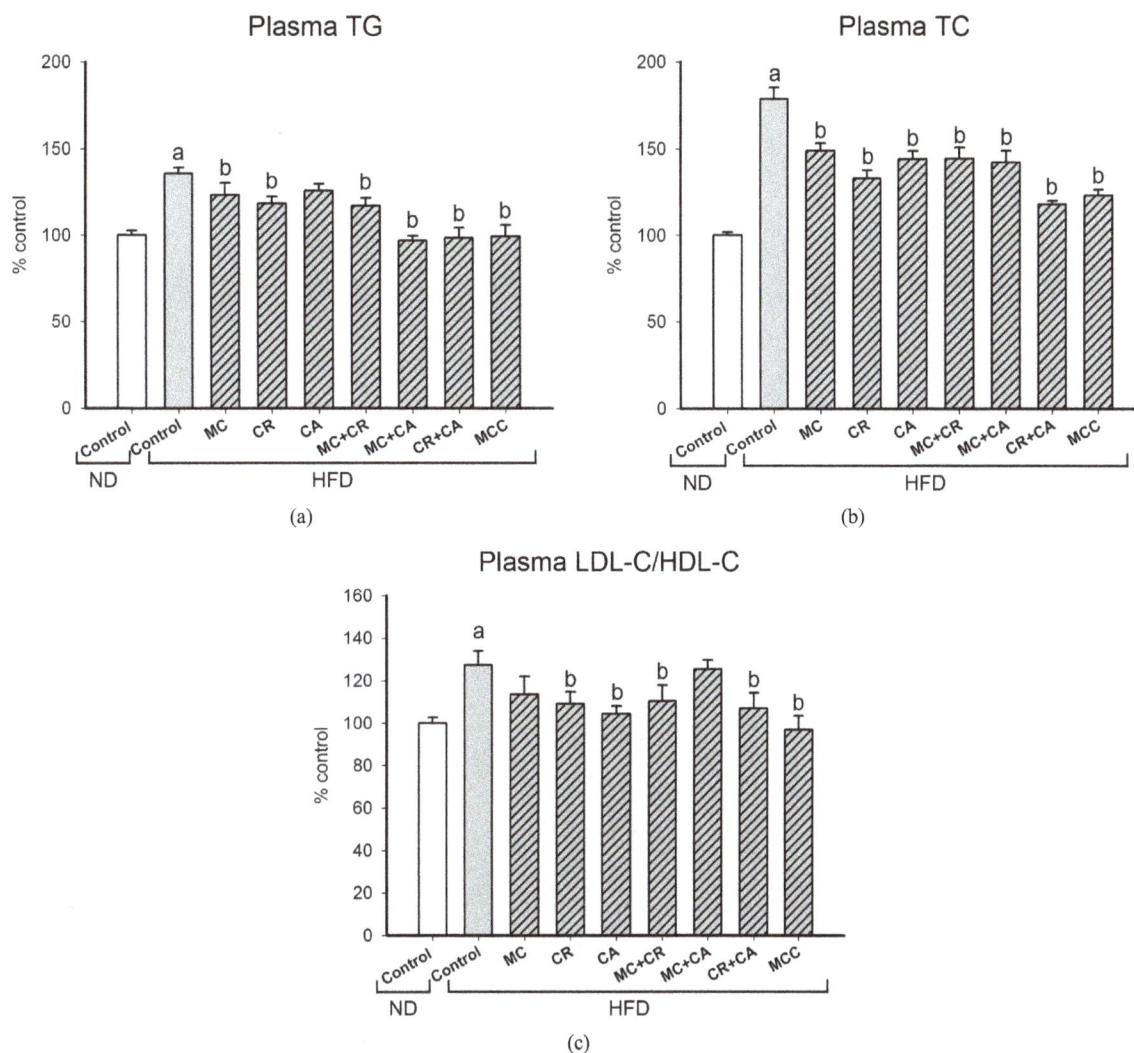

Figure 2. Effects of MCC and various combinations of its constituents on plasma lipid levels in HFD-fed mice. Mice were sacrificed at 24 h after the last dosing of MCC as described in Materials and Methods. Plasma triglyceride (TG) level (ND control = 59.0 ± 2.5 mg/dL), total lipoprotein cholesterol (TC) level (ND control = 146.3 ± 5.2 mg/dL) and ratio of low density lipoprotein cholesterol (LDL-C) to high density lipoprotein cholesterol (HDL-C) (ND control = 1.4 ± 0.11) were measured, as described in Materials and methods. Data were expressed as % control by normalizing with ND control. Value given are means ± SEM, with n = 10 - 15. [a]Significantly different from ND control; [b]Significantly different from HFD control.

skeletal muscle (**Table 3**). In addition, HFD increased the β-HAD activity (24%) and CPT activity (18%) of skeletal muscle in HFD-fed mice (**Table 3**). No detectable changes in CS activity of skeletal muscle in HFD-fed mice were observed. While MC, CR, CA and MC + CA partially reversed the HFD-induced reduction in PFK activity, CR, CA, MC + CR and MC + CA suppressed the CPT activity in HFD-fed mice.

3.6. Effects of MCC and Various Combinations of Its Constituents on Mitochondrial Coupling Efficiency of Skeletal Muscle in HFD-Fed Mice

HFD did not cause detectable change in mitochondrial coupling efficiency of skeletal muscle in HFD-fed mice. All single-component (MC, CR and CA) treatments decreased the coupling efficiency (36%, 19% and 31%, respectively), with the extent of reduction afforded by MC being most prominent (**Figure 4**). Among the 2-component combinations, only MC + CR and MC + CA decreased the mitochondrial coupling efficiency (28% and 20%, respectively) of skeletal muscle in HFD-fed mice. MCC did not affect the mitochondrial coupling effi-

Twenty four-hour fasting

(A)

Oral glucose tolerance test

(B)

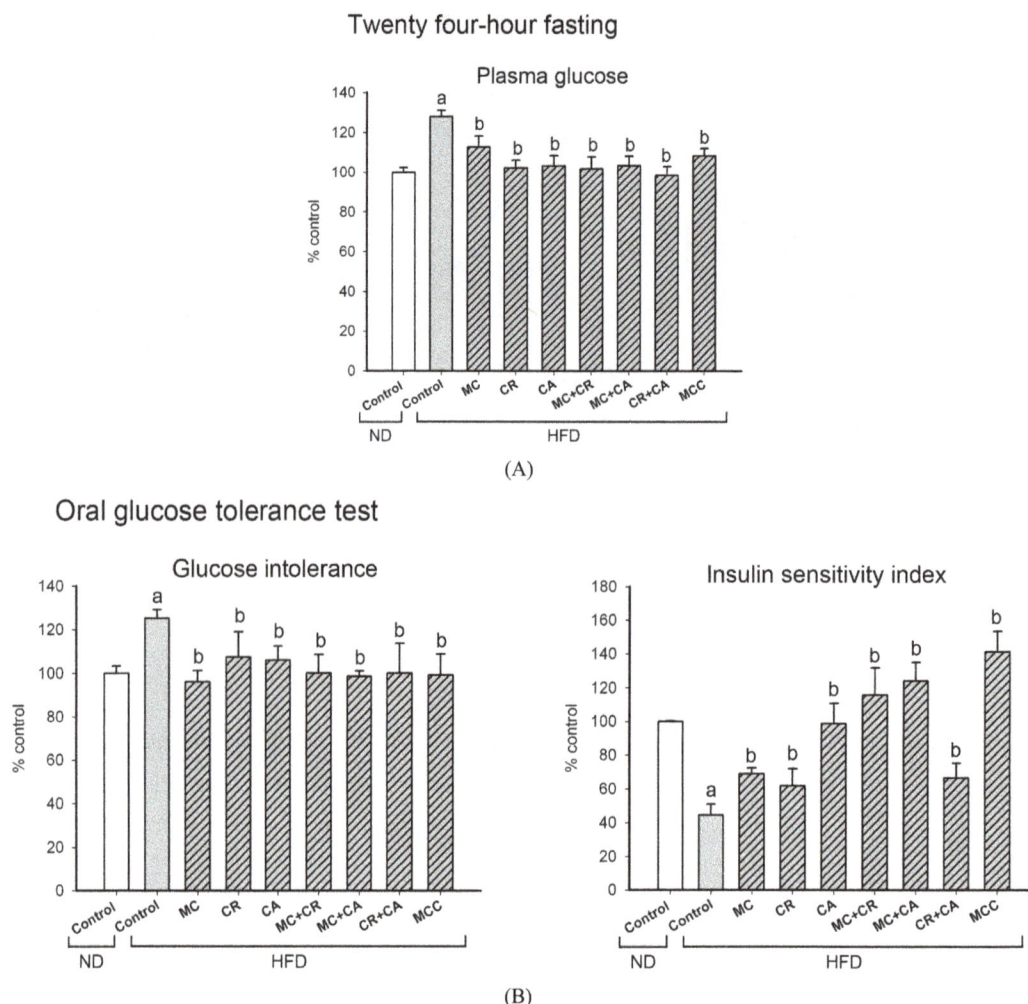

Figure 3. Effects of MCC and various combinations of its constituents on glucose homeostasis in HFD- fed mice. (A) Mice were sacrificed at 24 h after the last dosing of MCC as described in Materials and Methods. Plasma glucose level (ND control = 80.7 ± 4.2 mg/dL) was measured. (B) Mice were objected to oral glucose tolerance test at 24 h after the last dosing of MCC as described in Materials and Methods. Blood samples were collected at 15, 30, 60 and 120 min post-dosing of glucose. Plasma glucose and insulin levels were measured. Glucose intolerance was estimated by computing the area under the curve (AUC) plotting plasma glucose level against time and expressed in arbitrary unit (ND control = 1030 ± 40). Insulin sensitivity index (ISI) was estimated (ND control = 2623 ± 14), as described in Materials and Methods. Data were expressed as % control, by normalizing with ND control. Value given are means $\pm$ SEM, with n = 10 - 15. [a]Significantly different from ND control; [b]significantly different from HFD control.

ciency of skeletal muscle.

3.7. Effects of a Low Dose of MCC on Various Parameters in HFD-Fed Mice

The effects of MCC treatment at a low dose of 1.5 g/kg were also investigated in HFD-fed mice (**Table 4**). MCC (1.5 g/kg) reduced the HFD-induced body weight gain, with the degree of suppression being 64%. In contrast to the that of high dose of 6.0 g/kg, the weight reduction caused by the low dose of MCC was associated with decreases in total fat pad index (22%) as well as subcutaneous and mesenteric fat pad indices (36% and 66%, respectively) in HFD-fed mice. Consistent with this, MCC treatment also reduced the HFD-induced elevations of plasma TG and TC levels (by 65% and 72%, respectively) as well as plasma LDL-C to HDL-C ratio (127%). MCC also improved the glucose homeostasis in HFD-fed mice, as evidenced by the reversal of changes in fasting plasma glucose level (83%), glucose intolerance (100%) and insulin sensitivity (29%). Despite the fact

Table 3. Effects of MCC and various combinations of its constituents on various metabolic enzymes of skeletal muscle in HFD-fed mice.

Treatment	PFK	β-HAD	CS	CPT
ND				
Control	100 ± 2.6	100.0 ± 1.6	100.0 ± 1.3	100.0 ± 1.9
HFD				
Control	79.7 ± 1.6^a	124.3 ± 3.5^a	102.9 ± 3.0	117.9 ± 1.5^a
MC	95.1 ± 3.5^b	125.9 ± 1.8	101.1 ± 3.5	115.2 ± 2.8
CR	89.5 ± 4.8^b	119.7 ± 6.1	102.7 ± 2.7	103.9 ± 2.6^b
CA	91.4 ± 3.8^b	122.5 ± 5.3	108.8 ± 1.7	104.2 ± 3.7^b
MC + CR	88.1 ± 3.0	120.9 ± 4.2	108.2 ± 1.2	106.4 ± 3.5^b
MC + CA	93.0 ± 3.5^b	123.8 ± 3.6	107.3 ± 2.8	106.6 ± 4.2^b
CR + CA	82.8 ± 2.5	131.5 ± 4.6	96.4 ± 4.1	112.5 ± 3.7
MCC	85.7 ± 1.9	120.4 ± 3.6	$91.6 \pm 2.9^{a,b}$	112.1 ± 3.5

[a]Significantly different from ND control; [b]significantly different from HFD control.

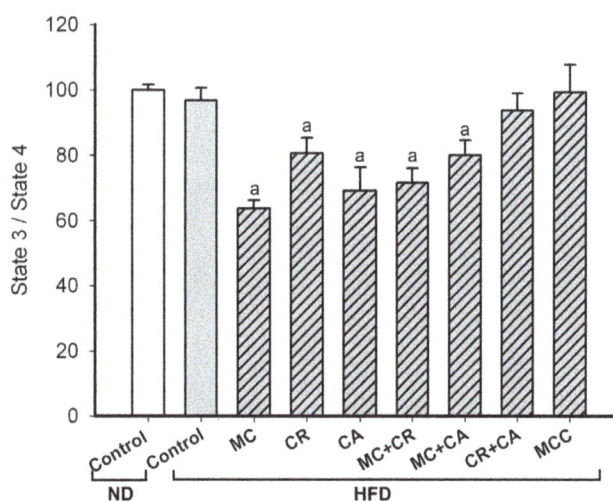

Figure 4. Effects of MCC and various combinations of its constituents on mitochondrial coupling efficiency of skeletal muscle in HFD-fed mice. Mice were sacrificed at 24 h after the last dosing of MCC as described in Materials and Methods. Mitochondrial respiratory of skeletal muscle was measured polarographically by a Clark-type oxygen electrode at 30°C. The respiratory control ratio (RCR) was estimated by calculating the ratio of state 3 to state 4 respirations. Data were expressed as % control, by normalizing with ND control. Values given are means ± SEM, with n = 10 - 15. [a]Significantly different from ND control; [b]significantly different from HFD control.

that MCC (1.5 g/kg) did not produce detectable changes in various metabolic enzyme activities (PFK, β-HAD and CS) of skeletal muscle, MCC decreased the CPT activity (56%) as well as the mitochondrial coupling efficiency (28%) of skeletal muscle in HFD-fed mice.

4. Discussion

HFD-fed mice, as observed in the present and other studies [12], showed increases in body weight, the degree of

Table 4. Effect of MCC (1.5 g/kg) on various parameters in HFD-fed mice.

MCC (1.5 g/kg)	% stimulation (+) or % suppression (−) VS HFD control
Body weight	
BW change	−64[a]
Fat pad indices	
Total fat pad index	−22[a]
Subcutaneous fat pad index	−36[a]
Gonadal fat pad index	No significant difference
Mesenteric fat pad index	−66[a]
Plasma lipid and leptin levels	
Plasma TG	−65[a]
Plasma TC	−72[a]
LDL to HDL ratio	−127[a]
Glucose homeostasis	
<u>24-h fasting</u>	
Plasma glucose	−83[a]
<u>Oral glucose tolerance test</u>	
Glucose intolerance	−100[a]
Insulin sensitivity index	+29[a]
Metabolic enzyme activities in skeletal muscle	
PFK	No significant difference
β-HAD	No significant difference
CS	No significant difference
CPT	−56[a]
Mitochondrial coupling efficiency in skeletal muscle	
Coupling efficiency	−25[a]

[a]Significantly different from ND control; [b]significantly different from HFD control.

adiposity and plasma lipid contents, as well as impairments in glucose homeostasis and metabolic status of skeletal muscle. It has been shown that HFD caused an increase in free fatty acid uptake in skeletal muscle, with a resultant insulin resistance [13], which is a well-established risk factor of diabetes and metabolic syndromes. In the present study, MCC and various combinations of its constituents reduced the weight gain in HFD-fed mice, which was accompanied with an improvement on glucose homeostasis. Our earlier study has suggested that the weight loss effect produced by MCC is likely due to a modulation of fatty acid absorption and/or metabolism [8]. In the present study, emodin, which was found to ameliorate metabolic dysfunctions in HFD-induced obese mice [14], was used as a positive control. Consistent with the recent findings, emodin reduced the weight gain, adiposity and plasma lipid contents in HFD-fed mice (data not shown), suggesting the validity of the mouse model of HFD-induce obesity in the present study. Varied effects of MCC and its constituents or their combinations on total and differential adiposity, plasma lipid contents and metabolic status of skeletal muscle were observed. We therefore sought to define the role of each constituent of MCC in producing the weight loss effect and the associated metabolic changes in HFD-induced obese mice.

Despite the fact that all constituents of MCC (MC, CA and CR) independently suppressed the HFD-induced weight gain in mice, MC seems to be the most effective. The MC/CA/CR-induced weight reduction in HFD-fed mice may be attributed to the improvement in metabolic status of skeletal muscle, as indicated by as a reversal increase in PFK activity and an induction of mitochondrial uncoupling, with the degree of improvement produced by MC being larger than those of CA and CR. However, only CA and CR, but not MC, significantly reduced the total adiposity and visceral adiposity (as assessed by mesenteric fat pad index) as well as plasma LDL-C to HDL-C ratio. On the other hand, MC, when being combined with CR or CA, could reduce the degree of visceral adiposity or the LDL-C to HDL-C ratio respectively, in addition to decreasing body weight. Given that an increased visceral adiposity and an elevated plasma LDL-C to HDL-C ratio are predisposing factors of metabolic disorders [2], the combination of MC with CR or CA may be beneficial for lowering the risk of metabolic disorders in obese individuals. This postulation was strengthened by the observation that among the 2-component combinations, MC + CA and MC + CR treatments were more effective than that of CA + CR in weight reduction, possibly due to the induction of mitochondrial uncoupling in skeletal muscle of mice. While MC + CA reduced the extent of visceral adiposity and stimulated the PFK activity of skeletal muscle, MC + CR decreased the plasma LDL-C/HDL-C ratio. Conceivably, MCC treatment may produce a multiple effect on weight reduction, visceral adiposity suppression and plasma LDL-C/HDL-C regulation in HFD-induced obese mice. Unexpectedly, the weight reduction afforded by MCC (6.0 g/kg) was not accompanied with the suppression of visceral adiposity and induction of mitochondrial uncoupling in skeletal muscle in HFD-induced obese mice. Since an inducer of mitochondrial uncoupling has been shown to cause a dose-dependent and biphasic response in round spermatids [15], the failure of MCC to induce mitochondrial uncoupling in skeletal muscle may be related to the high dose of treatment. This postulation is supported by the finding that the weight reduction afforded by MCC treatment at a lower dose (1.5 g/kg) was associated with an induction of mitochondrial uncoupling in skeletal muscle as well as a suppression of visceral adiposity and a reduction of LDL-C/HDL-C ratio in HFD-induced obese mice. While the ability of MCC to modulate the metabolism of cholesterol remains unclear, the suppression of visceral adiposity is likely causally related to mitochondrial uncoupling in skeletal muscle, which oxidizes excessive fatty acids in HFD-fed mice. As visceral adipose tissue contains a large number of mitochondria [16], we cannot exclude the possibility that MCC may also induce mitochondrial uncoupling in visceral adipose tissue, with a resultant mobilization of lipid reservoir in adipose tissue. As an excessive accumulation of visceral adipose tissue is associated with metabolic abnormalities such as insulin resistance and high blood lipid contents [17], the reduction of fat mass of visceral adipose tissue is therefore beneficial for preventing metabolic diseases such as metabolic syndromes and type 2 diabetes [18]. In this regard, MCC treatment was found to improve glucose tolerance and insulin sensitivity in HFD-fed mice.

Contemporary anti-obesity approaches have been targeted at the reduction of intestinal absorption [19], the enhancement of fatty acid metabolic status in skeletal muscle [20] and the induction of mitochondrial uncoupling in skeletal muscle [21]. An earlier study on the weight loss effect of MCC revealed that MCC treatment (5.1 g/kg) decreased the weight gain in HFD-fed mice, presumably due to the reduction of intestinal lipid absorption in HFD-fed mice [8]. In the present study, we have further demonstrated that a lower dose of MCC (1.5 g/kg) induces mitochondrial uncoupling in skeletal muscle of HFD-fed mice and thus provides an extended view on the biochemical mechanism underlying weight loss effect of MCC. In this connection, an induction of mitochondrial uncoupling in skeletal muscle was found to augment the energy expenditure in uncoupling protein 1 up-regulated mice [22].

5. Conclusion

In conclusion, MCC treatment at a dose of 1.5 g/kg was found to reduce the HFD-induced weight gain and the associated metabolic abnormalities in HFD-fed mice. The finding suggests that MCC may offer a promising prospect for ameliorating the diet-induced obesity and the associated metabolic disorders in humans.

References

[1] Ahima, R.S. and Lazar, M.A. (2013) The Health Risk of Obesity-Better Metrics Imperative. *Science*, **341**, 856-858. http://dx.doi.org/10.1126/science.1241244

[2] Fontana, L.J., Eagon, C., Trujillo, M.E., Scherer, P.E. and Klein, S. (2007) Visceral Fat Adipokine Secretion Is Associated with Systemic Inflammation in Obese Humans. *Diabetes*, **56**, 1010-1013. http://dx.doi.org/10.2337/db06-1656

[3] Manninen, V., Tenkanen, L., Koskinen, P., Huttunen, J.K., Mänttäri, M., Heinonen, O.P. and Frick, M.H. (1992) Joint Effects of Serum Triglyceride and LDL Cholesterol and HDL Cholesterol Concentrations on Coronary Heartdisease Risk in the Helsinki Heart Study. Implications for Treatment. *Circulation*, **85**, 37-45. http://dx.doi.org/10.1161/01.CIR.85.1.37

[4]   Wing, R.R. and Phelan, S. (2005) Long-Term Weight Loss Maintenance. *The American Journal of Clinical Nutrition*, **82**, 222S-225S.

[5]   Caveney, E., Caveney, B.J., Somaratne, R., Turner, J.R. and Gourgiotis, L. (2011) Pharmaceutical Interventions for Obesity: A Public Health Perspective. *Diabetes, Obesity and Metabolism*, **13**, 490-497. http://dx.doi.org/10.1111/j.1463-1326.2010.01353.x

[6]   Tseng, Y., Cypess, A.M. and Kahn, C.R. (2010) Cellular Bioenergetics as a Target for Obesity Therapy. *Nature Reviews Drug Discovery*, **9**, 465-482. http://dx.doi.org/10.1038/nrd3138

[7]   Thrush, A.B., Dent, R., McPherson, R. and Harper, M.E. (2013) Implications of Mitochondrial Uncoupling in Skeletal Muscle in the Development and Treatment of Obesity. *FEBS Journal*, **280**, 5015-5029. http://dx.doi.org/10.1111/febs.12399

[8]   Leong, P.K., Leung, H.Y., Wong, H.S., Chen, J., Ma, C.W., Yang, Y. and Ko, K.M. (2013) Long-Term Treatment with an Herbal Formula MCC Reduces the Weight Gain in High Fat Diet-Induced Obese Mice. *Chinese Medicine*, **4**, 63-71. http://dx.doi.org/10.4236/cm.2013.43010

[9]   Siddiqua, M., Hamid, K., Rashid, M.H.A., Akther, M.S. and Choudhuri, M.S.K. (2010) Changes in Lipid Profile of Rat Plasma after Chronic Administration of Laghobanondo Rosh (LNR)—An Ayurvedic Formulation. *Biology and Medicine*, **2**, 58-63.

[10]   Colberg, S.R., Simoneau, J.A., Thaete, F.L. and Kelley, D.E. (1995) Skeletal Muscle Utilization of Free Fatty Acids in Women with Visceral Obesity. *The Journal of Clinical Investigation*, **95**, 1846-1853. http://dx.doi.org/10.1172/JCI117864

[11]   Crescenzo, R., Mainieri, D., Solinas, G., Montani, J.P., Seydoux, J., Liverini, G., Iossa, S. and Dulloo, A.G. (2003) Skeletal Muscle Mitochondrial Oxidative Capacity and Uncoupling Protein 3 Are Differently Influenced by Semistarvation and Refeeding. *FEBS Letters*, **544**, 138-142. http://dx.doi.org/10.1016/S0014-5793(03)00491-5

[12]   Wang, C.Y. and Liao, J.K. (2012) A Mouse Model of Diet-Induced Obesity and Insulin Resistance. *Methods in Molecular Biology*, **821**, 421-433. http://dx.doi.org/10.1007/978-1-61779-430-8_27

[13]   Martins, R., Nachbar, R.T., Gorjao, R., Vinolo, M.A., Festuccia, W.T., Lambertucci, R.H., Cury-Boaventura, M.F., Silveira, L.R., Curi, R. and Hirabara, S.M. (2012) Mechanisms Underlying Skeletal Muscle Insulin Resistance Induced by Fatty Acids: Importance of the Mitochondrial Function. *Lipids in Health and Disease*, **11**, 30. http://dx.doi.org/10.1186/1476-511X-11-30

[14]   Feng, Y., Huang, S.L., Dou, W., Zhang, S., Chen, J.H., Shen, Y., Shen, J.H. and Leng, Y. (2010) Emodin, a Natural Product, Selectively Inhibits 11beta-Hydroxysteroid Dehydrogenase Type 1 and Ameliorates Metabolic Disorder in Diet-Induced Obese Mice. *British Journal of Pharmacology*, **161**, 113-126. http://dx.doi.org/10.1111/j.1476-5381.2010.00826.x

[15]   Nakamura, M., Ikeda, M., Suzuki, A., Okinaga, S. and Arai, K. (1988) Metabolism of Round Spermatids: Gossypol Induces Uncoupling of Respiratory Chain and Oxidative Phosphorylation. *Biology of Reproduction*, **39**, 771-778. http://dx.doi.org/10.1095/biolreprod39.4.771

[16]   Kraunsøe, R., Boushel, R., Hansen, C.N., Schjerling, P., Qvortrup, K., Støckel, P., Mikines, K.J. and Dela, F. (2010) Mitochondrial Respiration in Subcutaneous and Visceral Adipose Tissue from Patients with Morbid Obesity. *The Journal of Physiology*, **588**, 2023-2032. http://dx.doi.org/10.1113/jphysiol.2009.184754

[17]   Girard, J. and Lafontan, M. (2008) Impact of Visceral Adipose Tissue on Liver Metabolism and Insulin Resistance. Part II: Visceral Adipose Tissue Production and Liver Metabolism. *Diabetes & Metabolism*, **34**, 439-445. http://dx.doi.org/10.1016/j.diabet.2008.04.002

[18]   Knight, J.A. (2011) Diseases and Disorders Associated with Excess Body Weight. *Annals of Clinical & Laboratory Science*, **41**, 107-121.

[19]   Caveney, E., Caveney, B.J., Somaratne, R., Turner, J.R. and Gourgiotis, L. (2011) Pharmaceutical Interventions for Obesity: A Public Health Perspective. *Diabetes, Obesity and Metabolism*, **13**, 490-497. http://dx.doi.org/10.1111/j.1463-1326.2010.01353.x

[20]   Goto, T., Teraminami, A., Lee, J.Y., Ohyama, K., Fu-nakoshi, K., Kim, Y.I., Hirai, S., Uemura, T., Yu, R., Takahashi, N. and Kawada, T. (2012) Tiliroside, a Glycosidic Flavo-Noid, Ameliorates Obesity-Induced Metabolic Disorders via Activation of Adiponectin Signaling Followed by Enhancement of Fatty Acid Oxidation in Liver and Skeletal Muscle in Obese-Diabetic Mice. *The Journal of Nutritional Biochemistry*, **23**, 768-776. http://dx.doi.org/10.1016/j.jnutbio.2011.04.001

[21]   Costford, S., Gowing, A. and Harper, M.E. (2007) Mitochondrial Uncoupling as a Target in the Treatment of Obesity. *Current Opinion in Clinical Nutrition & Metabolic Care*, **10**, 671-678. http://dx.doi.org/10.1097/MCO.0b013e3282f0dbe4

[22] Adjeitey, C.N., Mailloux, R.J., Dekemp, R.A. and Harpe, M.E. (2013) Mitochondrial Uncoupling in Skeletal Muscle by UCP1 Augments Energy Expenditure and Glutathione Content While Mitigating ROS Production. *American Journal of Physiology—Endocrinology and Metabolism*, **305**, E405-E415. http://dx.doi.org/10.1152/ajpendo.00057.2013

List of Abbreviations

Analysis of variance (ANOVA); area under the curve (AUC); body mass index (BMI); L-carnitine (CA); carnitine palmitoyl CoA transferase (CPT); citrate synthase (CS); pericarpium of *Citri reticulate* (CR); fasting plasma insulin (FPI); fasting plasma glucose (FPG); β-hydroxyacyl-Co A dehydrogenase (β-HAD); high-density lipoprotein cholesterol (HDL-C); high fat diet (HFD); insulin sensitivity index (ISI); low-density lipoprotein cholesterol (LDL-C); the fruit of *Momordica charantia* (MC); normal diet (ND); oral glucose tolerance test (OGTT); phosphofructokinase (PFK); triglyceride (TG)

Effects of Rivastigmine Combined with Reinhartdt and Sea Cucumber Capsule in Patients with Mild-to-Moderate Parkinson's Disease Dementia: A Pilot Study

Yongxing Yan[1], Lizhen Liang[1*], Tao Xie[2], Yonghui Shen[1], Yanjing Cao[1]

[1]Department of Neurology, The Third People's Hospital of Hangzhou, Hangzhou, China
[2]Department of Neurology, University of Chicago Medicine, Chicago, USA
Email: [*]yuanyr@sohu.com

Abstract

Many patients with Parkinson's disease suffer cognitive impairment or dementia. Cholinesterase inhibitors (ChEIs) have positive effects on patients with Parkinson's Disease Dementia (PDD). But it is only improve symptoms. There is no etiological cure for PDD. So, In order to achieve the best outcomes, the combination of ChEIs and other therapeutic strategies is needed to study. In the present study, we investigate the efficacy and safety of rivastigmine combined with Reinhartdt and Sea Cucumber Capsule (RSC) in patients with mild-to-moderate PDD, and its effect on thyroid function. There were 52 patients were randomly assigned to receive either rivastigmine (3 mg/day) or rivastigmine plus RSC (2.7 g/day) treatment for 24 weeks. Efficacy was investigated by the change of the scores of Alzheimer's Disease Assessment Scale cognitive subscale (ADAS-Cog), Activities of Daily Life (ADL) and Unified Parkinson's Disease Rating Scale (UPDRS) part III (motor scale). Meanwhile, thyroid hormone levels were detected before and after 12 weeks, 24 weeks treatment in all patients. Results showed that the patients treated with rivastigmine plus RSC showed more improvement in the cognition and the daily life activities compared to those treated with rivastigmine alone. Significant difference was present after being treated for 12 weeks or more. However, no group difference was found on UPDRS part III, thyroid hormone level change and the incidence of adverse events (11.1% vs 16.0%) between the two groups of treatment. Adverse effects were nausea and vomiting which were the main reasons for the dropout. The finding suggests that Rivastigmine plus RSC may improves the treatment effects in cognition and the ADL of the patients with mild-to-moderate PDD, compared with the rivastigmine treatment alone. However, no effect was observed on the motor symptoms and thyroid hormone levels. In addition, this joint treatment is safe.

---

[*]Corresponding author.

Keywords

Parkinson's Disease, Cognitive Function, Rivastigmine, Reinhartdt and Sea Cucumber

1. Introduction

Parkinson's disease characterized by bradykinesia, tremor, rigidity, and postural instability is one of common neurodegenerative disease, its incidence of 14 per 100,000 [1] [2]. In China, the incidence rate is about 2% in the population of age ≥ 65-year old [3]. In addition to the typical motor symptoms of Parkinson's disease, it also have cognitive impairment or dementia [4]. Some studies have shown that about 30% of patients suffer dementia in Parkinson's disease [5] [6]. Parkinson's Disease Dementia (PDD) greatly affects functioning and quality of life. It can also increase caregiver burden, health-related costs, and duration of hospital stays etc [7]-[9].

In patients with PDD, cognitive changes are linked to disease-related disturbances of cholinergic activity [10]. Bohnen NI *et al.* found cholinergic deficits in PDD are more obvious in Alzheimer's disease, compared with similar levels of cognitive impairment [11]. Studies of cholinergic deficits in patients with PDD suggested that treatment of cholinesterase inhibitors (ChEIs) may effectively improve the impact of the disease on the cholinergic circuits. A Cochrane analysis supports the use of ChEIs in patients with PDD and shows that ChEIs have positive effects on cognitive function [12].

Although ChEIs have effects on PDD, up to date, many treatments all were symptomatic therapy. there is no etiological cure for PDD. In order to achieve the best treatment outcomes, the combination of ChEIs and other therapeutic strategies is widely studied. In China, some traditional herbs have been reported to improve cognitive function in dementia patients [13]-[15]. The combination of traditional herb and ChEIs suggested an obvious effect in treating the patients with Alzheimer's disease and vascular dementia [16] [17].

Reinhartdt and Sea Cucumber Capsule (RSC) has been used for many years in China to improve the cognition of Alzheimer's disease and vascular dementia [18] [19]. Here we hypothesize that RSC combined with a ChEIs rivastigmine may improve the treatment of mild-to-moderate PDD. the efficacy and tolerance of rivastigmine combined with RSC will be examined on the Alzheimer's Disease Assessment Scale cognitive subscale (ADAS-Cog), Activities of Daily Life (ADL) and Unified Parkinson's Disease Rating Scale (UPDRS) part III (motor scale) of the patients with mild-to-moderate PDD, and its effect on thyroid function axis.

2. Materials and Methods

2.1. Participants

Patients received a diagnosis of Parkinson's disease according to the clinical diagnostic criteria of the United Kingdom Parkinson's Disease Society Brain Bank [20] and a diagnosis of dementia due to Parkinson's disease based on criteria established by a Movement Disorders Society taskforce [21]. Patients had mild-to-moderately dementia as defined by a Mini-Mental State Examination (MMSE) score of 10 to 26. The vision, hearing and mental states of all patients were allowed cooperation to complete neuropsychological testing. All cases were in good nutritional status and had normal range of liver and kidney function in the blood. There was no history of thyroid disease, or drugs which can affect thyroid metabolism nearly a month.

Exclusion criteria included any causes of dementia other than Parkinson's disease; a history of a major depressive disorder; a history of hypersensitivity to ChEIs; the use of a cholinesterase inhibitor or other traditional herbal medicine which can interfere with the evaluation during the four weeks before randomization; serious abnormal heart, liver, kidney function; history of allergies and seafood allergy; a known or suspected history of alcoholism or drug abuse.

2.2. Study Design

In this 24-week, randomized, open-label and evaluator-blinded controlled study, all patients were informed and agreed to be consecutively enrolled in the study by their physicians. The random number table was used for randomized controlled trial design in the study. Basically, we randomly picked one number in the random number table for the first patient who was enrolled in the study. And the numbers following the first picked number in the random number table were consecutively assigned to other subjects according to the order of treatment. The subjects with singular number were treated with rivastigmine (Brand name: Exelon, Novartis Pharmaceutical Co., Switzerland) and the subjects with plural number were treated with rivastigmine plus Reinhartdt and Sea Cucumber Capsule (Brand name: Fufanghaishe, Hangkang Ocean Biological Pharmaceutical Co. Ltd., China).

During the treatment, all participants in rivasigmine group took rivastigmine orally at the doses of 3 mg/day, divided twice a day. In the combination treatment group, RSC was given at the dose of 0.9 g/time, three times a day orally. No other ChEIs or nootropics was taken by the patients in both groups during the treatment.

Patients were required to attend a regular interview every 4 weeks for the following evaluations. The following evaluations were routine physical and mental examination, psychometric tests (ADAS-Cog, ADL and UPDRS-III), and adverse events monitoring. Blood, urine, stool routine, liver and kidney function and Electrocardiography (ECG) were detected before and after 12 weeks and 24 weeks treatment in all patients. Thyroid hormone levels were also checked by immune chemiluminescence detection at the same time. Test box was provided by Bayer Co. Each normal reference values were: TT_3: 0.8 - 2.2 µg/L; TT_4: 42 - 135 µg/L; FT_3: 2.5 - 9.82 pmol/L; FT_4: 10 - 25 pmol/L; TSH: 0.2 - 7.0 mIU/L).

This study was conducted in accordance with the ethical standards of the responsible committee on human experimentation and with the Helsinki Declaration as revised in 1983.

2.3. Assessing Measurements

ADAS-Cog was used to measure the cognitive domains of PDD. The cognitive portion of the ADAS assesses orientation, memory, language, visuospatial, and praxis functions. Total scores ranged from 0 to 70, the higher the score, the greater the cognitive impairment. ADL was assessed with a standardized 20-item ADL scale. The scores ranged from 0 to 80 and a higher score, the greater less functional ability.

Changes in symptoms of Parkinson's disease were assessed by means of the motor section of the UPDRS (part III), for which scores can range from 0 to 108 points, with higher scores indicating more severe motor symptoms.

During the whole study, blinded and well trained evaluators performed the experiments to test MMSE, ADAS-Cog, ADL, UPDRS-III. All evaluators analyzed the data without any information about the patient group.

2.4. Statistical Analysis

Analyses were done on data from all patients who underwent randomization and who received at least one dose of study drug, applying the principle of intention-to-treat (ITT). We used the last-observation-carried-forward (LOCF) method to impute values if no follow-up information was available.

Statistical analyses were performed with the use of SPSS software, version 10.0. The basal comparison of characteristics in patients with two treatments was analyzed by a chi square test and student's t test. Changes from baseline in the ADAS-cog, ADL and UPRDS-III scores were assessed by means of analysis of covariance. Thyroid hormone levels data were expressed as mean ± standard deviation. Variance analysis (one-way ANOVA) was used in group while the Q test (post-hoc multiple comparisons between groups were made with Least-significant difference) was used between groups. A p-value < 0.05 was considered statistically significant.

3. Results

3.1. Patient Disposition

A total of 58 eligible patients were enrolled to attend the study. During the study, 3 patients previously took cholinesterase inhibitors, 2 patients quitted the study and 1 patient had severe renal dysfunction. Those 6 patients were excluded from our randomized study for treatment. The Consolidated Standards of Reporting Trias (CONSORT)-like flowchart was showed in **Figure 1**. The rest of 52 subjects were randomly divided into two treatment group. One group of 25 patients (11 males and 14 females) of aged 69.7 ± 4.2 years old (from 60 to 76

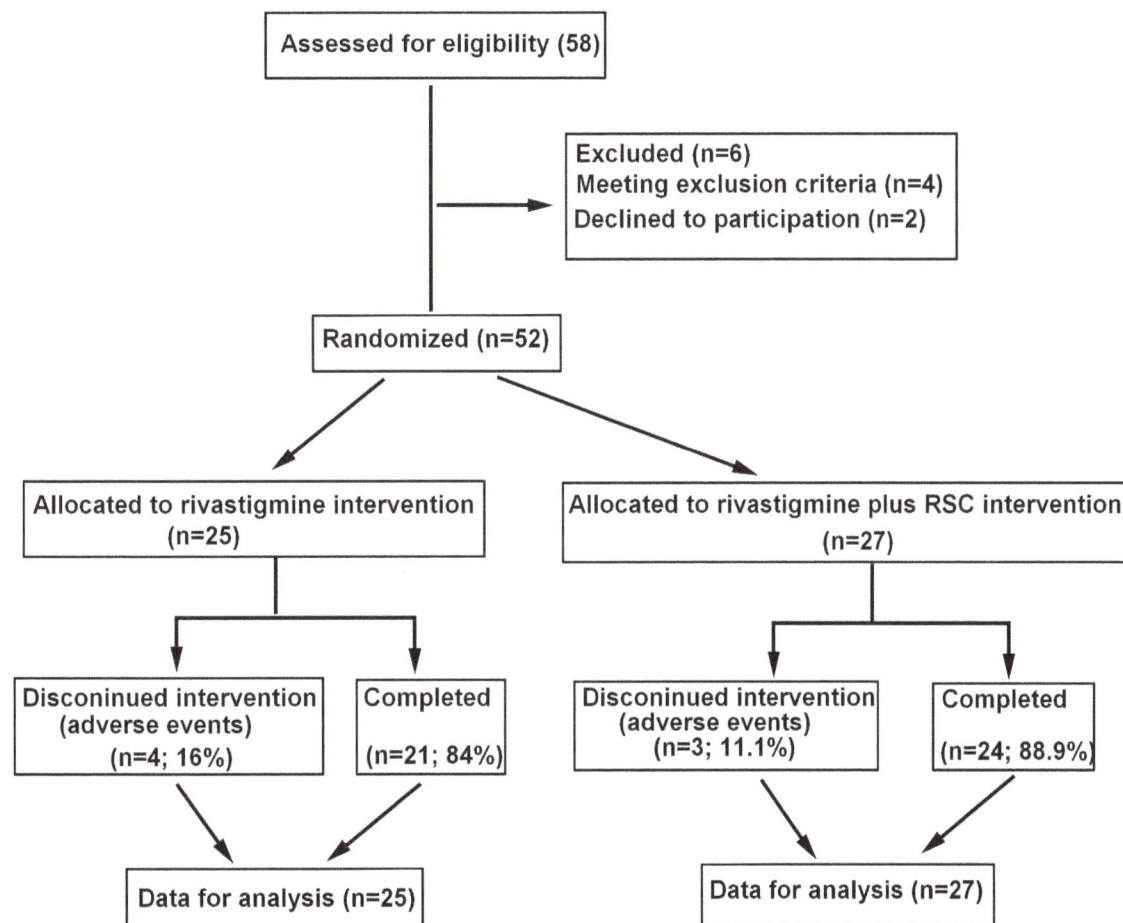

Figure 1. The CONSORT-like flowchart of patients.

years old) were treated with rivastigmine alone. The average duration of PDD for those patients was 1.6 ± 0.9 years. Another group of 27 patients (16 males and 11 females) of aged 70.6 ± 6.9 years (from 58 to 82 years old) were treated with rivastigmine plus RSC. The average duration of PDD was 1.6 ± 0.8 years. The results did not show any significant difference between the two groups in baseline data, the characteristics of two groups were shown in **Table 1**.

All patients with PDD from the two groups were also administered the following concomitant medications (single rivastigmine treatment vs rivastigmine plus RSC): levodopa agents (96.0% vs 92.6%), dopamine agonists agents (76.0% vs 81.5%), Amantadine (36.0% vs 25.9%), Comtan (catechol-O-methyltransferase inhibitor; Entacapone) (16.0% vs 11.1%), antidepressants (28.0% vs 22.2%), antianxiety agents (32.0% vs 37.0%),and antipsychotic agents (32.0% vs 33.3%). There were no significant differences between two groups ($p > 0.05$) in most common concomitant medications.

3.2. Efficacy

The ADAS-Cog scores declined at the beginning of the treatment in both groups. This meant the cognition of the patients improved after the treatments. Compared to the rivastigmine treatment alone group, rivastigmine plus RSC group had significantly more reduction in ADAS-Cog scores and ADL scores. The ADAS-Cog scores in the combined group had an obvious decrease ($p < 0.05$ at 12weeks, $p < 0.01$ after 16 weeks) and the patients displayed much better cognition since the 12th week (**Figure 2**). The ADL scores also significantly decreased in rivastigmine plus RSC treatment group from the 12th week to the end of the study as compared with rivastigmine treatment alone (**Figure 3**). There is no difference was observed in the UPDRS part III score between two groups at each time (**Figure 4**).

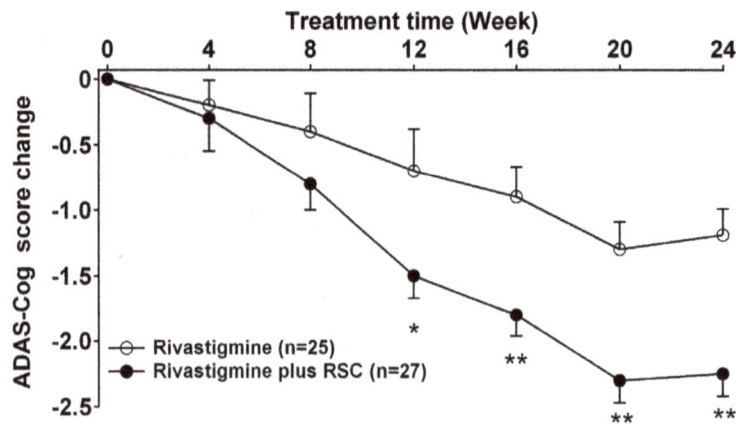

Figure 2. The change of the scores of ADAS-Cog in each group (mean ± SD). *: $p < 0.05$, **: $p < 0.01$ between the rivastigmine treatment and the rivastigmine plus RSC treatment.

Table 1. The characteristics of the patients in each group.

Parameter	Rivastigmine, N = 25	Rivastigmine plus RSC, N = 27	Statistic values
Sex (male/female)-no.	11/14	16/11	$x^2 = 1.211$; $p = 0.271$
Age (mean ± SD)	69.7 ± 4.2	70.6 ± 6.9	$t = 0.571$; $p = 0.570$
Education (mean ± SD)	9.1 ± 2.1	8.9 ± 3.1	$t = 0.316$; $p = 0.753$
Duration of PD (mean ± SD)	7.9 ± 1.9	7.8 ± 2.4	$t = 0.292$; $p = 0.771$
Duration of PDD (mean ± SD)	1.6 ± 0.9	1.6 ± 0.8	$t = 0.044$; $p = 0.965$
MMSE score (mean ± SD)	20.8 ± 3.9	19.8 ± 3.8	$t = 0.283$; $p = 0.778$
ADAS-cog score (mean ± SD)	25.4 ± 9.4	26.2 ± 9.1	$t = 0.320$; $p = 0.750$
ADL score (mean ± SD)	42.6 ± 9.3	42.1 ± 11.0	$t = 0.173$; $p = 0.863$
UPDRS part III score (mean ± SD)	33.6 ± 11.1	33.3 ± 12.5	$t = 0.092$; $p = 0.927$
Medications used-no. (%)			
Levodopa	24 (96%)	25 (92.6%)	$x^2 = 0.277$; $p = 0.599$
Dopamine agonists	19 (76.0%)	22 (81.5%)	$x^2 = 0.234$; $p = 0.629$
Amantadine	9 (36.0%)	7 (25.9%)	$x^2 = 0.618$; $p = 0.432$
Comtan	4 (16.0%)	3 (11.1%)	$x^2 = 0.266$; $p = 0.606$
Antidepressants	7 (28.0%)	6 (22.2%)	$x^2 = 0.231$; $p = 0.631$
Antianxiety agents	8 (32.0%)	10 (37.0%)	$x^2 = 0.146$; $p = 0.703$
Antipsychotic agents	8 (32.0%)	9 (33.3%)	$x^2 = 0.010$; $p = 0.918$

Thyroid hormone levels of the two groups of patients were evaluated before and after 12 weeks, 24 weeks treatment, but no statistical difference was found between the each time period ($p > 0.05$, **Table 2**).

3.3. Safety

The main treatment-related adverse events were nausea and vomiting in this study. Three participants (2 patients vomiting, 1 patient nausea) in the rivastigmine plus RSC and four subjects (1 patient vomiting, 3 patients nausea) in the single rivastigmine group experienced mild-to-moderate adverse events related to nausea and vomiting. They all failed to complete the study due to the adverse events. No serious adverse events were occurred during the study. The statistical results found no significant difference in the laboratory and auxiliary examination (blood, urine, stool routine, liver and kidney function, ECG). The discontinuation rate was similar in two groups

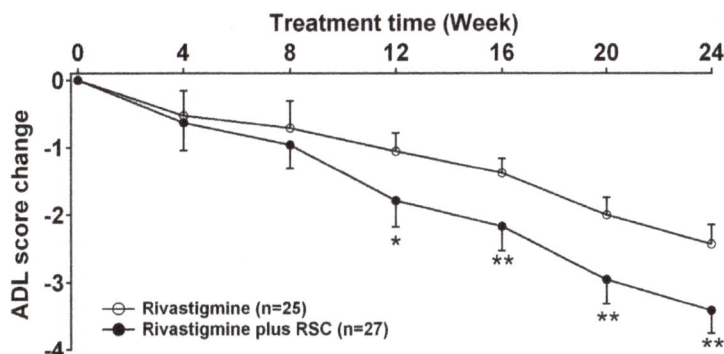

Figure 3. The change of the scores of ADL in each group (mean ± SD). *p < 0.05, **p < 0.01 between the rivastigmine treatment and the rivastigmine plus RSC treatment.

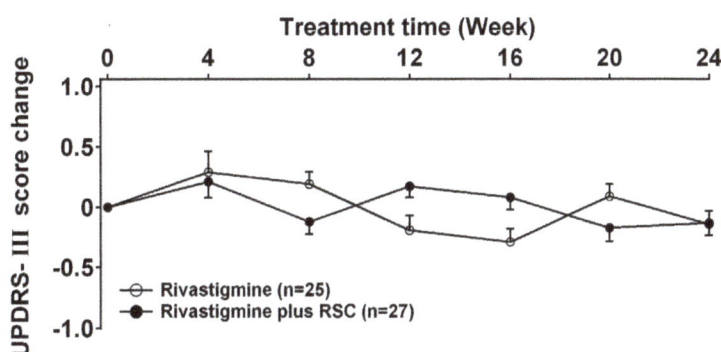

Figure 4. The change of the scores of UPDRS-III in each group (mean ± SD). There is no difference between two groups at each time.

Table 2. Thyroid hormone levels before and after treatment in each group (mean ± SD).

Groups	No.	Period	TSH (mIU/L)	TT_3 (μg/L)	TT_4 (μg/L)	FT_3 (pmol/L)	FT_4 (pmol/L)
Rivastigmine	25	Before treatment	4.0 ± 0.9	1.6 ± 0.3	76.1 ± 10.7	5.8 ± 2.1	18.0 ± 3.5
	25	After 12 weeks	4.0 ± 0.9	1.7 ± 0.2	74.6 ± 9.3	5.7 ± 1.7	17.7 ± 2.9
	25	After 24 weeks	4.2 ± 0.8	1.7 ± 0.3	76.6 ± 8.1	5.6 ± 1.8	17.9 ± 2.9
Rivastigmine plus RSC	27	Before treatment	4.1 ± 0.9	1.7 ± 0.3	78.2 ± 10.7	6.0 ± 1.3	17.8 ± 3.7
	27	After 12 weeks	4.1 ± 1.0	1.7 ± 0.3	79.2 ± 9.6	5.7 ± 1.3	18.1 ± 3.2
	27	After 24 weeks	4.2 ± 0.9	1.6 ± 0.2	78.0 ± 9.7	6.1 ± 1.3	16.9 ± 3.3

(11.1% in rivastigmine plus RSC group; 16.0% in rivastigmine alone group). No difference was observed between two groups in reasons for discontinuation (p > 0.05).

4. Discussion

Dementia in Parkinson's disease is linked to disease-related disturbances of cholinergic activity [10]. Cholinergic neuron loss as the main feature of non-dopaminergic neurons dysfunction was an important pathophysiological mechanism in Parkinson's disease dementia [10] [11]. The main neuropathological change was that the Lewy bodies widely appear in the basal ganglia and the limbic system [22]-[24]. Thus, base on the pathophysiological mechanism, many scholar think that mechanism-based treatments can improve cognition in Parkinson's disease. The first study about ChEIs treatment PDD in 1996, it showed the cognition of patients with PDD improved after treated with tacrine [25]. Although only seven patients with PDD in the study, the result of this study provided the rationale for large randomized controlled trials of ChEIs in PDD. EXPRESS study which a

24-week randomized placebo-controlled trial, showed that rivastigmine significantly improved cognition and clinical outcomes compared with placebo [26]. Meanwhile ,The results of extension phase also showed that rivastigmine might provide sustained benefits for up to 48 weeks [27].when the patients with PDD were treated with rivastigmine, amplified brain perfusion on Single-photon Emission Computed Tomography and increased α-activity on quantitative EEG in frontal regions were found [28] [29]. Now, rivastigmine is widely approved for clinical use in the treatment of PDD [30]. In this study, we observed obvious improvement in cognition and the daily activities of patients with mild-to-moderate PDD after taking rivastigmine 3 mg/d for 24 weeks. In China, some traditional herbal medicine can improve cognitive function in dementia patients [13]-[15]. RSC is one of traditional Chinese medicine which improves the cognition of Alzheimer's disease and vascular dementia and has been used for many years in China [18] [19]. RSC is a natural product which is made of Hainan semirings sea snakes, Yuzu sea cucumber and polygala tenuifolia by biological engineering technology. The main ingredients were sea snakes, sea cucumbers, Polygala and stone calamus. Researches about RSC in cell and molecular level indicated that it could significantly increase the content of acetylcholine and superoxide dismutase in the brain, and reduce the glutamic acid and lipid peroxide levels. The mechanism for improving cognitive and memory function is changing a variety of brain neurotransmitters and biochemical factors [31]-[33]. ChEIs was also reported to treat the patients with Alzheimer's disease and vascular dementia with a certain effect [17] [34]. In the present study, we observed more improvement in cognition and the daily activities of patients after 24-weeks treatment with rivastigmine plus RSC group compared with rivastigmine alone treatment group. Significant difference was found in ADAC-cog, ADL scores at the 12-weeks. Patients showed better cognitive and behavior abilities with rivastigmine plus RSC treatment. These results suggest that rivastigmine plus RSC treatment has a better effect on improving the cognitive deficit in PDD patients than rivastigmine alone treatment. It also indicated the potency of RSC in delaying the cognitive decline in PDD when treated with rivastigmine simultaneously. In our study, the improvement of the cognition and the daily function of the patients in the combined treated group may be due to the improvement of acetylcholine content in the brain. The improvement of daily living function may be due to the improvement in cognition, as the motor function remains unchanged after the treatment.

Thyroid hormone plays an important role in the central nervous system development and normal function [35] [36]. Slight change in thyroid hormone level even in the normal range may be associated with the elderly emotional and cognitive function change. Previous studies have shown that thyroid hormone levels were closely linked with Alzheimer's disease. Thyroid hormone levels were reported to be changed in Alzheimer's disease patients after cholinesterase inhibitor therapy [37] [38]. Our previous study also found that the RSC combined with donepezil therapy in patients with Alzheimer's disease and vascular dementia raised its T_3, T_4 level, synergistically improving cognitive function [17] [34]. However, in present study, no change about thyroid hormone levels was found before and after 12 weeks and 24 weeks in either single rivastigmine treatment or rivastigmine plus RSC treatment. It is consistent with previous researches that thyroid hormone levels were not correlated to the severity of Parkinson's disease [39] [40].

The predominant adverse events caused by cholinergic disorder are nausea,vomiting, tremor, diarrhea, anorexia, etc. Most of these adverse events were reversible, and were mild to moderate. Although tremor may occurred during the initial treatment period, the analysis about rivastigmine effect on motor effects showed that Parkinson's disease did not get worse during 48 weeks in the EXPRESS study [41]. Adverse events were not observed to be different in UPDRS motor scores including tremor-related items between the control groups and treatment group [24]. Compared to the treatment in previous studies, the combination treatment in our study indicated a lower incidence of side effects (13.5%, 7 cases). The side effect is the reason for withdrawing from the study. It mainly showed nausea (3 cases), vomiting (4 cases), and symptoms improved after withdraw. No tremor and other movement disorders aggravation were observed. There was no difference in UPDRS motor scores. It may be related to rivastigmine used in small dosage (3 mg/day) in our study.

Of cause, some limitations are still present in our study. First, these results may partly reflect a normal clinical treatment, not a double-blind, randomized, controlled trial. Second, the sample size is still small, due to the strict inclusion and exclusion criteria. A better rigorous research with more patients needs to be performed in the future.

5. Conclusion

In conclusion, our results show that rivastigmine plus RSC treatment has a better effect in improving the symptoms of the patients with mild-to-moderate PDD than rivastigmine treatment alone. The formula was safe and it had no effect on thyroid hormone levels in PDD patients.

Competing Interests

The authors have declared that no competing interest exists.

References

[1] Jankovic, J. (2008) Parkinson's Disease: Clinical Features and Diagnosis. *Journal of Neurology, Neurosurgery & Psychiatry*, **79**, 368-376. http://dx.doi.org/10.1136/jnnp.2007.131045

[2] Hirtz, D., Thurman, D.J., Gwinn-Hardy, K., Mohamed, M., Chaudhuri, A.R. and Zalutsky, R. (2007) How Common Are the "Common" Neurologic Disorders? *Neurology*, **68**, 326-337. http://dx.doi.org/10.1212/01.wnl.0000252807.38124.a3

[3] Zhang, Z.X., Roman, G.C., Hong, Z., Wu, C.B., Qu, Q.M., Huang, J.B., Zhou, B., Geng, Z.P., Wu, J.X., Wen, H.B., Zhao, H. and Zahner, G.E. (2005) Parkinson's Disease in China: Prevalence in Beijing, Xian, and Shanghai. *Lancet*, **365**, 595-597. http://dx.doi.org/10.1016/S0140-6736(05)17909-4

[4] Galvin, J.E., Pollack, J. and Morris, J.C. (2006) Clinical Phenotype of Parkinson Disease Dementia. *Neurology*, **67**, 1605-1611. http://dx.doi.org/10.1212/01.wnl.0000242630.52203.8f

[5] Aarsland, D., Zaccai, J. and Brayne, C. (2005) A Systematic Review of Prevalence Studies of Dementia in Parkinson's Disease. *Movement Disorders*, **20**, 1255-1263. http://dx.doi.org/10.1002/mds.20527

[6] Riedel, O., Klotsche, J., Spottke, A., Deuschl, G., Förstl, H., Henn, F., Heuser, I., Oertel, W., Reichmann, H., Riederer, P., Trenkwalder, C., Dodel, R. and Wittchen, H.U. (2010) Frequency of Dementia, Depression, and Other Neuropsychiatric Symptoms in 1449 Outpatients with Parkinson's Disease. *Journal of Neurology*, **257**, 1073-1082. http://dx.doi.org/10.1007/s00415-010-5465-z

[7] Winter, Y., von Campenhausen, S., Arend, M., Longo, K., Boetzel, K., Eggert, K., Oertel, W.H., Dodel, R. and Barone, P. (2011) Health-Related Quality of Life and Its Determinants in Parkinson's Disease: Results of an Italian Cohort study. *Parkinsonism & Related Disorders*, **17**, 265-269. http://dx.doi.org/10.1016/j.parkreldis.2011.01.003

[8] Vossius, C., Larsen, J.P., Janvin, C. and Aarsland, D. (2011) The Economic Impact of Cognitive Impairment in Parkinson's Disease. *Movement Disorders*, **26**, 1541-1544. http://dx.doi.org/10.1002/mds.23661

[9] Fletcher, P., Leake, A. and Marion, M.H. (2011) Patients with Parkinson's Disease Dementia Stay in the Hospital Twice as Long as Those without Dementia. *Movement Disorders*, **26**, 919. http://dx.doi.org/10.1002/mds.23573

[10] Klein, J.C., Eggers, C., Kalbe, E., Weisenbach, S., Hohmann, C., Vollmar, S., Baudrexel, S., Diederich, N.J., Heiss, W.D. and Hilker, R. (2010) Neurotransmitter Changes in Dementia with Lewy Bodies and Parkinson Disease Dementia *in Vivo*. *Neurology*, **74**, 885-892. http://dx.doi.org/10.1212/WNL.0b013e3181d55f61

[11] Bohnen, N.I., Kaufer, D.I., Ivanco, L.S., Lopresti, B., Koeppe, R.A., Davis, J.G., Mathis, C.A., Moore, R.Y. and DeKosky, S.T. (2003) Cortical Cholinergic Function Is More Severely Affected in Parkinsonian Dementia Than in Alzheimer Disease: An *in Vivo* Positron Emission Tomographic Study. *Arch Neurol*, **60**, 1745-1748. http://dx.doi.org/10.1001/archneur.60.12.1745

[12] Rolinski, M., Fox, C., Maidment, I. and McShane, R. (2012) Cholinesterase Inhibitors for Dementia with Lewy Bodies, Parkinson's Disease Dementia and Cognitive Impairment in Parkinson's Disease. *Cochrane Database of Systematic Reviews*, **3**, CD006504. http://dx.doi.org/10.1002/14651858.CD006504.pub2

[13] Wu, T.Y., Chen, C.P. and Jinn, T.R. (2011) Traditional Chinese Medicines and Alzheimer's Disease. *Taiwanese Journal of Obstetrics and Gynecology*, **50**, 131-135. http://dx.doi.org/10.1016/j.tjog.2011.04.004

[14] Lin, H.Q., Ho, M.T., Lau, L.S., Wong, K.K., Shaw, P.C. and Wan, D.C. (2008) Anti-Acetylcholinesterase Activities of Traditional Chinese Medicine for Treating Alzheimer's Disease. *Chemico-Biological Interactions*, **175**, 352-354. http://dx.doi.org/10.1016/j.cbi.2008.05.030

[15] Kim, H.G. and Oh, M.S. (2012) Herbal Medicines for the Prevention and Treatment of Alzheimer's Disease. *Current Pharmaceutical Design*, **18**, 57-75. http://dx.doi.org/10.2174/138161212798919002

[16] Li, D.Q., Zhou, Y.P. and Yang, H. (2012) Donepezil Combined with Natural Hirudin Improves the Clinical Symptoms of Patients with Mild-to-Moderate Alzheimer's Disease: A 20-Week Open-Label Pilot Study. *International Journal of Medical Sciences*, **9**, 248-255. http://dx.doi.org/10.7150/ijms.4363

[17] Yan, Y.X., Liang, L.Z. and Zhou, Z.L. (2007) Clinical Study of Combined Treatment with Compound Reinhartdt and Sea Cumber Capsule and Donepezil for Vascular Dementia. *Chinese Journal of Integrated Traditional and Western Medicine*, **27**, 887-890.

[18] Wang, C.F., Ma, Y.X., Gu, Y.D., Xie, S.Z., Yu, Z.Y. and Yang, J.Y. (2000) A Double-Blind Clinical Study on the Reinhardt and Sea Cucumber Capsule in Treating Dementia in the Aged. *Geriatrics & Health Care*, **6**, 11-15.

[19] Kang, J. (2009) Research of Compound Reinhartdt and Sea Cumber Capsule Treating Encephalopathy. *World Chinese Medicine*, **4**, 58-59.

[20] Gibb, W.R. and Lees, A.J. (1988) The Relevance of the Lewy Body to the Pathogenesis of Idiopathic Parkinson's Disease. *Journal of Neurology, Neurosurgery & Psychiatry*, **51**, 745-752. http://dx.doi.org/10.1136/jnnp.51.6.745

[21] Emre, M., Aarsland, D., Brown, R., Burn, D.J., Duyckaerts, C., Mizuno, Y., Broe, G.A., Cummings, J., Dickson, D.W., Gauthier, S., Goldman, J., Goetz, C., Korczyn, A., Lees, A., Levy, R., Litvan, I., McKeith, I., Olanow, W., Poewe, W., Quinn, N., Sampaio, C., Tolosa, E. and Dubois, B. (2007) Clinical Diagnostic Criteria for Dementia Associated with Parkinson's Disease. *Movement Disorders*, **22**, 1689-1707. http://dx.doi.org/10.1002/mds.21507

[22] Hurtig, H.I., Trojanowski, J.Q., Galvin, J., Ewbank, D., Schmidt, M.L., Lee, V.M., Clark, C.M., Glosser, G., Stern, M.B., Gollomp, S.M. and Arnold, S.E. (2000) Alpha-Synuclein Cortical Lewy Bodies Correlate with Dementia in Parkinson's Disease. *Neurology*, **54**, 1916-1921. http://dx.doi.org/10.1212/WNL.54.10.1916

[23] Aarsland, D., Perry, R., Brown, A., Larsen, J.P. and Ballard, C. (2005) Neuropathology of Dementia in Parkinson's Disease: A Prospective, Community-Based Study. *Annals of Neurology*, **58**, 773-776. http://dx.doi.org/10.1002/ana.20635

[24] Braak, H., Rüb, U., Jansen Steur, E.N., Del Tredici, K. and de Vos, R.A. (2005) Cognitive Status Correlates with Neuropathologic Stage in Parkinson Disease. *Neurology*, **64**, 1404-1410. http://dx.doi.org/10.1212/01.WNL.0000158422.41380.82

[25] Hutchinson, M. and Fazzini, E. (1996) Cholinesterase Inhibition in Parkinson's Disease. *Journal of Neurology, Neurosurgery & Psychiatry*, **61**, 324-325. http://dx.doi.org/10.1136/jnnp.61.3.324-a

[26] Emre, M., Aarsland, D., Albanese, A., Byrne, E.J., Deuschl, G., De Deyn, P.P., Durif, F., Kulisevsky, J., van Laar, T., Lees, A., Poewe, W., Robillard, A., Rosa, M.M., Wolters, E., Quarg, P., Tekin, S. and Lane, R. (2004) Rivastigmine for Dementia Associated with Parkinson's Disease. *The New England Journal of Medicine*, **351**, 2509-2518. http://dx.doi.org/10.1056/NEJMoa041470

[27] Poewe, W., Wolters, E., Emre, M., Onofrj, M., Hsu, C., Tekin, S. and Lane, R., EXPRESS Investigators (2006) Long-Term Benefits of Rivastigmine in Dementia Associated with Parkinson's Disease: An Active Treatment Extension Study. *Movement Disorders*, **21**, 456-461. http://dx.doi.org/10.1002/mds.20700

[28] Ceravolo, R., Volterrani, D., Frosini, D., Bernardini, S., Rossi, C., Logi, C., Manca, G., Kiferle, L., Mariani, G., Murri, L. and Bonuccelli, U. (2006) Brain Perfusion Effects of Cholinesterase Inhibitors in Parkinson's Disease with Dementia. *Journal of Neural Transmission*, **113**, 1787-1790. http://dx.doi.org/10.1007/s00702-006-0478-6

[29] Fogelson, N., Kogan, E., Korczyn, A.D., Giladi, N., Shabtai, H. and Neufeld, M.Y. (2003) Effects of Rivastigmine on the Quantitative EEG in Demented Parkinsonian Patients. *Acta Neurologica Scandinavica*, **107**, 252-255. http://dx.doi.org/10.1034/j.1600-0404.2003.00081.x

[30] van Laar, T., De Deyn, P.P., Aarsland, D., Barone, P. and Galvin, J.E. (2011) Effects of Cholinesterase Inhibitors in Parkinson's Disease Dementia: A Review of Clinical Data. *CNS Neuroscience & Therapeutics*, **17**, 428-441. http://dx.doi.org/10.1111/j.1755-5949.2010.00166.x

[31] Wang, C.F., Ma, Y.X., Xie, S.Z., Li, W.B., Zhang, B.L. and Tao, G.S. (1999) The Study of Reinhartdt and Sea Cucumber Capsule on the Efficacy and Mechanism of Action in the Dementia Model. In: Ma, Y.X., Wang, C.F. and Shi, F,Y., Eds., *New Progress of Aging and Geriatrics*, 1st Edition, FU Dan University Press, Shanghai, 477-487.

[32] Lv, J., Jia, H., Jiang, Y., Ruan, Y., Liu, Z., Yue, W., Beyreuther, K., Tu, P. and Zhang, D. (2009) Tenuifolin, an Extract Derived from Tenuigenin, Inhibits Amyloid-Beta Secretion *in Vitro*. *Acta Physiologica*, **196**, 419-425. http://dx.doi.org/10.1111/j.1748-1716.2009.01961.x

[33] Jia, H., Jiang, Y., Ruan, Y., Zhang, Y., Ma, X., Zhang, J., Beyreuther, K., Tu, P. and Zhang, D. (2004) Tenuigenin Treatment Decreases Secretion of the Alzheimer's Disease Amyloid Betaprotein in Cultured Cells. *Neuroscience Letters*, **367**, 123-128. http://dx.doi.org/10.1016/j.neulet.2004.05.093

[34] Zhou, Z.L., Liang, L.Z. and Yan, Y.X. (2007) Clinical Study of Reinhartdt and Sea Cucumber Capsule Combined with Donepezil in Treating Alzheimer's Disease. *Chinese Journal of Integrated Traditional and Western Medicine*, **27**, 110-113.

[35] Jahagirdar, V. and McNay, E.C. (2012) Thyroid Hormone's Role in Regulating Brain Glucose Metabolism and Potentially Modulating Hippocampal Cognitive Processes. *Metabolic Brain Disease*, **27**, 101-111. http://dx.doi.org/10.1007/s11011-012-9291-0

[36] Carreón-Rodríguez, A. and Pérez-Martínez, L. (2012) Clinical Implications of Thyroid Hormones Effects on Nervous System Development. *Pediatric Endocrinology Reviews*, **9**, 644-649.

[37] Bauer, M., Goetz, T., Glenn, T. and Whybrow, P.C. (2008) The Thyroid-Brain Interaction in Thyroid Disorders and

Mood Disorders. *Journal of Neuroendocrinology*, **20**, 1101-1114. http://dx.doi.org/10.1111/j.1365-2826.2008.01774.x

[38] Bunevicius, R. (2009) Thyroid Disorders in Mental Patients. *Current Opinion in Psychiatry*, **22**, 391-395. http://dx.doi.org/10.1097/YCO.0b013e328329e1ae

[39] Schaefer, S., Vogt, T., Nowak, T. and Kann, P.H., German KIMS board (2008) Pituitary Function and the Somatotmphie System in Patients with Idiopathic Parkinson's Disease under Chronic Dopaminersic Therapy. *Journal of Neuroendocrinology*, **20**, 104-109. http://dx.doi.org/10.1111/j.1365-2826.2007.01622.x

[40] Bonuccelli, U., D'Avino, C., Caraccio, N., Del Guerra, P., Casolaro, A., Pavese, N., Del Dotto, P. and Monzani, F. (1999) Thyroid Function and Autoimmunity in Parkinson's Disease: A Study of 101 Patients. *Parkinsonism & Related Disorders*, **5**, 49-53. http://dx.doi.org/10.1016/S1353-8020(99)00010-3

[41] Oertel, W., Poewe, W., Wolters, E., De Deyn, P.P., Emre, M., Kirsch, C., Hsu, C., Tekin, S. and Lane, R. (2008) Effects of Rivastigmine on Tremor and Other Motor Symptoms in Patients with Parkinson's Disease Dementia: A Retrospective Analysis of a Double-Blind Trial and an Open-Label Extension. *Drug Safety*, **31**, 79-94. http://dx.doi.org/10.2165/00002018-200831010-00007

3

Evaluation of Acute and Repeated Dose Toxicity of the Polyherbal Formulation Linkus Syrup in Experimental Animals

Allah Nawaz[1,2], Saira Bano[1], Zeeshan Ahmed Sheikh[1], Khan Usmanghani[1,3*], Iqbal Ahmad[4], Syed Faisal Zaidi[5], Aqib Zahoor[1], Irshad Ahmad[6,7]

[1]Research and Development Department, Herbion Pakistan (Pvt.) Limited, Karachi, Pakistan
[2]First Department of Internal Medicine, Faculty of Medicine, Graduate School of Medical & Pharmaceutical Sciences, University of Toyama, Toyama, Japan
[3]Jinnah University for Women, Karachi, Pakisntan
[4]Baqai Institute of Pharmaceutical Sciences, Baqai Medical University, Karachi, Pakistan
[5]Department of Basic Medical Sciences, College of Medicine, King Saud bin Abdulaziz University of Health Sciences, Jeddah, KSA
[6]Department of Pharmacy, The Islamia University of Bahawalpur, Bahawalpur, Pakistan
[7]Clinical Pharmacy and Health Care, Jinnah University for Women, Karachi, Pakistan
Email: *usman.ghani@herbion.com, *ugk_2005@yahoo.com

Abstract

The objective of the present study was to evaluate the pre-clinical efficacy and toxicity of polyherbal cough syrup Linkus. Method: Animals (healthy Wistar albino rats; (150 - 250 g) of either sex) were housed under standard environmental conditions; *i.e.* 25°C ± 1°C and 12 h dark/light cycle. Food and water were available *at libitum*. The rats were treated orally with the recommended doses of the test drug (Linkus). After 15 minutes, they were individually placed in a closed Plexiglas chamber (20 × 10 × 10 cm) and exposed to citric acid (0.1 g/ml) inhalation for 7 minutes. The cough reflexes were produced and counted for the last 5 minutes and compared with those of the control animals. The following studies were conducted to evaluate the toxicity of the test drug in healthy Wistar albino rats: lethal dose$_{50}$ (LD$_{50}$); rats of either sex (n = 10/sex) were treated orally with doses (1 or 5 g/kg) of the test drug. Mortality and behavioral changes were observed for 1 week. Repeated dose toxicity on the healthy Wistar albino rats of both sexes (n = 5/dose/sex) was treated orally with doses of 20 mg/kg (adult human dose = ~1400 mg), 500 mg/kg (adult human dose = ~35,000 mg) and 1000 mg/kg (adult human dose = ~70,000 mg) of test drug (Linkus) for 14

---

*Corresponding author.

days. Additionally, the control animals were treated orally with water for 14 days. Results: In female rats, the test drug (Linkus) at the dose of 300 mg/kg caused significant ($p < 0.01$) reduction in the cough reflexes as compared to the control. However, in male rats, a significant reduction was observed at the tested dose of 200 mg/kg ($p < 0.05$) and 300 mg/kg ($p < 0.01$). The test product did not cause mortality in rats at the given doses of 1 or 5 g/kg. Other signs of toxicity like hair loss and weight reduction were not observed. In female and male rats, the test drug (Linkus) at different doses did not show any abnormal effects on complete blood count profile of rats. Serum enzyme markers, *i.e.* alanine aminotransferase (ALT), alakaline phosphatase, gamma glutamyle transferase (GGT), direct bilirubin, creatinine, and proteins were also observed and found that the test drug at a higher dose did not cause any of the abnormality and had shown significant p value as compared to the control. Conclusion: The test drug (Linkus) could be an effective and safe cough syrup because it did not show any of the side effects or toxicity on experimental animals.

Keywords

Cough Expectorant, Alanine Amino Transferase (ALT), Polyherbal, Gamma Glutamyl Transferase (GGT), Toxicity

1. Introduction

Cough is defined as the process by which foreign material and mucus from the lungs and upper airway passage are removed. The expelled out mucus during cough is called as phlegm or sputum. It is a most common problem for which the person or patients seeks medical attention; if medical treatment is not started at an earlier stage, it may progress intensely so as to disturb the quality of life. If left untreated, it may lead to vomiting, miscarriage, fever, abdominal pain, headache, seizure, and chest pain etc. [1]. In the social life coughing condition generally causes the embarrassment and self-consciousness and those suffering feeling difficulty in speaking or to speak loud [2]. It has been cited in the literature that the herbal medicines are frequently utilized to cure cough mlaise. In the developed and developing countries there has been expanded use of the medicinal plants and their parts in the complementary and alternative medicine for the treatment of different cough ailments because of their safety, accessibility and efficacy [3] [4]. A major concern regarding the use of herbal medicines is the lack of the preclinical studies for safety evaluation [5]. Many medicinal plants such as *Ocimum sanctum* [6], *Passiflora incarnate* [7], *Adhatoda vasica* [8], *Glycyrrhiza glabra* [9], *Zingiber officinale* [10], *Asparagus racemosus* [11], *Trichodesma indicum* [12], *Asparagus racemosus* [13] and *Emblica officinalis* [14] have been cited in the literature for their antitussive activity. Previous work *in vitro* in experimental model has been done by Keter and coworkers on combination of herbal components on Wister rats for antitussive activity and the result demonstrated significant activity [15]. In another study Gupta and associates tested antitussive activity of combination of herbal drugs formulation and induced cough model in mice and formulation proved to be useful in alleviating cough [16]. In general concept it is commonly observed that many of the well-known herbal or eastern and natural supplements have not been thoroughly evaluated as western medicine to confirm their safety and efficacy. On the other hand, the text of associated products and food supplements had a chronic delusion. There is diversity found in the same brand of medicine claims on label, but from past 12 to 14 years the clinical and pharmacological interests in the efficacy and safety of herbal remedies were started but we found very rare complete study on mixture of herbs for alleviating the cough in experimental animals and to evaluate acute toxicity as well. Many people who frequently use the herbal medicine as self-medication were driven by the realization that, particularly complementary and alternative medicine offers a failure to treat chronic disease as cancer, diabetes, autoimmune disease, and persistent infection [17] [18]. It is worthwhile importance that these medicines cure the different ailments as claimed by different manufacturers and also physician practicing herbal or natural medicine for management of various disorders at their clinic but there is lack of evidence behind their theory to prove their efficacy and safety in scientific logic basis. It is a general concept from many centuries that herbal medicine is considered safe because these originated from natural sources but scientist and researchers have proven that many of the herbal medicinal plants are very toxic even at minor dose; for example toxic herbal product is the leaves of *Atropa belladonna*, *Aconitum* and *Digitalis pursuer* [19] which cause severe toxicities if taken without precautionary measures. In the current study, we followed the acute oral toxicity test in evaluating the toxicity and efficacy of the Linkus syrup. We conducted this study in two parts: first was to administer the Linkus syrup with different doses to evaluate acute and repeated does toxicity and in second we administered this test drug to animals for efficacy study by observing cough reflexes in comparison with control and Hydryllin (**Hydryllin** (Searle): [Aminophylline Plus Compound Syrup] + Active Ingredients: Aminophylline 32 mg, Ammonium chloride 30 mg, Diphenylhydramine 8 mg, Menthol 0.98 mg). Indications: productive cough, smokers' cough, cough associated with asthma and cough due to bronchitis and due to other respiratory diseases. Contraindication Hydryllin should not be given to patients with active peptic ulcers or acute myocardial infarction. It should not be used in patients with hypersensitivity to its components. Because of its diphenhydramine component, Hydryllin should be used in caution and in consultation with physician in asthmatic patients.

The tested animals were then monitored for 16 days for any sign of pathologic and behavioral toxicities detailed are given in methodology section. In market few combined Aherbal formulation study on antitussive activity so far reported. So in this scenario the dosage form design of Linkus consists of some of these herbal drugs but as such to the best of our knowledge no such work on the stated poly herbal as antitussive herbs is reported. Linkus syrup is a polyherbal formulation used for treating patients having complaints of cough in Pakistan and abroad. The Linkus syrup comprises of the following *Adhatoda vasica* (AV)—Bansa, *Piper longum* L. (PL)—Filfil Daraz, *Cordia latifolia* Roxb. (CL)—Sapistan, *Glycyrrhiza glabra* L. (GG)—Mulathi, *Hyssopus officinalis* L. (HO)—Zufa, *Alpinia galangal* Willd. (AG)—Khulanjan, *Viola odorata* L. (VO)—Banafsha, *Althea officinalis* L. (AO)—Khatmi, *Zizyphus vulgaris* Lam. (ZV)—Unnab, *Onosma bracteatum* Wall. (OB)—Gaozaban and excipients. Although herbal supplements may be considered to be safe, some are known to be toxic at high doses and others may have potentially adverse effects after prolonged use. The pre-clinical toxicological studies are necessary to be conducted on these herbal medicines to assess their efficacy and find out side or adverse effects. This product was developed in research and development department, Herbion Pakistan Private Limited, and it is intended to be used as remedy for alleviating cough symptoms.

2. Material and Method

2.1. Preparation of Linkus Extract and Syrup

The medicinal plants in test drug (Linkus) were purchased from Insaf Karyana Store Jodia Bazar, Karachi and authenticity of the samples was kindly carried out by Pro. Dr. Iqbal Azhar, Department of Pharmacognosy University of Karachi. The voucher specimens were deposited in Quality Control Herbarium Sections with identities as AV = B18, PL = F1, CL = S9, GG = M4, HO = Z1, AG = K2, VO = B2, AO = K3, ZV = U3, OB = B13.

Linkus syrup batch manufacturing size was of 2500.0 liters and the finished packs realized in 20,833 units, whereas pack size was of 120 ml in primary packaging in amber colored glass bottle. The details of Linkus ingredients and process of extraction are given in the **Table 1**.

The detailed method of preparation of Linkus syrup is given as under:

STEP I:

Grinding

Individual herbs were taken into the grinder according to the quantities mentioned above and were sieved through 60 # mesh to get the desired particle size.

STEP II:

Extraction

a) Individual grinded herbs were taken into extractor and water as solvent was added to the grinded herbs in the ratio of 1:10 with herb:solvent;

b) The extractors were heated with steam for 2 - 3 hours to get the desired extract in the form of decoction (individual liquid extract);

c) The decoctions were than filtered and transferred to evaporators to remove the extra solvent and to get the desired moisture content *i.e.* not more than 25%. The individual extracts were stored in the form of thick extracts;

Table 1. The herbs, extraction solvent and extraction yield of Linkus syrup.

Herb			Quality of Raw Herb (kg)	Solvent	Herb/Solvent Ratio	Extract Obtained (kg)
Botanical Name	Vernacular Name	English Name				
Adhatoda vasica	Bansa	Malabar Nut	150	Water	1.10	20
Glycyrrhiza glabra	Mulaithi	Licorice	100	Water	1.10	15
Piper longum	Filfil Draz	Lomg Papper	25	Water	1.10	5
Coredia latifolia	Sapistan	Sabestan	25	Water	1.10	5
Althea officinalis	Khatmi	Marshmello	25	Water	1.10	5
Zizyphus vulgaris	Unnab	Jujube	25	Water	1.10	5
Borago officinalis	Gaozaban	Sedge	25	Water	1.10	5
Hyssopus officinalis	Zufa	Hyssopus	12.50	Water	1.10	250
Alpinia galangal	Khulanjan	Galangal	12.50	Water	1.10	250
Viola odorata	Banafsha	Sweet Violet	6.250	Water	1.10	125

Excipients

Ingredients	Functions
Sugar	Sweetening and Bulking Agent
Citric Acid	Buffering (pH Maintaining) Agent
Sodium Benzoate	Anti-Microbial Preservative
Potassium Sorbate	Anti-Microbial Preservative
Glycerin	Humectant
Pippermint Oil	Flavoring Agent
Purified Water	Bulking Agent

d) Quality Control (QC) sampling was done of all the individual extracts to check the quality of the extracts. The following tests, such as pH, density, volume variations, and microbiological purity along with qualitative and quantitative estimations of polysaccharides, tanning agents, ascorbic acid and total alkaloides have been carried out.

STEP III:

Syrup manufacturing

a) Water as vehicle and bulking agent was added in a syrup manufacturing tank and heated to boil;

b) Sugar was then added in portions with continuous stirring;

c) Individual thick extracts were then added to the above one-by-one with continuous stirring;

d) Glycerin was then added to the above with continuous stirring;

e) Anti-microbial preservatives were then added by first dissolving and filtering in warm water and then added to the above with continuous stirring;

f) The syrup was then allowed to cool to reach the room temperature through chilled water circulation;

g) Flavor was then added to the syrup to get the bulk product;

h) Final filtration was done;

i) QC sampling was done to check the quality of the product.

STEP IV:

Syrup packaging

a) After QC release, the product was transferred to packaging hall through S.S. water pumps;

b) Syrup was filled automatically into 120 ml amber colored glass bottle;

c) Bottles were automatically labeled, punt into unit cartons along with leaf inserts;

d) QC sampling was done to check the quality of the finished product;

e) After QC release, the bottles were packed in master carton and finally to the pallets to shift them to finished goods store.

2.2. Experimental Animals

Healthy Wistar albino rats of both sexes weighing from 150 g to 250 g, were obtained from Animal Laboratory of Herbion Pakistan (Pvt.) Limited. They were housed in a cross-ventilated room and kept under standard environmental conditions, *i.e.* 25°C ± 1°C and 12/12 h dark/light cycle. Food and water were available *ad libitum*. They were divided into four groups of 10 rats per group. Each group comprised of five male and five female rats respectively. They were individually placed in a closed plexiglass chamber (20 × 10 × 10 cm) fed with standard rat pellet and water *ad libitum*. They were allowed to adaptation for 7 days to the laboratory conditions before the experiment. The experiments were performed in accordance with the ICH and FDA guidelines [20] [21].

2.2.1. Acute Toxicity Test (Lethal Dose$_{50}$ (LD$_{50}$))
Healthy Wistar albino rats of either sex (n = 5/sex) weighing between 150 - 250 g were treated orally with doses (1 or 5 g/kg) of the test product, maintained under standard laboratory conditions and used for the acute toxicity test. A total of 10 animals of equal numbers of male and female rats were used and each received a single oral-dose of 1000 mg/kg body weight of the test drug (Linkus). Animals were kept overnight fasting prior to the drug administration by oral gavage. After administration of the drug sample, food was withheld for further 3 - 4 h. Animals were observed individually at least once during the first 30 min after dosing, periodically during the first 24 h (with special attention during the first 4 h) and daily, thereafter, for a period of 7 days. Mortality and behavioral changes were observed for 1 week. Daily observations on the changes in skin and fur, eyes and mucus membrane (nasal), respiratory rate, circulatory signs (heart rate and blood pressure), autonomic effects (salivation, lacrimation, perspiration, piloerection, urinary incontinence and defecation) and central nervous system (ptosis, drowsiness, gait, tremors and convulsion) were noted.

2.2.2. Repeated Dose Toxicity
Healthy Wistar albino rats of both sexes (n = 5/dose/sex) were treated orally with doses of 20 mg/kg (adult human dose = ~1400 mg), 500 mg/kg (adult human dose = ~35,000 mg) and 1000 mg/kg (adult human dose = ~70,000 mg) of the test drug for 14 days. Additionally, the control animals were treated orally with water for 14 days.

3. Efficacy Study

The following animal model of cough was used to investigate the antitussive potential of Linkus:

3.1. Citric Acid Induced Cough

Healthy Wistar albino rats were treated orally with the recommended doses of Linkus. After 15 minutes, they were individually placed in a closed plexiglass chamber (20 × 10 × 10 cm) and exposed to citric acid inhalation (0.1 g/ml) for 7 minutes. The cough reflexes were counted for the last 5 minutes and compared with those of the control animals.

3.2. Measurement of Body Weight

The body weights of the treated animals were evaluated at 0, 7 and 14 day of the doses before analysing the tests.

3.3. Specimen Collection

At the last day of treatment all the treated rats were individually housed in metabolic cages for 24 h to collect the urine sample. On 15th day, *i.e.* 24 h after the last treatment, the urine sample was collected and following parameters were noted in the urine using urine analyzer (Uriscan) with the aid of urine-strips, *i.e.* glucose, blood cells, pH, protein, specific gravity and volume. For hematological analysis the blood was collected from the aforementioned control and the treated animals on the last day of treatment and then the samples were transferred to vacutainers and sent to the diagnostic facility of Dr. Panjwani Center for Molecular Medicine & Drug Research (PCMD), Karachi, for Complete Blood Count (CBC) testing. On 15th day, *i.e.* 24 h after the last treatment, the blood was collected from the treated animals and transferred to the test tubes. The heparinized blood was centrifuged within 5 min of the collection at 3000 rpm for 10 minutes. After centrifugation the serum has collected in ependdorf tubes and was used to observe any changes in the blood chemistry. The following parameters (prioritized parameters mentioned in Red Book updated 2007, FDA) were measured using chemical analyzer (Microlab, Merck) with the aid of commercially available kits *i.e.* alanine aminotransferases (ALT), alkaline phosphatase, gamma-glutamyl transpeptidase, total bilirubin, direct bilirubin, glucose, protein (total), urea and creatinine.

4. Statistical Analysis

The experimental results were subjected to were presented as mean ±Standard Error Mean (SEM). Differences between various means were evaluated by one way ANOVA followed by Least Significant Difference (LSD), by using SPSS version 18.0.

5. Results

The test product (Linkus) did not cause any mortality in Wistar albino rats at the given doses of 1 or 5 g/kg. Other signs of toxicity like hair loss and weight reduction were also not observed. In the female and male rats, the test drug at doses of 20, 500 and 1000 mg/kg did not cause any change on complete blood count and gave significant p value as compared to the control (**Table 2**).

The ALT levels were observed to be within the normal range at the administered dose of 1000 mg/kg. In the male rats, a significant reduction in ALP ($p < 0.05$).

In female rats, the creatinine level was significantly declined at the 20 mg/kg (**Table 3**) as compared to the control, protein ($p < 0.005$), urea ($p < 0.005$) and creatinine ($p < 0.05$) was noted at the three different doses *i.e.* 20, 500, 1000 mg/kg (**Table 4**).

In female rats, none of the tested parameters for urine analysis was significantly altered as compared to the control (**Table 4**). In male rats, at 20 mg/kg, the WBC ($p < 0.005$), ketones ($p < 0.05$) and protein ($p < 0.05$) were significantly reduced as compared to the control. At 1000 mg/kg, a significant increase in pH ($p < 0.05$) and specific gravity ($p < 0.05$), where as reduction in ketones ($p < 0.05$) and protein ($p < 0.05$) were observed. By comparing the test drug efficacy with the control drug (ADM), it was observed that in both male and female rats, the test drug at a dose of 300 mg/kg caused significant ($p < 0.01$) reduction in cough reflexes as compared to the control. The standard or control antitussive drug (Hydryllin syrup) also significantly reduced (500 mg/kg, $p < 0.05$) the cough reflexes as compared to the control as shown in **Table 5(a)** and **Table 5(b)** and **Figure 1**.

Table 2. Complete blood count of rats at different doses of Linkus syrup.

Rats	Dose (mg/kg)	Complete Blood Count							
		Hb (g/dl)	RBC (Million/µL)	Hct/Pev (%)	MCV (fl)	MCH (pg])	MCHC (g/dl)	WBC (10^9/L)	Platelets Count
Female	Control	13 ± 0.1	7 ± 0.1	39 ± 0.4	57 ± 1	19 ± 0.3	33 ± 0.2	6 ± 1	873 ± 31
	20	12 ± 0.8	7 ± 0.2	38 ± 0.7	60 ± 1	20 ± 1.4	33 ± 1.7	4 ± 1	871 ± 50
	500	13 ± 0.5	7 ± 0.2	38 ± 0.4	56 ± 1	19 ± 1	34 ± 0.5	4 ± 1	829 ± 6
	1000	13 ± 1	7 ± 0.1	38 ± 0.2	57 ± 1	18 ± 0.2	31 ± 0.3	4 ± 1	892 ± 44
Male	Control	14 ± 0.2	8 ± 0.2	44 ± 0.5	57 ± 13	19 ± 0.5	32 ± 0.3	8 ± 1	960 ± 67
	20	14 ± 0.2	8 ± 0.2	43 ± 0.8	57 ± 0.5	17 ± 0.2	33 ± 0.1	7 ± 1	911 ± 39
	500	15 ± 0.2	8 ± 0.7	46 ± 0.4	58 ± 2	19 ± 0.07	32 ± 0.4	8 ± 1	853 ± 28
	1000	14 ± 0.2	8 ± 0.1	45 ± 0.8	57 ± 1	18 ± 0.3	32 ± 0.2	6 ± 1	834 ± 48

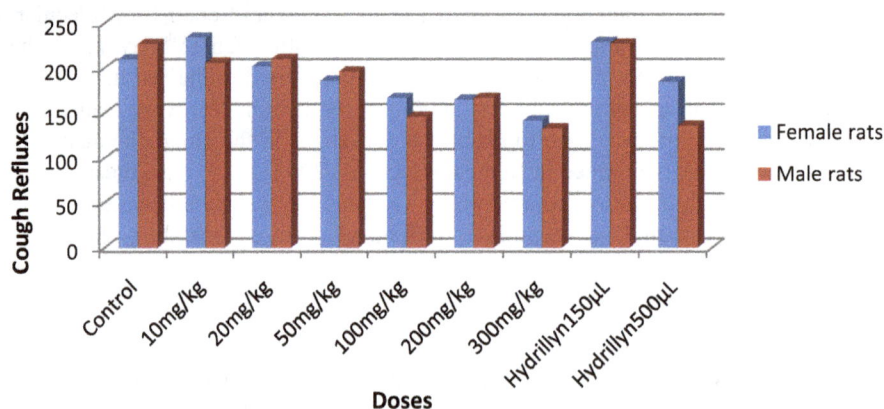

Figure 1. Cough reflexes of rats with test and control drugs.

Table 3. Urine analysis of rats at different doses of Linkus syrup.

Rats	Dose (mg/kg)	Urine Detail Report									
		pH	Gluc	SPG	RBC	WBC	Nit	Bili	Urobil	Ket	Prot
Female	Control	8 ± 0.4	15 ± 0	1 ± 0.001	20 ± 0	18 ± 0	13 ± 2	20 ± 0	25 ± 0	18 ± 0	76 ± 16
	20	8 ± 0.2	15 ± 0	1 ± 0.001	20 ± 0	25 ± 4	11 ± 2	20 ± 0	28 ± 3	21 ± 3	83 ± 8
	500	7 ± 0.3	15 ± 0	1 ± 0.002	20 ± 0	14 ± 2	13 ± 2	20 ± 0	25 ± 0	21 ± 3	51 ± 4
	1000	8 ± 0.3	15 ± 0	1 ± 0.002	20 ± 0	23 ± 8	11 ± 2	20 ± 0	25 ± 0	20 ± 2	92 ± 20
Male	Control	6 ± 0.2	15 ± 0	1 ± 0.001	20 ± 0	43 ± 5	10 ± 0	20 ± 0	28 ± 3	25 ± 9	130 ± 0
	20	6 ± 0.2	15 ± 0	1 ± 0.001	20 ± 2	40 ± 3	12 ± 1	20 ± 0	25 ± 0	27 ± 4	125 ± 25
	500	6 ± 0.3	15 ± 0	1 ± 0.002	20 ± 0	39 ± 4	10 ± 0	20 ± 0	25 ± 0	31 ± 4	130 ± 0
	1000	7 ± 0.5	15 ± 0	1.1 ± 0.002	20 ± 0	35 ± 0	12 ± 1	23 ± 3	32 ± 7	33 ± 3	79 ± 21

Table 4. Blood chemistry of rats at different doses of Linkus syrup.

Rats	Dose (mg/kg)	Blood Chemistry							
		ALT	ALP	GGT	T-bilib	D-bilib	Prot	Urea	Creat
Female	Control	38 ± 5	213 ± 9	1.4 ± 1	0.2 ± 0.03	0.6 ± 0.1	4 ± 0.4	26 ± 6	1.1 ± 0.1
	20	35 ± 6	127 ± 4	1 ± 1	0.3 ± 0.04	0.4 ± 0.01	4 ± 0.3	22 ± 2	0.7 ± 1
	500	40 ± 5	261 ± 57	1.2 ± 0.5	0.4 ± 0.03	0.3 ± 0.04	5 ± 0.5	30 ± 4	1.1 ± 0.1
	1000	33 ± 6	192 ± 22	1.2 ± 0.2	0.4 ± 0.2	0.4 ± 0.03	4 ± 0.04	28 ± 3	1.1 ± 0.01
Male	Control	46 ± 5	238 ± 24	2 ± 1	0.2 ± 0.04	0.5 ± 0.2	5.7 ± 0.8	28 ± 4	0.7 ± 0.1
	20	47 ± 4	217 ± 17	1 ± 0.2	0.4 ± 0.03	0.6 ± 0.2	4.6 ± 0.2	30 ± 3	0.5 ± 0.1
	500	49 ± 4	180 ± 10	2.4 ± 0.4	0.3 ± 0.04	0.6 ± 0.1	4.7 ± 0.4	30 ± 4	0.6 ± 0.1
	1000	45 ± 13	241 ± 14	1 ± 0.4	0.4 ± 0.1	0.3 ± 0.2	5.17 ± 2	28 ± 3	0.7 ± 0.1

Table 5. (a) Cough reflexes of rats with test drug; (b) Cough reflexes of rats with control drugs.

(a)

Rats	Cough Reflexes/5min						
	Control	10 mg/kg	20 mg/kg	50 mg/kg	100 mg/kg	200 mg/kg	300 mg/kg
Female	210 ± 23	234 ± 24	202 ± 28	186 ± 60	167 ± 6	165 ± 11	142 ± 13[**]
Male	227 ± 25	206 ± 31	210 ± 22	196 ± 18	146 ± 11	167 ± 5[*]	133 ± 19[***]

(b)

Treatment	Cough Reflexes/5min		
	Control	190.5 mg/kg	635.3 mg/kg
Hydrillin	211 ± 23	227 ± 18	136 ± 14

6. Discussion

The different studies on cough have been carried out to evaluate antitussive activity by utilizing the medicinal plants. In one of the citation the experiments have been conducted on *Glycyrrhiza glabra* and *Adhatoda vasica* by using a cough model induced by sulphur dioxide gas in mice. The effect of the ethanol extracts of *Glycyrrhiza glabra* and *Adhatoda vasica* on SO_2 gas induced cough in experimental animals have very significant effects at the level of $p < 0.01$ in inhibiting the cough reflex at a dose of 800 mg/kg and 200 mg/kg body wt p.o., in comparison with the control group. Mice showed an inhibition of 35.62%, in cough on treatment with *Glycyrrhiza glabra* and 43.02% inhibition on treatment with *Adhatoda vasica* within 60 min of the experiment. The antitussive activity of the extract was comparable to that of codeine sulphate (10, 15, 20 mg/kg body wt), a standard antitussive agent. Codeine sulphate, as a standard drug for suppression of cough, produced 24.80%, 32.98%, and 45.73% inhibition in cough at a dose of 10 mg/kg, 15 mg/kg and 20 mg/kg respectively, whereas, codeine sulphate (20 mg/kg) showed maximum 45.73% ($p < 0.001$) inhibition at 60 min of the experiment [22]. Polysaccharide fraction of *Althaea officinalis* mimics the intensity and frequency of cough by aqueous extract of its root and the anti-tussive activity is more effective than prenoxdiazine [23].

Marshmallow root extract and isolated mucilage polysaccharide were tested for antitussive activity in un-anaesthetized cats of both sexes at oral doses of 50 to 100 mg/kg body weight, in a cough induced by mechanical stimulation, in comparison with the cough-suppressing effects of Althaea syrup (1000 mg/kg), prenoxdiazine (30 mg/kg), dropropizine (100 mg/kg) and codeine (10 mg/kg). Both the extract and isolated polysaccharide significantly reduced the intensity and the number of cough efforts from laryngopharyngeal and tracheobronchial areas. The root extract was less effective than the isolated polysaccharide. The antitussive activity was found to be lower than that of codeine, but higher than those of prenoxdiazine and dropropizine. Polysaccharides of Marshmallow exhibited statistically significant cough-suppressing activity, which was noticeably higher than that of the non-narcotic drug used in clinical practice to treat coughing. By testing many plants, the most expressive antitussive activity was observed with the polysaccharide from marshmallow, containing the highest proportion of the uronic acid constituent. In a double blind clinical study, Rouhi and Ganji used *Althaea officinalis* in patients with hypertension who had been developed cough during taking of angiotensin converting enzyme inhibitors. The patients received 40 mg of *Althaea officinalis* three times daily as 20 drops for four weeks. The mean scores of the severity of the cough in the group which have been treated by *Althaea officinalis* had a significant change from the score of 2/66 + 0.958 (to) 1/23 + 1.006. Eight patients in the *Althaea officinalis* group showed almost complete cough abolition [24].

The cough in guinea pigs was induced by 0.3 M Citric Acid (CA) aerosol for 3 min interval, in which total number of cough efforts (sudden enhancement of expiratory flow accompanied by cough movement and sound) was counted. Specific airway resistance and its changes induced by citric acid aerosol were considered as an indicator of the *in vivo* reactivity changes. The results showed 1) *Althaea officinalis* polysaccharide rhamnogalacturonan dose-dependently inhibits cough reflex in unsensitized guinea pigs. Simultaneously, plant polysaccharide shortened the duration of antitussive effect when it was been tested in inflammatory conditions. 2) Rhamnogalacturonan did not influence airways reactivity *in vivo* conditions expressed as specific resistance values neither sensitized nor unsensitized groups of animals. 3) The antitussive activity of codeine (dose 10 mg/kg (−1) b.w. orally) tested under the same condition was comparable to higher dose of rhamnogalacturonan in unsensitized animals. 4) The characteristic cellular pattern of allergic airways inflammation was confirmed by histopathological investigations. Rhamnogalacturonan isolated from *Althaea officinalis* mucilage possesses very high cough suppressive effect in guinea pigs test system, which is shortened in conditions of experimentally induced air ways allergic inflammation [25].

The pre-clinical study was conducted on both the test (Linkus) and the control (Hydryllin) drugs on healthy albino rats. Generally, there was no test drug related mortality observed at the highest tested dose of 5 g/kg (2001). It was found that no acute toxicity observed in all the treated rats and according to statement that any of the tested substance with LD_{50} determined that dose greater than 1000 mg/kg could be considered as safe and low toxic [26]. In the light of this view the test drug at a higher dose of 5 g/kg did not show toxicity and mortality, hence considered safe. It was suggested that LD_{50} may not be considered as a biological constant due to the difference from one animal species to the other species, strains, gender, cage environment and the duration of treatment [27]. The data so generated on the efficacy and toxicity (lethal dose (LD_{50})), and the repeated toxicity dose was analyzed by using SPSS version 18.0. The test drug did not show any toxicity even at a dose of 1 or 5 g/kg as compared to the control. In repeated dose toxicity determination, the test drug was given at three different doses *i.e.* 20, 500 and 1000 mg/kg and the parameters assessed, included CBC, blood chemistry and urine analysis. The test product did not show any of the abnormality and pathology observed by assessing these parameters at a maximum dose of 1000 mg/kg. At higher doses no change in CBC profile of rats and blood chemistry and urine analysis were observed. The ALT levels were normal at the administered dose of 1000 mg/kg. In the male rats, a comparing the test drug efficacy with the control drug (Hydryllin), it was observed that in both male and female rats, the test drug at a dose of 300 mg/kg caused significant ($p < 0.01$) reduction in cough reflexes as compared to the control. The standard or control antitussive drug (Hydryllin syrup) also significantly reduced (635.5 mg/kg, $p < 0.05$) the cough reflexes as compared to the control. In addition the test drug (Linkus) cough reflexes and blood profile displayed significant performance. Different herbs in Linkus have been combined so as to relieve different form of cough ailments. The selection of an herbal combination of Linkus is primarily based on the wide ethnomedical use as well as literature search. The mixing of individuals extracts of the given medicinal plants in the Linkus components causes significant difference in reducing cough in the animal model. From the experiment carried out and the data generated, Linkus syrup has shown good promise to control cough and has found greater acceptability in this respect and it was safe by observing acute and repeated dose toxicity. Linkus syrup did not show any mortality even at the doses of 1 to 5 gm/kg of body weight. Even by repeated dose toxicity, effects on urine, the blood profile and Liver Functions Test (LFT), the test drug has been found to be quite safe and there was no change in the highlighted signs in rats during 14 days *in vivo* study. There is an increasing use of herbal or traditional medicine in all over the developing countries due to their popularity and safety on long term use [28]-[30]. Even though these types of medicines are being used for centuries, in this modern world, there are safety concerns that these medicines may or may not produce affect on liver, brain or kidneys and thus cause abnormality [31] [32]. There are various herbal medicines available, but very few have been taken for clinical and preclinical trial studies to confirm their safety and efficacy [33]. Antitussive activity: aqueous and methonolic extract of Ocimum sanctum was studied for antitussive activity in guinea pigs at the doses of 1.55 gms and 0.875 gms/kg body wt respectively. Cough was induced by exposure to the aerosol of citric acid (7.5% w/v). The study showed that both the test extracts posses significant antitussive activity and aqueous extract showed a higher activity than the methonolic extract. The potential mechanism has not explored for this study. The body weight over the experimental time course before and during treatment did not change (see **Table 6**).

In the present *in vivo* study, it was observed that the test drug has not shown any acute and repeated dose toxicity even at higher doses.

Table 6. 14 days treatment (body weights means).

S. NO.	Dose (mg/kg)	Sex	Body Weight (g)		
			Day 1st	Day 7th	Day 14th
1	Control	Female	266	268	268
2	190.5	Female	275	273	271
3	635.3	Female	238	237	235
4	1270.0	Female	373	371	368.8
5	Control	Male	300	302	302
6	190.5	Male	346	345	341.8
7	635.3	Male	289	288	286
8	1270.0	Male	374.8	373.6	370

7. Conclusion

Acute toxicity test (LD$_{50}$) Wistar albino rats 10 in number weighing from 150 to 250 g received a single oral dose of 1000 mg/kg body weight of the test drug (Linkus). Animals were observed individually at least once during the first 30 min after dosing, periodically during the first 24 h, then first 4 h and finally for 7 days. Mortality and behavioral changes observed in skin and fur, eyes and mucus membrane (nasal), respiratory rate, circulatory signs (heart rate and blood pressure), autonomic effects (salivation, lacrimation, perspiration, piloerection, urinary incontinence and defecation) and central nervous system (ptosis, drowsiness, gait, tremors and convulsion) were noted. Dose toxicity was repeated in rats with doses of 20 mg/kg (whereas equivalent adult human dose = 1400 mg), 500 mg/kg (whereas equivalent adult human dose = 35,000 mg) and 1000 mg/kg (whereas equivalent adult human dose = 70,000 mg) of the test drug for 14 days. Usually cough is induced by citric acid but all coughs are not induced by it. It was concluded that test drug (Linkus) exhibited effectiveness as compared to the control drug (Hydryllin syrup) in alleviating the cough and has shown no toxicity or adverse reactions in experimental models.

Acknowledgements

This study was funded by Herbion Pakistan (Pvt) Limited, Karachi, Pakistan. The authors are thankful to Mr. Nadeem Khalid, CEO and Mr. Abid Mumtaz, COO as well as other colleagues for their support and contribution.

References

[1]   Irwin, R.S. and Madison, J.M. (2000) The Diagnosis and Treatment of Cough. *New England Journal of Medicine*, **343**, 1715-1721. http://dx.doi.org/10.1056/NEJM200012073432308

[2]   French, C.L., Irwin, R.S., Curley, F.J. and Krikorian, C.J. (1998) Impact of Chronic Cough on Quality of Life. *Archives of Internal Medicine*, **158**, 1657-1661. http://dx.doi.org/10.1001/archinte.158.15.1657

[3]   Irwin, R.S., Boulet, L.P. and Cloutier, M.M. (1998) Managing Cough as a Defense Mechanism and as a Symptom. *Chest*, **114**, 133S-181S. http://dx.doi.org/10.1378/chest.114.2_Supplement.133S

[4]   Salawu, O.A., Chindo, B.A., Tijani, A.Y., Obidike, I.C., Salawu, T.A. and Akingbasote, A.J. (2009) Acute and Sub-Acute Toxicological Evaluations of the Methanolic Stem Bark Extract of *Crossopteryx febrifuga* in Rats. *African Journal of Pharmacy and Pharmacology*, **3**, 621-626.

[5]   Angell, M. and Kassierr, J.P. (1998) Alternative Medicine—The Risk of Untested and Unregulated Remedies. *New England Journal of Medicine*, **339**, 839-841. http://dx.doi.org/10.1056/NEJM199809173391210

[6]   Nadig, P.D. and Laxmi, S. (2005) Study of Anti-Tussive Activity of Ocimum Sanctum Linn in Guinea Pigs. *Indian Journal of Physiology and Pharmacology*, **49**, 243-245.

[7]   Dhawan, K. and Sharma, A. (2002) Antitussive Activity of the Methanol Extract of *Passiflora incarnate* Leaves. *Fitoterapia*, **73**, 397-399. http://dx.doi.org/10.1016/S0367-326X(02)00116-8

[8]   Dhule, J.N. (1999) Antitussive Effect of Adhatoda Vasica Extract on Mechanical or Chemical Stimulation-Induced Coughing in Animals. *Journal of Ethnopharmacology*, **67**, 361-365. http://dx.doi.org/10.1016/S0378-8741(99)00074-4

[9]   Chang, H.M. and Butt, P.P.H. (1986) Pharmacology and Applications of Chinese Materia Medica. Vol. 1, World Scientific, Singapore, 304. http://dx.doi.org/10.1142/0284

[10]   Suekawa, M., Ishige, A., Yuasa, K., Sudo, K., Aburada, M. and Hosoya, E. (1984) Pharmacological Studies on Ginger. I. Pharmacological Actions of Pungent Constitutents, (6)-Gingerol and (6)-Shogaol. *Journal of Pharmacobio-Dynamics*, **7**, 836-848. http://dx.doi.org/10.1248/bpb1978.7.836

[11]   Mandal, S.C., Kumar, C.K.A., Mohana Lakshmi, S., Sinha, S., Murugesan, T., Saha, B.P. and Pal, M. (2000) Antitussive Effect of *Asparagus racemosus* Root against Sulfur Dioxide-Induced Cough in Mice. *Fitoterapia*, **71**, 686-689.

[12]   Srinath, K., Murugesan, T., Kumar, C.A., Suba, V., Das, A.K., Sinha, S., Arunachalam, G. and Manikandan, L. (2002) Effect of *Trichodesma indicum* Extract on Cough Reflex Induced by Sulphur Dioxide in Mice. *Phytomedicine*, **9**, 75-77. http://dx.doi.org/10.1078/0944-7113-00086

[13]   Mandal, S.C., Ashok-Kumar, C.K., Lakshmi, S.M., Sanghamitra, S., Murugesan, T., Saha, B.P. and Pal, M. (2000) Antitussive Effect of *Asparagus racemosus* Root against Sulfur Dioxide-Induced Cough in Mice. *Fitoterapia*, **71**, 686-689. http://dx.doi.org/10.1016/S0367-326X(00)00151-9

[14]   Nosál'ová, G., Mokrý, J. and Hassan, K.M. (2003) Antitussive Activity of the Fruit Extract of *Emblica officinalis* Gaertn. (Euphorbiaceae). *Phytomedicine*, **10**, 583-589. http://dx.doi.org/10.1078/094471103322331872

[15] Keter, L.K., Mwikwabe, N.M., Mbaabu, M.P., Sudhee, H.M., Tolo, F.M., Dhanani, P. and Orwa, J.A. (2013) Valida-tion of Safety and Efficacy of Antitussive Herbal Formulations. *African Journal of Pharmacology and Therapeutics*, **2**, 26-31.

[16] Gupta, Y.K., Kaytyal, J., Kumar, G., Mehla, G., Katiyar, C.K., Sharma, N. and Yav, S. (2009) Evaluation of Antitus-sive Activity of Formulations with Herbal Extracts in Sulphur Dioxide (SO_2) Induced Cough Model in Mice. *Indian Journal of Physiology and Pharmacology*, **53**, 61-66.

[17] Calixto, J.B. (2000) Efficacy, Safety, Quality Control, Marketing and Regulatory Guidelines for Herbal Medicines (Phytotherapeutic Agents). *Brazilian Journal of Medical and Biological Research*, **33**, 179-189. http://dx.doi.org/10.1590/S0100-879X2000000200004

[18] Firenzuoli, F. and Gori, L. (2007) Herbal Medicine Today: Clinical and Research Issues. *Evidence-Based Complemen-tary and Alternative Medicine*, **4**, 37-40. http://dx.doi.org/10.1093/ecam/nem096

[19] Greenblatt, D.J. and Shader, R.I. (1971) Uses and Toxicity of Belladonna Alkaloids and Synthetic Anticholinergics. *Seminars in Psychiatry*, **3**, 449-476.

[20] Red Book (2007) Guidance for Industry and Other Stakeholders Toxicological Principles for the Safety Assessment of Food Ingredients. Revised Edition, Chapter IV, 000045. http://www.cfan.fda.gov/guidance.html

[21] ICH Harmonized Tripartite Guideline (2002) Guidance for Good Clinical Practice. E6 (R1); PMP/ICH/135/95. Euro-pean Agency, London.

[22] Yasmeen, I. and Siddiqui, H. (2012) Study of the Antitussive Potential of *Glycyrrhiza glabra* and *Adhatoda vasica* Using a Cough Model Induced by Sulphur Dioxide Gas in Mice. *International Journal of Pharmaceutical Sciences and Research*, **3**, 1668-1674.

[23] Nosal'ova, G., Saab, B.R., Pashayan, N. and El, C.S. (1992) Antitussive Efficacy of the Complex Extract and the Po-lysaccharide of Marshmallow (*Althaea officinalis* L. var. Robusta). *Pharmazie*, **47**, 224-226.

[24] Al-Snafi, A.I. (2013) The Pharmaceutical Importance of *Altahea officinalis* and *Althaea rosea*. *International Journal of PharmTech Research*, **5**, 1378-1385.

[25] Sutovska, M., Capek, P., Franova, S., Joskova, M., Sutovsky, J., Marcinek, J. and Kalman, M. (2011) Antitussive Ac-tivity of *Althaea officinalis* L. Polysaccharide Rhamnogalacturonan and Its Changes in Guinea Pigs with Ovalbumine-Induced Airways Inflammation. *Bratislavské lekárske listy*, **112**, 670-675.

[26] Clarke, M.L. and Clarke, E.G.C. (1967) Veterinary Toxicology. Bailliere Tindall, London.

[27] Zbinden, G. and Roversi, F. (1981) Significance of the LD_{50} Test for the Toxicological Evaluation of Chemical Sub-stances. *Archives of Toxicology*, **47**, 77-99. http://dx.doi.org/10.1007/BF00332351

[28] Daswani, G.P., Brijesh, S. and Birdi, J.T. (2006) Preclinical Testing of Medicinal Plants: Advantages and Approaches. *Workshop Proceedings on Approaches towards Evaluation of Medicinal Plants Prior to Clinical Trial*, Foundation for Medical Research at Yashwantrao Chavan Academy of Development Administration (YASHADA), 60-77.

[29] Ogbonnia, S.O., Mbaka, G.O., Anyika, E.N., Osegbo, O.M. and Igbokwe, N.H. (2010) Evaluation of Acute Toxicity in Mice and Subchronic Toxicity of Hydro-Ethanolic Extract of *Chromolaena odorata* (L.) King and Robinson (Fam. Asteraceae) in Rats. *Agriculture and Biology Journal of North America*, **1**, 859-865. http://dx.doi.org/10.5251/abjna.2010.1.5.859.865

[30] Stewart, M.J., Moar, J.J., Steenkamp, P. and Kokot, M. (1999) Findings in Fatal Cases of Poisoning Attributed to Tra-ditional Remedies in South Africa. *Forensic Science International*, **101**, 177-183. http://dx.doi.org/10.1016/S0379-0738(99)00025-0

[31] Saad, B., Azaizeh, H., Abu-Hijleh, G. and Said, O. (2006) Safety of Traditional Arab Herbal Medicine. *Evidence-Based Complementary and Alternative Medicine*, **3**, 433-439. http://dx.doi.org/10.1093/ecam/nel058

[32] Colson, C.R. and De Broe, M.E. (2005) Kidney Injury from Alternative Medicines. *Advances in Chronic Kidney Dis-ease*, **12**, 261-275. http://dx.doi.org/10.1016/j.ackd.2005.03.006

[33] Cheng, C.W., Bian, Z.X. and Wu, T.X. (2009) Systematic Review of Chinese Herbal Medicine for Functional Consti-pation. *World Journal of Gastroenterology*, **15**, 4886-4895. http://dx.doi.org/10.3748/wjg.15.4886

4

Efficacy of Yiqi Fumai (Freeze-Dried Powder) on Ischemic Diastolic Heart Failure

Dalin Song[1,2]*, Mengfen Hu[2], Tongliang Han[1], Hua Zhang[1], Yongjun Mao[2], Tao Tian[3]*

[1]Department of Geriatric Cardiology, Geriatric Institute, Qingdao Municipal Hospital, Qingdao, China
[2]Qingdao University, Qingdao, China
[3]Department of Geriatric Cardiology, Linyi People's Hospital, Linyi, China
Email: *dsong55cn@aliyun.com

Abstract

Objective: To evaluate the efficacy of Yiqi Fumai freeze-dry powder (YFP) on ischemic diastolic heart failure. Methods: 100 patients diagnosed with unstable angina accompanying ischemic diastolic heart failure (IDHF) were selected randomly. 52 patients with TCM syndrome of qi-yin deficiency were divided into Chinese and Western combination therapy group. 48 patients have no TCM syndrome of qi-yin deficiency, and were treated with standard western medicine. After treatment, Seattle Angina Questionnaire Evaluation, ECG, conventional and stress echocardiography (SE) index, NT-proBNP were compared between before and after treatment. Results: The differences of PL, TS, DP between before and after treatment by YFP were statistically significant ($P < 0.05$). SE parameters of LVEF, E/A were significantly increase; E/e' decreased. The differences were statistically significant. However, echocardiography parameters showed no significant differences after treatment. After the combination treatment, NT-proBNP level had negative correlation with LVEF, E/A ($r = -0.432, -0.643$, both $P < 0.01$). Conclusion: Yiqi Fumai freeze-dry powder is safe and effective to patients with ischemic diastolic heart failure. Stress echocardiography can improve the diagnostic of ischemic diastolic heart failure, and maybe an effectively predict treatment response.

Keywords

Yiqi Fumai (Freeze-Dried Powder), Diastolic Heart Failure, Seattle Angina Questionnaire (SAQ) Evaluation, Stress Echocardiography

1. Introduction

Cardiovascular events are major fatal disease in China. Acute myocardial infarction (AMI) and ischemic heart

---

*Corresponding authors.

failure (IHF) are the most common and most serious stage in cardiac development. Unstable angina is one type of the acute coronary syndrome and its pathogenesis is unstable coronary plaque that plaque rupture may develop acute myocardial infarction. Myocardial ischemia and wide degeneration, necrosis and fibrosis caused by coronary artery disease can result in myocardial systolic and (or) diastolic dysfunction. Diastolic function occurs prior to systolic function. Diastolic heart failure (DHF) can be further developed to systolic heart failure, which has serious impact on cardiac function and quality of life of patients. Therefore, combination treatment of standardized western medicine joint proprietary Chinese medicine has been increasingly accepted by clinicians.

Coronary heart disease is divided into two categories, thoracic obstruction and angina pectoris, in traditional Chinese medicine (TCM). Both types of coronary disease are severe and require urgent intervention. The pathogenesis of coronary heart disease mainly involves heart vessel blockage or stasis. Delay in the treatment of this chronic disease may cause damage to Yin and Yang as well as Qi and Yin, according to TCM theory. The Yiqi Fumai freeze-dry powder (YFP) was here prepared based on the TCM formula of pulse-activating powder using modern production technology refined for formulation of modern Chinese medicine. The pulse-activating powder formula was taken from a comprehensive TCM book called *Medicine Origin*. It is one of the more famous TCM formulas for pulse activation. It consists of three active ingredients: ginseng, Mai Dong, and Chinese magnoliavine fruit. YFP has a beneficial impact on the replenishment of Qi and pulse activation. It also well nourishes Yin and promotes glandular secretion in TCM theory. Integrative Medicine may bring good results for those patients with Qi and Yin deficiency. However, there is still a lack of reliable clinical studies to prove the efficacy of this treatment. In this study, the Seattle Angina Scale (SAQ), ECG, stress echocardiography (stress echocardiography, SE) and amino-terminal pro-brain natriuretic peptide precursor (NT-proBNP) were used to assess the efficiency of YFP which was based on pulse-activating powder.

2. Materials and Methods

2.1. Ethics

This study was approved by hospital of Qingdao Municipal Hospital and Linyi People's Hospital Committee, and conformed to the guidelines of the National Institutes of Health for the care.

2.2. Study Design

100 patients diagnosed with unstable angina [1] (unstable angina pectoris, UAP) were selected randomly from 2011 to 2012 in both hospitals. Inclusion criteria of UAP cases: >18 years old; diagnosed with coronary heart disease (previous myocardial infarction, or revascularization history, at least one major vascular diameter stenosis > 50% by coronary angiography); or patients with the positive results of stress electrocardiogram test (male), radionuclide or stress echocardiography test; episode of angina; angina (seizure frequency, extent and level of incentives induced angina) has been stable for at least one at entrance; the Canadian Cardiovascular Society angina class I - IV grade. Exclusion criteria of UAP: patients developed acute myocardial infarction in less than three months; postoperative of revascularization (PCI or CABG) in less than three months, so 78 male patients and 22 female patients met these criteria. They were in line with the diagnostic criteria of ischemic diastolic heart failure (IDHF) [2]. Exclusion criteria of IDHF: patients with heart failure caused by non-coronary artery disease; heart failure symptoms aggravated due to digitalis poisoning.

All following patients were excluded: patients with severe hepatic or renal dysfunction (serum ALT levels > 3 times the upper limit of the normal value, serum creatinine level ≥ 442 μmol/L); uncontrolled hypertension (systolic blood pressure ≥ 180 mmHg, diastolic blood pressure ≥ 100 mmHg); Diabetic with glycemic level not controlled satisfactorily; previous history of allergy to ginseng, Ophiopogon japonicus, Schisandra chinensis; pregnant or lactating women.

All subjects signed the informed consent form. Grouping diagrammatic drawing was shown in **Figure 1**. 52 patients with TCM syndrome of qi-yin deficiency were accessed into Chinese and Western combination therapy group (chinese and western medicine treatment group, CWMTG) with 32 male and 20 female, and their ages were from 62 to 74 (average years were 69.5). 48 patients have no TCM syndrome of qi-yin deficiency including 8 females and 40 males with age from 57 to 70 (average years were 65.0 ± 9.0) were treated with standard western medicine (western medicine treatment group, WMTG).

UAP: unstable angina pectoris; TCM: raditional Chinese medicine; MTG: chinese and western medicine

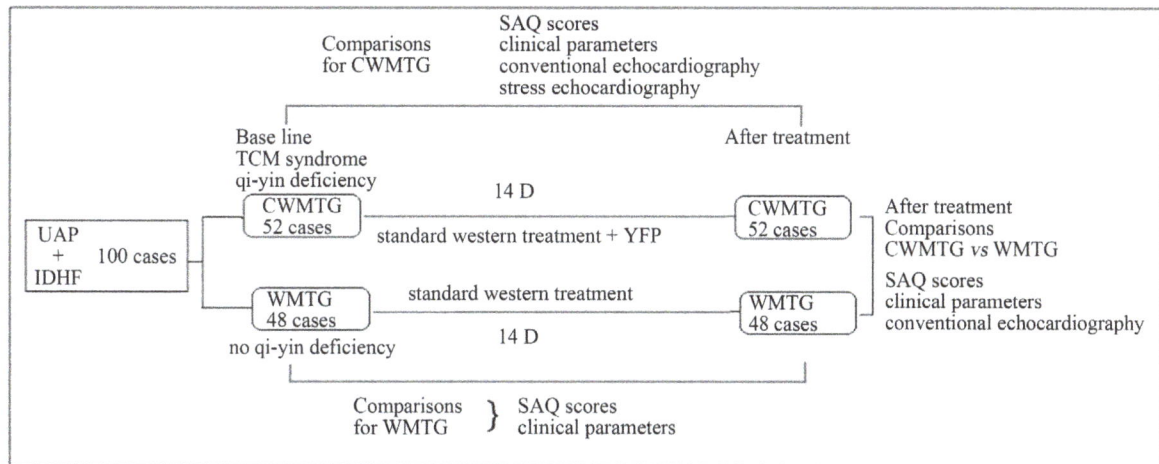

Figure 1. Study design and grouping.

treatment group; WMTG: western medicine treatment group; IDHF: ischemic diastolic heart failure; SAQ: seattle angina questionnaire.

2.3. Treatment

The standard western treatment includes the principles of conventional treatment of IDHF with diuretics, β-blockers, angiotensin-converting enzyme inhibitors (ACEI), angiotensin II receptor blockers (ARB); as well as standard ASC drugs such as aspirin, clopidogrel, isosorbide dinitrate and stantins. Patients in WMTG were given standard western treatment. On the basis of western medicine treatment, patients in CWMTG were given Yiqi Fumai dry powder (Tianjin Tasly Pharmaceutical Co., Ltd. Specification: 0.65 g/bottle. Approval Number: Z20060463). Dosage and Administration: 5.2 g each time, namely 8 bottles at a time, one time per day. The drugs were dissolved in 250 - 500 ml 5% glucose injection or saline intravenous injection and were injected at the rate of about 40 drops per minute for 14 days).

2.4. Seattle Angina Questionnaire (SAQ) Evaluation

With the necessary explanations of SAQ by the doctor before and after treatment, patients independently completed the questionnaire. Seattle Angina scale evaluate the efficiency from following five aspects: physical limitation level (PL, Question 1), angina steady state (AS, Question 2), angina frequency (AF, Questions 3 - 4), treatment satisfaction (TS, Questions 5 - 8), disease perception (DP, Questions 9 - 11), one by one score, the total score is 100 points, the higher the score, the better the patient's quality of life and organism function [3].

2.5. ECG Evaluation

After treatment, disappearance of ischemic manifestation indicated in resting ECG or negative treadmill exercise test were considered markedly effective; that ST segment rebounded 0.05mV, inverted T wave become shallow more than 50% or the inverted, low T wave become upright was effective; ST - T no change was invalid; ST segment descend, or T wave inversion deepens was aggravating.

2.6. Stress Echocardiography

Used Philips IE 33 ultrasonic diagnostic apparatus, X3-1 probe, 1-3MHz frequency, we recorded the left ventricular diastolic diameter (LVDd), interventricular sepal thickness at the end of diastolic (IVSd), left ventricular posterior wall thickness (LVPWd), left atria diameter (LAD). We measured the LVEF, the left ventricular output (CO) and cardiac index (CI) by biplane Simpson on the parasternal long-axis under the resting standard state. Double-blind method was applied. All data measured repeatedly three times. The mean value was reserved. Patients that underwent stress echocardiography were asked to do treadmill exercise until their heart rates were stable at 110/min. After 1 min, the test was terminated, and the indices were recorded at the same site. Indicators of cardiac Doppler echocardiography included cardiac systolic function LVEDV, LVESV, SV, CO, CI, EF, diastolic function E/A etc. All patients completed the test with satisfying results.

2.7. NT-proBNP

N-terminal pro brain natriuretic peptide (NT-proBNP) was detected by euzymelinked immunosorbent assay (biomelieux SA kit).

2.8. Statistical Analysis

SPSS11.5 statistical software was applied. All quantitative data were reported as mean ± S.D. $\left(\bar{x} \pm s\right)$. Indicators between before and after treatment were compared using paired t-test, non-continuous variables between groups were compared using t-test. The continuous variables and rates were compared using X^2 test. Non-parametric continuous variables were represented as the median (minimum - maximum). Paired Wilcoxon test was applied for comparisons before and after treatment; correlation between variables were analyzed using Pearson correlation analysis and independent factors were analyzed using multiple regression. P < 0.05 was as statistically significant.

3. Results

3.1. SAQ Scores

There were no significant differences of clinical general characteristics between two groups. Life quality of patients before and after treatment: scores of PL, AS, AF, TS, and DP are shown in **Table 1**. The results showed that the differences of PL, TS, DP between before and after treatment by YFP were statistically significant (P < 0.05), indicating that combination of YFP can improve physical limitation extent in patients with unstable angina, and can improve patients' satisfaction and their perception of the disease, making the patient's conditions to be stabilizing. The rate of nitrates use, ECG indicators, SAQ and symptoms were significant different before and after treatment (P = 0.05). Patients' satisfaction and disease perception in CWMTG were significantly decreased (P = 0.05) and the proportion of ineffectiveness in CWMTG was significantly decreased (P = 0.02) (**Figure 2** and **Table 1**).

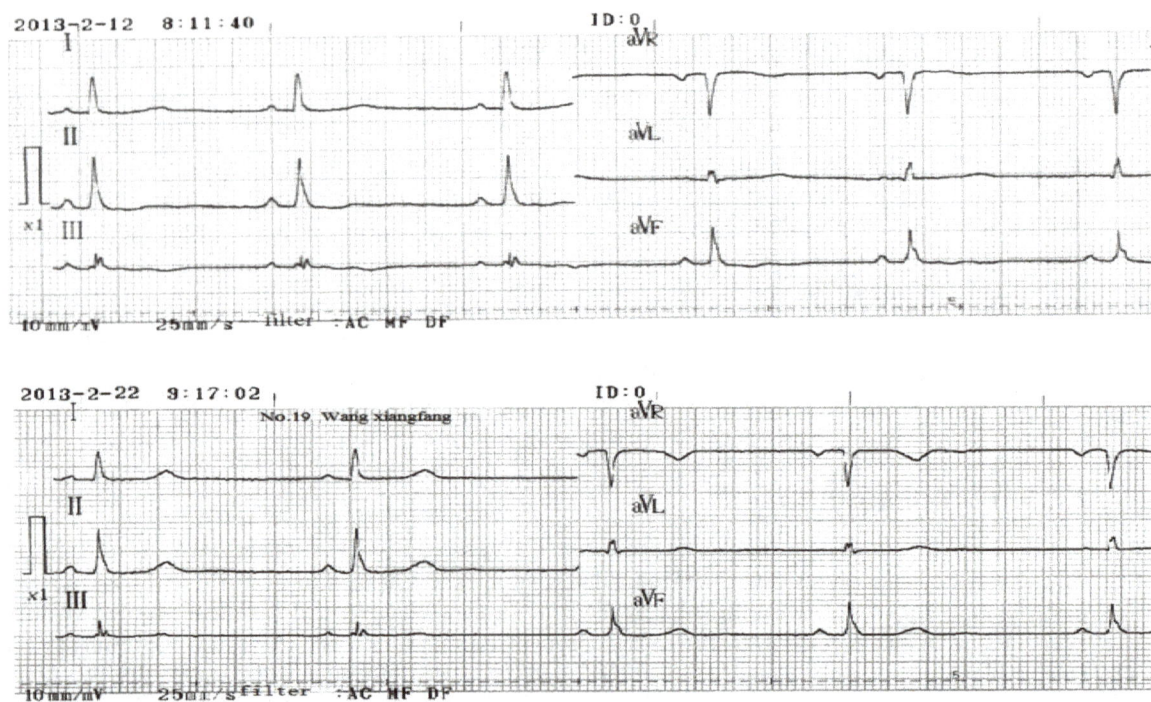

Figure 2. Changes of ECG of patients with IDHF before and after treatment.

Table 1. Seattle angina questionnaire (SAQ) scores of two groups before and after treatment.

	CWMTG (n = 52)			WMTG (n = 48)			P*
	Before treatment	After treatment	P	Before treatment	After treatment	P	
General clinical characteristics							
Age (years)	65.2 ± 9.7			65.0 ± 9.0			0.55
Male (%)	76.4			78.9			0.21
Diabetes (%)	28.2			29.0			0.89
Hypertension (%)	39.5			38.8			0.66
Hyperlipidemia (%)	60.5			61.2			0.75
Symptoms efficacy							
Markedly	59.2			56.9			0.22
Effective	24.4			20.2			0.21
Ineffectiveness	16.4			22.9			0.02
Treatment							
Anti-platelet (%)	91.2	90.5	0.75	94.2	94	0.66	0.07
β-blockers (%)	65.9	62.2	0.91	64.9	64.2	0.94	0.85
statins (%)	88.4	84	0.45	88.9	86.4	0.28	0.75
ACEI/ARB (%)	57.2	56.9	0.91	61.2	60.5	0.75	0.05
Nitrates (%)	65.6	34.4	0.001	60.5	39.5	0.009	0.05
SAQ							
PL	64 ± 22	54 ± 25	0.02	65 ± 23	60 ± 24	0.05	0.04
AS	40 ± 34	37 ± 31	0.05	39 ± 30	33 ± 20	0.05	0.55
AF	66 ± 27	59 ± 27	0.03	67 ± 26	61 ± 25	0.03	0.75
TS	89 ± 18	96 ± 16	0.001	88 ± 16	90 ± 17	0.004	0.05
DP	42 ± 22	48 ± 23	0.05	44 ± 24	49 ± 22	0.05	0.05

P: Comparisons of each group before and after treatment; P*: Comparisons of the two groups after treatment.

3.2. Comparisons of Clinical Baseline Data of Patients with IDHF before and after Treatment

Clinical baseline characteristics of patients in CWMTG before and after treatment are shown in **Table 2**. After treatment, plasma NT-proBNP levels and the rate of β-blocker's use were decreased, the exercise tolerance increased. The differences were statistically significant. The rate of diuretics and lipid-lowering drugs use reduced without statistical significance. Plasma NT-proBNP levels of patients in CWMTG decreased significantly after treatment (70.5 (62.0 - 79.0) ng/L vs 74.0 (65.0 - 84.0) ng/L, P < 0.05). After treatment, plasma NT-proBNP levels of patients in WMTG were not significantly changed (**Table 2**).

3.3. Changes of Echocardiography of Patients with IDHF before and after Treatment

Comparisons of echocardiography parameters of 52 patients with DHF before and after combination therapy were shown in **Table 3**. The results showed that after treatment, SE parameters of LVEF, E/A were significantly increase; E/e' decreased. The differences were statistically significant. However echocardiography parameters showed no significant differences after treatment (**Figure 3** and **Table 3**).

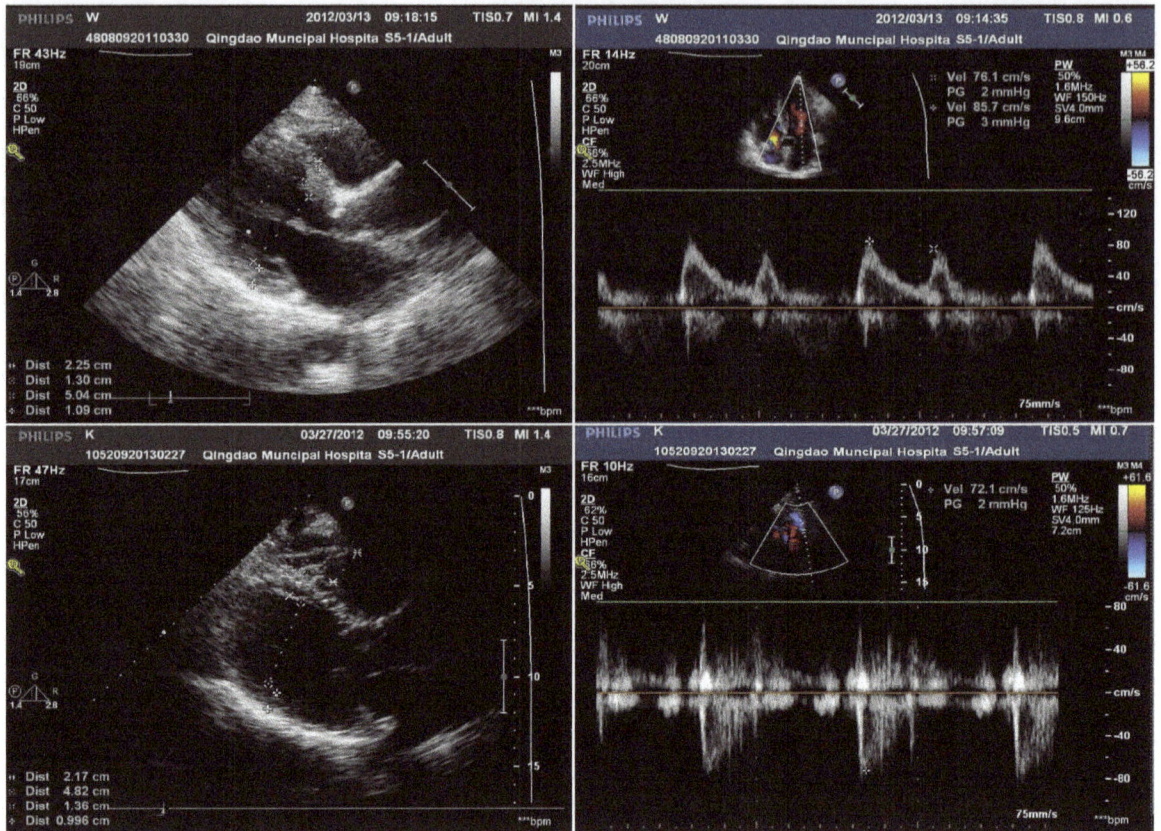

Figure 3. Changes of echocardiography of patients with IDHF before and after treatment.

Table 2. comparisons of clinical parameters of 52 patients with ischemic diastolic heart failure patients before and after treatment.

Clinical parameters	Before treatment	After treatment	P
Demographic characteristics			
Age	69. (62.0 - 74.0)	—	—
Male (%)	32 (61.5%)	—	—
Hypertension (%)	33 (63.5%)	—	—
Diabetes (%)	12 (23.1%)	—	—
Hyperlipidemia (%)	35 (67.3%)	—	—
Fat (%)	19 (36.5%)	—	—
BMI (kg/m^2)	29.5 (26.0 - 33.0)	—	—
Treatment			
Diuretics (%)	27 (52.6%)	20 (38.5%)	0.737
β-blockers (%)	40 (76.3 %)	40 (54.7%)	0.032
Lipid-lowering drugs (%)	33 (63.2%)	27 (52.8%)	0.325
ACEI/ARB (%)	36 (68.4%)	35 (67.9%)	0.960
NT-proBNP (ng/L)	250.7 (167.5 - 544.0)	94.3 (67.0 - 151.5)	<0.001
Hemodynamic			
Heart rate (bpm)	70.5 (62.0 - 79.0)	74.0 (65.0 - 84.0)	0.045
Systolic blood pressure (mmHg)	130.0 (120.0 - 150.0)	130.0 (120.0 - 140.0)	0.042
Diastolic blood pressure (mmHg)	82.5 (80.0 - 95.0)	80.0 (80.0 - 90.0)	0.158
Muscle testing			
Exercise tolerance (s)	387.0 (305.0 - 482.0)	463.0 (382.0 - 527.0)	<0.001

P: Comparisons of before and after treatment.

Table 3. Comparisons of conventional and stress echocardiography index of 52 patients with ischemic diastolic heart failure patients before and after treatment.

The indexes	Before treatment Echo	After treatment Echo	After treatment SE	P
Two-dimensional echocardiography				
EDVI (mL/m^2)	45.0 (39.0 - 54.0)	45.0 (39.9 - 50.0)	45.0 (40.5 - 49.5)	0.717
ESVI (mL/m^2)	16.0 (12.0 - 21.0)	15.2 (12.0 - 18.9)	14.0 (11.0 - 16.5)	0.167
LVEF (%)	54.0 (50.0 - 60.0) a	58.0 (70.0 - 66.0) a	69.5 (66.5 - 73.0) b	0.000
LVMI (g/m^2)	102.5 (88.0 - 123.0) a	101.4 (83.0 - 110.6) a	89.0 (72.0 - 93.5) b	<0.001
LAVI (mL/m^2)	36.0 (29.0 - 41.0) a	34.0 (28.0 - 37.9) a	28.0 (24.0 - 32.0) b	0.001
LVDd	54.7 (50.2 - 55.0)	53.5 (49.7 - 54.1)	51.0 (46.2 - 53.0)	0.03
Left ventricular				
Doppler				
E (cm/s)	77.5 (67.0 - 94.0)	76.0 (65.0 - 96.3)	70.0 (61.5 - 80.0)	0.179
E-exe (cm/s)	107.5 (94.0 - 126.0) a	105.2 (92.3 - 120.2) a	96.0 (83.5 - 102.5) b	0.005
A (cm/s)	92.0 (79.0 - 105.0) a	90.1 (72.2 - 101.4) a	72.0 (65.0 - 79.0) b	<0.001
A-exe (cm/s)	103.0 (92.0 - 121.0) a	101.3 (90.8 - 118.7) a	97.5 (87.0 - 109.5) a,b	0.041
E/A	0.8 (0.7 - 1.0) a	0.8 (0.5 - 1.1) a	1.0 (0.9 - 1.1) b	0.016
E-exe/A-exe	1.0 (0.9 - 1.2)	1.0 (0.8 - 1.2)	0.9 (0.8 - 1.1)	0.826
DT (ms)	189.0 (167.0 - 208.0) a	181.2 (161.2 - 203.0) a	159.5 (149.5 - 189.0) b	0.017
Ard–Ad (ms)	−10.0 (−30.5 - (−1.5))	−11.3 (−30.0 - (−2.2))	−10.5 (−17.0 - (−5.0))	0.640
e' (cm/s)	7.1 (6.3 - 8.4) a	7.9 (6.9 - 9.2) a	9.4 (8.8 - 10.5) b	<0.001
e'-exe (cm/s)	9.3 (8.1 - 10.8) a	9.8 (9.5 - 12.9) a	12.9 (12.0 - 14.3) b	<0.001
a' (cm/s)	9.8 (8.4 - 11.0) a	10.2 (8.9 - 11.7) a	11.2 (9.6 - 12.6) b	0.012
a'-exe (cm/s)	11.1 (9.2 - 13.3) a	12.5 (10.9 - 14.2) a	14.4 (13.0 - 16.5) c	<0.001
s' (cm/s)	7.6 (7.0 - 8.2) a	7.9 (7.8 - 8.6) a	8.8 (8.0 - 9.3) b	<0.001
s'-exe (cm/s)	9.5 (8.8 - 10.3) a	10.5 (8.9 - 13.2) a	13.9 (12.5 - 15.5) c	<0.001
E/e'	10.6 (9.4 - 12.7) a	10.4 (9.0 - 10.9) a	7.0 (6.0 - 8.9) b	<0.001
E-exe/e'-exe	11.0 (9.9 - 12.5) a	10.0 (8.9 - 11.2)	7.2 (6.5 - 7.7) b	<0.001

3.4. Main Echocardiography Parameters of CWMTG Patients and NT-proBNP Correlation Analysis

After the combination treatment, NT-proBNP level had negative correlation with LVEF, E/A, r = −0.432, −0.643, both P < 0.01. After treatment, multiple stepwise regression analysis of NT-proBNP and cardiac function indexes showed that the left ventricular end-diastolic diameter (LVDd), left ventricular ejection fraction (LVEF), early diastolic mitral flow velocity (E), DT, left ventricular isovolumic relaxation time (IVRT), E/A were independent relevant factors of NT-proBNP (**Table 4**).

4. Discussions

In TCM, heart failure is divided into the categories of edema, palpitation, gasp syndrome, phlegm and fluid retention, and blood stasis. Therapy combining Chinese and Western medicine may have pronounced efficacy in the treatment of patients with unstable angina who have been diagnosed with Yin and Qi deficiencies by TCM differentiation. However, there are a few of studies confirming the efficacy of this combination therapy. Studies focusing on objective indicators of improved myocardial function, such as the evaluation index of DHF, regardless of self-reported symptoms of the patients, would be especially useful. In the present work, the SAQ, ECG, stress echocardiography (SE), and the NT-proBNP were all used to assess the efficacy of YFP, which was prepared based on the TCM formula of pulse-activating powder. Assessment of SAQ suggested that treatment with CWMTG brought about significant improvements, including reduced number and severity of angina attacks, and improved the quality of life. In addition, ECG analysis indicated that CWMTG had a more pronounced curative effect than isosorbide denigrate treatment. The results of the SE demonstrated that all patients had symptoms of heart failure and that their LVEF was >50% and the ration of early (E) and late (A) transmittal diastolic velocity

Table 4. Multiple stepwise regression analysis of NT-proBNP and cardiac function indexes of 52 patients after treatment.

Indexes	Non-standardized coefficients	Standardized coefficients	t	P
Two-dimensional echocardiography				
LVEF	1.972°	0.147 b	3.487	0.001
LVDd	8.651	0.131	3.399	0.001
Left ventricular Doppler				
E	6.150°	0.254 a,b	6.260	0.000
E/A	0.104	0.097 b	2.616	0.009
DT	2.296	0.168	3.498	0.001

a: compared with before treatment, P < 0.05. b: compared with conventional echocardiography, P < 0.05.

(E/A ratio) was <1, suggesting that the patients suffered from DHF. After treatment with CWMTG, the relative number of irregular inter-ventricular sepal (IVS) and LVPW movements was significantly went down. LVEF, CO and CI were significantly increased and the patients showed enhanced diastolic function (E/A ratio). All of these indicated that the LVMI was reduced. Systolic function and diastolic function were improved, and stress echocardiography is more sensitive than conventional echocardiography for evaluating the therapeutic effect of diastolic heart failure.The blood levels of NT-proBNP in the patients of the CWMTG were significantly lower than that in controls. The patients also showed improved exercise tolerance and some of them were able to reduce their doses of diuretics and lipid-lowering drugs.

Clinical symptoms of UAP are chest tightness and pain, chest pain involving the back, back pain involving the chest, shortness of breath, gasping, and restlessness. In severe cases, the disease may lead to death within hours of the initial onset of symptoms. The etiological factors are mainly invasion of pathogenic cold, eating disorders, mental stress and extreme changes in emotional state, disorders of the internal organs caused by fatigue, and old age. The location of the disease is mainly the heart and pathogenesis is heart vessel blockage stasis. In the TCM symptom classification system, patients with the mild form of the disease have hypo function of Yang-Qi in the chest, excessive cold syndrome, and blockage of Qi. Patients with severe form of the disease have accumulation of blood-phlegm, congestion in the chest, and blockage of Qi. Delays in treatment may cause damage to Yin and Yang and deficiencies in Qi and Yin, according to TCM theory. The active ingredients of YFP include *Radix Ginseng Rubra* (Panax ginseng or red ginseng), *Radix Ophiopogonis* (Mai Dong), and *Fructus Schisandrae* (Chinese magnoliavine fruit). Red ginseng reinforces vital energy of body, improves lung function, and promotes glandular secretion. It also provides fixation and hidroschesis. It also provides the principle curative action (sovereign drug). The effects of Mai Dong can nourish Yin and relieve dryness of the body. Combination of this herb with red ginseng may notify both Qi and Yin. Mai Dong is also used as minister drug. Chinese magnoliavine fruit can astringe Yin to stop sweating. Combinations of this herb with red ginseng and Mai Dong may consolidate Qi and glandular secretion to prevent leakage and promote recovery from wastage of Qi and Yin. For this reason, it is also termed an assistant drug, an adjuvant drugs that increases the efficacy or potency of sovereign and minister drugs in TCM. These three herbs are combined: to resolve Qi deficiency using red ginseng as a basis; to prevent Qi leakage using Chinese magnoliavine fruit as a standard; and to replenish Yin using Mai Dong. This eventually allows primordial Qi to be ventilated in the lungs, Yin to be restored, and the pulse to be normalized.

Modern pharmacological research has confirmed that the active ingredients of ginseng extracts (panaxosides or ginsenosides) promote DNA and RNA syntheses, increasing hypoxia tolerance, enhancing myocardial contractility, increasing plasma levels of cyclic adenosine monomphsopate (cAMP) and the synthesis of prostaglandin I_2, or PGI_2, thus inhibiting platelet aggregation and improving myocardial cell metabolism [4]. Mai Dong stabilizes myocardial cell membranes with a positive inotropic effect and eliminates free radicals [5]. Chinese magnoliavine fruit strengthens myocardial contractions, improves microcirculation and inhibits lipid peroxidatiuon. Combinations of these three herbs may enhance myocardial contractility, improve left ventricular function and tolerance of myocardial hypoxia, and protect the injured myocardial ultrastructure [6]. YFP injection can tonify Qi and activate blood circulation; reduce plasma viscosity: promote fibrinolysis; inhibit thrombosis; improve abnormal hemorheology, thereby relieving angina and improving self-reported symptoms [7].

Inhibition of Na^+-K^+-ATPase activity affects Na^+-K^+ and Na^+-Ca^{2+} exchange, thereby increasing Ca^{2+} influx and Ca^{2+} concentration. This promotes the interaction of Ca^{2+} with cardiac troponin, resulting in increases in myocardial contractility and cardiac output [8]. Clinical studies published by Zhong et al. demonstrated that pulse-activating injection enhances the capacity of myocardial contraction in patients with ischemic heart disease [9]-[11]. These patients also showed improvement in myocardial compliance and coordination, increased perfusion pressure, and a higher myocardial survival rate and ejection fraction. In the present study, patients' LVEF values were significantly increased and their plasma levels of NT-proBNP were significantly reduced after YFP treatment, suggesting that YFP treatment efficiently improves cardiac function. In addition, these findings are consistent with those of other studies performed using in vivo models. In these studies, pulse-activating injection enhanced patients' myocardial contractility and vasodilation but did not increase the heart rate (all regimens either reduced the heart rate or left it unchanged) [12] [13].

It is not subject to the insufficiencies of more commonly used quality of life scales, which do not sufficiently address the specific conditions or psychology of CAD patients, lack internal consistency in some areas, and have poor response to treatment intervention [14]. Repeated assessments involving the SAQ scale has demonstrated its strong reproducibility. In TCM, efficacy is assessed mostly via clinicians' observations of improvements and patient recovery after the examination through TCM's four diagnostic methods of TCM, observation, auscultation and olfaction, interrogation, and assessments of pulse and palpation. However, these assessments do not consider the quality of life of the patients (e.g., patient's comfort, subjective feelings, and degree of life satisfaction). Quality of life does not only represent and integrate personal values with judgment of health status and life satisfaction but also reveals the patient's expectations with respect to the efficacy of the treatment and improvements in function [15].

The SAQ shows that YFP effectively reduces the frequency of clinical attacks of UAP and facilitates significant improvements in UAP self-reported symptoms, quality of life, and patient satisfaction. However, most of the clinical research to date has only focused on adjuvant TCM therapy on the basis of conventional Western medicine. The lack of evidence-based medicine that can be used to assess the clinical efficacy of an individual TCM regimen or TCM regimen used in place of standard UAP drug therapy complicates the assessment of specificity and definite efficacy of TCM treatment. In addition, the standard treatment for UAP has a standardized duration of follow-up after drug administration. However, there are no published reports addressing the long-term use of TCM and duration of TCM administration in this disease. The present work study confirmed that YFP was associated with improvements in patients' self-reported symptoms of UAP and in patients' satisfaction after treatment. It showed efficacy superior to that of a treatment with Western medicine, so it may be possible to use YFP to compensate for some of the insufficiencies of conventional Western medicine.

During myocardial ischemia, abnormalities in cardiac diastolic function occur prior to systolic dysfunction. Left ventricular diastole includes isovolumetric relaxation (early diastole) and ventricular filling phases. The isovolumetric relaxation phase and rapid filling phase involve active energy-consuming processes; but in the slow filling phase and atria systole phase, the ventricle was passively diastole, which was dependent on the stiffness of the left ventricular myocardial muscle. Conventional echocardiography is not sensitive enough to facilitate prognosis or assessment of the efficacy of treatment. This can lead to misdiagnosis and missed diagnoses. In this way, conventional echocardiography has significant limitations. Stress echocardiography (SE) is a new technique that combines a treadmill exercise stress test and an echocardiography analysis. It is a functional test that involves allowing the patient to exercise to increase myocardial oxygen consumption, which induces pronounced homodynamic changes and increases the detection rate of coronary heart disease while maintaining high sensitivity, specificity, and accuracy for the detection of myocardial ischemia. Because of its noninvasiveness, convenience, repeatability, and ability to determine the homodynamic changes in patients, SE can be used to guide treatment and perform prognosis. In this way, it is one of the more reliable and objective tests to have achieved widespread use in clinical settings in recent years. Although all of the patients in this study had DHF with normal systolic function, SE still demonstrated the changes in myocardial systolic function after YFP treatment. LVEF and LVMI changed significantly after YFP treatment, suggesting enhancement of systolic function and further illustrating that SE allows for a comprehensive evaluation of the therapeutic effect. However, evaluation with left ventricular Doppler flow spectrum was affected by heart rate, preload (left atria pressure) and after load (aortic pressure). Exercise increases heart rate, which may affect the results of left ventricular Doppler flow spectrum and may merit further analysis. In this way, SE also has some limitations. The key to improve the sensitivity of SE is correct detection of load-induced segmental wall motion abnormalities (SWMAs). SWMAs occur only during myocardial ischemia. Sometimes, even under circumstances involving severe coronary artery stenosis, SWMAs can remain undetected if myocardial ischemia is not induced by load. In addition, the limitations of traditional tissue Doppler imaging include inability to measure myocardial motions at different sites at the same time and an inability to detect myocardial velocity gradient. These issues should be addressed in future studies.

Modern medicine suggests that heart failure is not only related to homodynamic abnormalities but also associated with the activation of the neuroendocrine system. The NT-proBNP is a cardiac neurohormone. In the human body, it plays a role in diuresis, natriuresis, and vasodilatation. Declined cardiac output, increased tension of the ventricular wall, and overloaded pressure induce the secretion of NT-proBNP, and levels of NT-proBNP can be indicative of the overall situation of circulatory congestion. There is a positive correlation between the NT-proBNP value and the severity of heart failure, indicating that compensatory pathophysiological changes have taken place. The NT-proBNP value is a marker of the state of restoration of the balance of circulation in human body, and it is negatively correlated with the quality of cardiac function [16]. This study suggested that the NT-proBNP is negatively correlated with LVEF and E/A (r = −0.432 and −0.643). Left ventricular diastolic dysfunction (LVDd), LVEF, E, diastolic (D wave) flow velocity, isovolumic relax-action time (IVRT), and E/A ratio were found to be independent factors associated with NT-proBNP, suggesting that the increase of left ventricular end-systolic pressure (LVESP) and the diastolic dysfunction may result in increased production of NT-proBNP. The changes in NT-proBNP levels may represent the systolic and diastolic functions of the heart. These results are consistent with the SE evaluation of the severity of heart failure. However, NT-proBNP can distinguish neither the cause of heart failure nor the type of heart failure; whereas SE can compensate this inadequacy, that is to say, SE can distinguish the cause and the type of heart failure. This study examined the comprehensive evaluation of cardiac function using patients' SE and plasma NT-proBNP levels. These methods were found to facilitate diagnosis of chronic heart failure and evaluation of its severity in a more reasonable and accurate manner than other methods. These methods were also used to diagnose the underlying heart conditions of the patients, suggesting that the evaluation in these patients using SE and plasma NT-proBNP index was reliable and sensitive.

This study confirmed that YFP treatment improves self-reported symptoms, increases the degree of satisfaction, and makes up for the drawbacks of standard Western medical regimen. It was here confirmed that SAQ is sensitive and suitable for evaluation of the curative effects of TCM, as been shown in a previous study [17].

Stress echocardiography provides some parameters for evaluation of the changes in IDHF and can serve as a quantitative indicator of the clinical efficacy of YFP treatment. The present study confirmed that YFP treatment is reliable and can improve cardiac function and the exercise tolerance in patients. In this study, we didn't discuss whether YFP is effective to all patients with ischemic diastolic heart failure or just effective to ischemic diastolic heart failure patients with with TCM syndrome of qi-yin deficiency. Besides, the sample cases were too little, we should increase the cases to make the results reliable.Improvements in the SE index, levels of NT-proBNP and clinical symptoms in the patients remained consistent throughout this study, suggesting that the combination of these methods may be helpful for research into integrative therapy involving TCM and Western medicine.

References

[1]   Cardiovascular Medicine Branch of Chinese Medical Doctor Association, Evidence-Based Medicine Branch of Chinese Medical Doctor Association Commition (2007) Guidelines and Consensus on Prevention and Treatment of Cardiovascular Diseases 2007[M]. People's Medical Publishing House, Beijing, 37-39.

[2]   Young, M.N., Shoemaker, M.B., Kurtz, E.G., et al. (2012) Heart Failure with Preserved Left Ventricuiar Function: Diagnosticand Therapeutic Challenges in Patients with Diastolic Heart Failure. The American Journal of the Medical Sciences.

[3]   Spertus, J.A., Winders, J.A., Dewhurst, T.A., et al. (1995) Development and Alidation of the Seattle Angina Questionnaire: Journal of the American College of Cardiology, 25, 333-341. http://dx.doi.org/10.1016/0735-1097(94)00397-9

[4]   Yang, W.M. and Zhou, Y.X. (1997) Clinical Observation on Treatment of Chronic Congestive Heart Failure with Shenmai Injection: 62 Cases. Practical Journal of Integrated Traditional Chinese and Western Medicine, 10, 1446.

[5]   Wang, J.H. (1994) Handbook of Commonly Used Traditional Chinese Medicine [M]. The Golden Shield Press, Beijing, 112.

[6]   Xu, L.H. (2009) Therapeutic Effect of Yiqi Fumai in Patients with Chronic Congestive Heart Faliure. *Clinical Medicine*, **22**, 2418-2419.

[7]   Yuan, C.L. and Du, S.L. (2012) Efficacy of Yi Qi Fu Mai Injection on Heart Failure Complicated with Angina Pectoris in Patients with Coronary Heart Disease. *Chinese Journal of New Drugs*, 1774-1777.

[8]   Mao, J.Y., Zhang, B.L. and Wang X.L. (2006) Progress in Mechanism of Shenmai Injection in the Treatment of Heart Failure. *Chinese Traditional Patent Medicine*, **28**, 1801-1803.

[9]   Dong, Q.Z., Chen, K.Y. and Tu, X.H. (1984) Hemodynamic Effects of Shengmai Injection in the Treatment of Acute Myocardial Infarction. *Chinese Journal of Cardiology*, **12**, 5-6.

[10]   Zhong, Y.S. (1998) Effect of Shengmai Injection on Left Ventricular Volume and Function of Patients with Heart Failure after Acute Myocardial Infarction. *Journal of Wuhan Postgraduate Medical College*, **26**, 1-2.

[11]   Zhuang, A.L. and Guan, E.J. (1997) Effect of "Sheng Mai" Injection on Cardiac Function of Patients with Ischemic Heart Disease. *Chinese Journal of Integrated Traditional and Western Medicine in Intensive and Critical Care*, **4**, 310-311.

[12]   Department of Chest Emergency Coordination Group of the State Administration of Traditional Chinese Medicine Medical Administration. (1995) Clinical and Experimental Studies of Shenmal Injection for Treatment of 219 Cases of Angina Pectoris of CHD. *Journal of Emergency in Traditional Chinese Medicine*, **4**, 152-155.

[13]   Meng, Q.Y. (2000) Preliminary Study on Rapid Injection of Shengmai Injection in the Treatment of Hypertensive Emergencies. *Hebei Medicine*, **6**, 133-134.

[14]   Xing, W.H. and Chen, X.M. (2004) Feasibility of SF-8 Short Scale for Testing Health Related Quality of Life in Patients with Coronary Heart Disease. *Foreign Medical Sciences (Section of cardiovascular)*, **5**, 181-184.

[15]   Hao, Y.T., Fang, J.Q., Li, C.X., *et al.* (1999) World Health Organization. WHOQOL and Its Chinese Version. *Foreign Medical Sciences (Section of Social Medicine)* **16**, 118-122.

[16]   Wang, L., Hu, Y.S., Wu, X., *et al.* (2010) Significances of NT-proBNP and hs-CRP in Heart Failure. *National Medical Journal of China*, **90**, 1635-1636.

[17]   Liu, T.X., Kong, S.P., Liao, Z.Y., *et al.* (1997) Assessment Study on Physical Function and the Quality of Life for CHD Patients with SAQ. *Chinese Journal of Behavioral Medical Science*, **6**, 127-129.

Abbreviation

IHF: ischemic heart failure
YFP: Yiqi Fumai freeze-dry powder
TCM: traditional Chinese medicine
IDHF: ischemic diastolic heart failure
CWMTG: Chinese and western medicine treatment group
WMTG: western medicine treatment group
SAQ: Seattle Angina Questionnaire
AMI: acute myocardial infarction
DHF: diastolic heart failure
SE: stress echocardiography
UAP: unstable angina pectoris
ACS: acute coronary syndrome
PCI: percutaneous transluminal coronary intervention
CABG: Coronary artery bypass grafting
ACEI: angiotensin-converting enzyme inhibitors
ARB: angiotensin II receptor blockers
LVDd: left ventricular diastolic diameter
IVSd: interventricular sepal thickness at the end of diastolic
LVPWd: left ventricular posterior wall thickness
LAD: left atria diameter
LVEF: left ventricular ejection fraction
CO: left ventricular output

CI: cardiac index
IVS: inter-ventricular sepal
SWMAs: segmental wall motion abnormalities
IVRT: isovolumic relax-action time
LVESP: left ventricular end-systolic pressure
LAVI: left atrial volume index
EDVI: left ventricular end-diastolic volume
ESVI: systolic volume index;
LVMI: left ventricular mass index
E: early diastolic two mitral flow velocity
A: late diastolic mitral flow velocity
E / e ': early diastolic mitral flow velocity and early diastolic mitral annular velocity ratio
DT: mitral E wave deceleration Time
Ard - Ad: aortic root diameter.
Echo: conventional echocardiography
SE: stress echocardiography
ECG: electrocardiogram
NT-proBNP: N-terminal pro brain natriuretic peptide

5

Clinical Study of Sulfotanshinone Sodium Injection in Treating Non-Ischemic Retinal Vein Occlusion

Bingwen Lu, Xingwei Wu*

Ophthalmology Department, Shanghai First People's Hospital, Shanghai, China
Email: *704487389@qq.com

Abstract

Objectives: To study the effect of sulfotanshinone sodium (SS) injection in the treatment of non-ischemic retinal vein occlusion (RVO). Methods: Sixty-two RVO patients treated in our hospital between Jan. 2013 and Oct. 2014 were randomly divided into Control Group (30 patients; Bendazol tablets) and Treatment Group (32 patients, Bendazol tablets + SS injections), each with a follow-up period of 6 months. Statistical analysis was then performed on changes in visual acuity, central retinal thickness (CRT) and retinal circulation time (RCT) before and after the treatment. Results: After treatment, both Control Group and Treatment Group witnessed an improvement on visual acuity (Control Group: $t = 2.103$, $p = 0.044$; Treatment Group: $t = 8.021$, $p = 0.000$). Visual acuity could be greatly improved in Treatment Group when compared with Control Group, with significant differences ($p < 0.01$). Macular edema could be greatly relieved in Treatment Group measured by CRT ($t = 2.571$, $p = 0.007$) while the difference was of no statistical significance in Control Group ($t = 1.016$, $p = 0.070$). RCT were remarkably shortened in both groups (Control Group: $t = 43.83$, $p = 0.000$; Treatment Group: $t = 27.34$, $p = 0.000$), and when compared with Control group, the changes in Treatment Group were more significant ($p < 0.05$). Conclusion: SS injection could effectively improve the therapeutic effect in patients with non-ischemic retinal vein occlusion.

Keywords

Sulfotanshinone Sodium Injection, Non-Ischemic Retinal Vein Occlusion

1. Introduction

Retinal vein occlusion (RVO) is the second most common retinal vascular disorder after diabetic retinopathy

---
*Corresponding author.

with significant morbidity, including branch retinal vein occlusion (BRVO) and central retinal vein occlusion (CRVO) as well as their ischemic and non-ischemic subtypes [1]. Major causes of vision loss include macular edema and neovascularization with secondary vitreous hemorrhage and/or neovascular glaucoma [2]. Until recently, effective treatment options for RVO were limited, including grid laser photocoagulation, intravitreal injections of triamcindion acetonide and intravitreal injections of anti-vascular endothelial growth factor (VEGF) agents [3].

Tanshinone IIA (TSA) is an herbal monomer with a clear chemical structure, isolated from Danshen (Salvia miltiorrhiza). In Traditional Chinese Medicine (TCM), Danshen is considered to promote blood circulation for removing blood stasis and improve microcirculation, which thus has been widely used to treat cardiovascular diseases for more than 2000 years in China [4]. Over the last decade, interest in the mechanism of its versatile protective effects on neurodegenerative diseases, metabolic abnormalities, and ischemic damages has been growing [5]-[7]. Up till now, few studies have reported on its clinical use in the area of retinal ischemic diseases. This prospective clinical study was designed to assess the safety and efficacy of TSA in treating RVO patients.

2. Materials and Methods

2.1. Research Objects and Grouping

This prospective, open-label, comparative case series study was conducted at Ophthalmology department of Shanghai First People's Hospital from Jan. 2013 to Oct. 2014. Consecutive cases of RVO patients who could come for regular follow-up visits were invited to participate in the study.

The study group comprised patients who met the eligibility criteria as follows: 1) age of at least 18 years with RVO; 2) best-corrected visual acuity (BCVA) of 30 letters to 90 letters using the ETDRS charts; 3) color fundus photography documented thin retinal artery, dilated vein, posterior pole retinal edema and hemorrhage; 4) fundus fluorescence angiography (FFA) featured delayed arterial filling, delayed retinal arterial branches filling, delayed laminar flow in large retinal veins, and no filling or only retrograde filling in retinal vein branches. No capillary non-perfusion (NP) was present in non-ischemic RVO.

Patients were excluded from the study if they had undergone any other treatment for RVO within 3 months, such as laser therapy or intravitreal injections. Patients with age-related macular degeneration, diabetic retinopathy, uncontrolled glaucoma, or ocular inflammation that could compromise visual acuity were excluded. Patients with uncontrolled hypertension, diabetic mellitus, myocardial infarction, or cerebrovascular accident within three months of presentation were also excluded.

Informed consent was obtained from the patients before enrollment in the study. Ethical approval was obtained from the Shanghai First People's Hospital Research Center.

2.2. Experiment Medicine

Sixty-two RVO patients were randomized into two groups: Control Group receiving Bdazol tablets only (10 mg each time, three times daily), Treatment Group receiving Bendazol tablets (10 mg each time, three times daily) + sulfotanshinone sodium (SS) injections (20 mg per day, one week consecutively in one month).

SS injection (5 mg/ml) manufactured by the First Biochemical Pharmaceutical Co. Ltd., Shanghai, China, is now the clinically available TSA agent, approved by State Food and Drug Administration of China. The dosage for administration of SS injection is 20 mg per day. SS injection is given diluted at the point of treatment in 250 mL 5% glucose injection for intravenous administration.

In addition to the treatment medicines, usages of any other traditional Chinese medicine or modern western medicine that affects blood circulation during the 6 months follow-up were prohibited.

2.3. Experiment Methods

A detailed history was taken to ascertain each patient's demographics and chief complaints, including duration of the symptom and presence of systemic diseases, such as hypertension, diabetes mellitus, cardiac diseases and hyperlipidemia.

Each patient underwent BCVA measurement with the ETDRS chart. Clinical examination included slit-lamp examination, intraocular pressure measurement using noncontact tonometer (NCT) (Nikon, Japan). Baseline central retinal thickness (CRT) was measured with Optical Coherence Tomography (OCT) (Zeiss, Germany). A fluorescein angiogram (FFA) (Heidelberg, Germany) was performed to identify the presence of non-ischemic RVO and record the retinal circulation time (RCT).

All patients underwent monthly BCVA testing, intraocular pressure measurement and OCT scans. FFA was carried out again at the 6 month.

A flow diagram of the entire trial was presented (**Figure 1**).

2.4. Statistical Analysis

Test results were represented by x ± s using the SPSS 18.0 software. Statistical methods such as t-test for independent samples, paired sample t-test and analysis of variance were used for testing and analysis. P values less than 0.05 were considered statistically significant in this study.

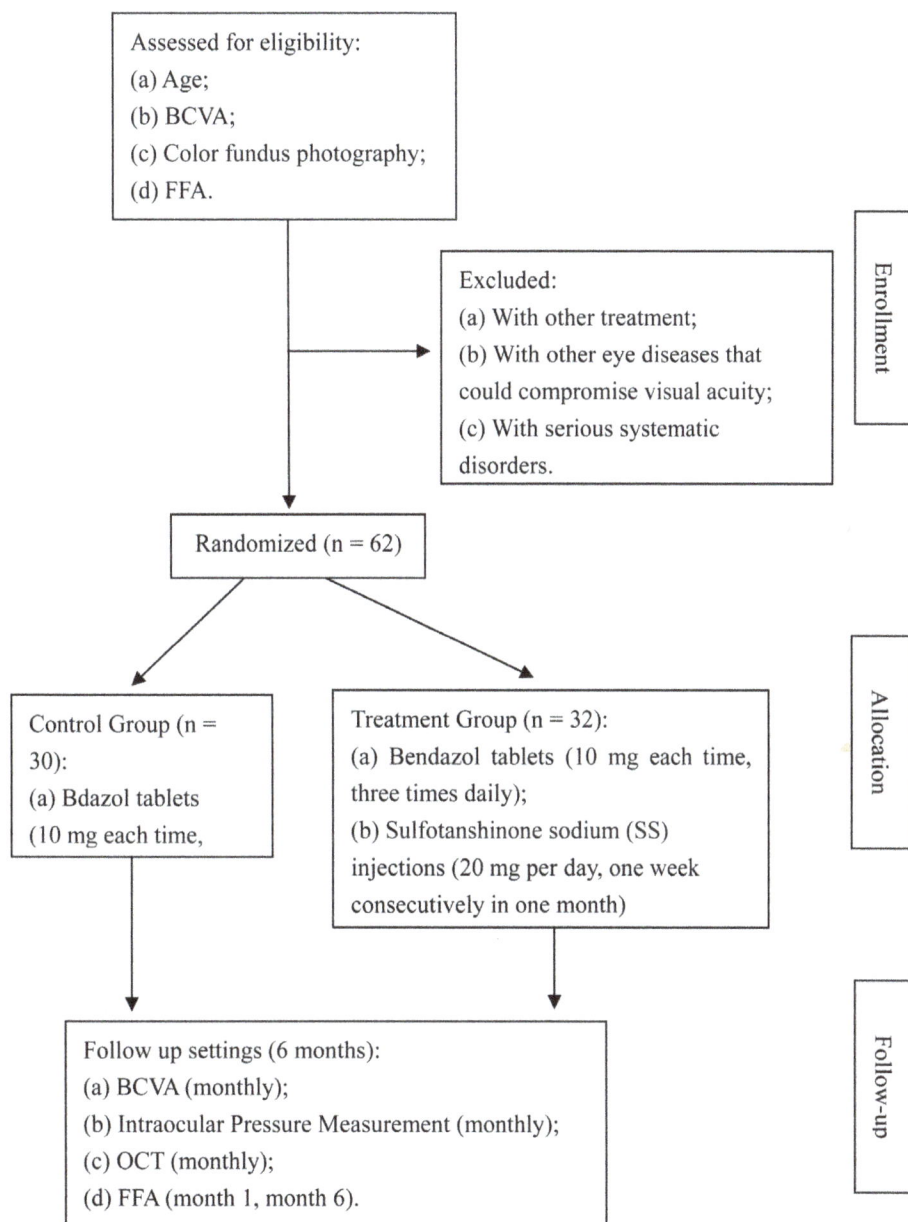

Figure 1. Flow diagram of the progress through the phases of a randomized trial (enrollment, intervention allocation, and follow-up). BCVA: Best-Corrected Visual Acuity; FFA: Fluorescein Angiogram; OCT: Optical Coherence Tomography.

3. Results

3.1. Patient Demographics and Baseline Characteristics

A total of 62 eyes of 62 consecutive patients (20 men and 42 women) were included in the study. The mean age of the study population was 62 ± 7 years (range 50 - 80). The mean duration of symptoms prior to presentation was 2.8 ± 1.8 months with a range of 0.2 months to 6 months. Eighteen eyes had CRVO, and 44 eyes had BRVO. Concurrent systemic hypertension was found in 30 cases (48.3%), and nine patients (14.5%) had diabetic mellitus. Sixty-two patients were randomized into Control Group and Treatment Group. **Table 1** summarizes the clinical characteristics of the two groups. Demographic date revealed no statistical difference.

3.2. Visual Acuity

RVO patients in Treatment Group had a mean BCVA of 64 ± 14 letters before treatment. After the initial 3 months, mean BCVA improved signigicantly, and this gain was maintained at 6 months. Final BCVA was 74 ± 10 letters, which was significantly better than the acuity at baseline (t = 8.021, p = 0.000). RVO patients in Control Group had a mean BCVA of 65 ± 13 before treatment and a final BCVA of 67 ± 13 letters. Visual acuity did not significantly improve between baseline and 6 months (t = 2.103, p = 0.044). The improvement of visual acuity was better in Treatment Group when compared with Control group (p < 0.01). **Table 2** summarizes the changes of BCVA of the two groups (x ± s, letters).

3.3. Central Retinal Thickness (CRT)

The mean CRT of RVO patients in Treatment Group at baseline was 406.3 ± 23.3 μm and 338.4 ± 20.7 μm at 6 months. The changes in CRT from baseline were statistically significant (t = 2.571, p = 0.007). The mean CRT of RVO patients in Control Group at baseline was 385.3 ± 8.3 μm and 342.7 ± 19.2 μm at 6 months. The changes in CRT from baseline were of no statistical importance (t = 1.016, p = 0.07). The changes of CRT of the two groups were summarized in **Table 3**.

3.4. Retinal Circulation Time (RCT)

Prolonged RCT was found in both CRVO and BRVO patients. After treatment, the RCT in RVO patients in Treatment Group were reduced to 3.04 ± 0.14 sec from 5.11 ± 0.29 sec. The changes in RCT from baseline were statistically significant (t = 43.83, p = 0.000). The mean RCT of RVO patients in Control Group at baseline was 5.15 ± 0.21 sec and 3.81 ± 0.13 at 6 months. Although the changes were also of statistical importance (t = 27.34, p = 0.000). When compared with Control Group, the changes in Treatment Group were more significant (p < 0.05). The changes of RCT of the two groups were summarized in **Table 4**.

3.5. Safety

There were no major ocular or systemic problems, such as increased intraocular pressure, retinal detachment, intraocular inflammation, or vascular events during the 6 months follow-up in both groups.

Table 1. Demographics and clinical characteristics of the two groups.

	Control Group	Treatment Group
Number of patients	30	32
Age, years	62 ± 7	62 ± 7
Sex (male/female)	10/20	10/22
Duration of symptoms prior to presentation, months	2.5 ± 1.9	3.0 ± 1.4
BCVA, letters	65 ± 13	64 ± 14
CRT, μm	385.3 ± 8.3	406.3 ± 23.3
RCT, sec	5.15 ± 0.21	5.11 ± 0.29

Data are mean ± SD; BCVA: Best-Corrected Visual Acuity; CRT: Central Retinal Thickness; RCT: Retinal Circulation Time.

Table 2. Changes of BCVA of the two groups (x ± s, letters).

	BCVA Results		t	p
	Baseline	6 months		
Treatment Group	64 ± 14	74 ± 10	8.021	0.000
Control Group	65 ± 13	67 ± 13	2.103	0.044

Data are mean ± SD; BCVA: Best-Corrected Visual Acuity.

Table 3. Changes of CRT of the two groups (x ± s, μm).

	OCT Results		t	p
	Baseline	6 months		
Treatment Group	406.3 ± 23.3	338.4 ± 20.7	2.571	0.007
Control Group	385.3 ± 8.3	342.7 ± 19.2	1.016	0.07

Data are mean ± SD; CRT: Central Retinal Thickness; OCT: Optical Coherence Tomography.

Table 4. Changes of RCT of the two groups (x ± s, sec).

	RCT Results		t	p
	Baseline	6 months		
Treatment Group	5.11 ± 0.29	3.04 ± 0.14	43.83	0.000
Control Group	5.15 ± 0.21	3.81 ± 0.13	27.34	0.000

Data are mean ± SD; RCT: Retinal Circulation Time.

4. Discussion

Retinal vascular occlusive disorders constitute one of the major causes of blindness and impaired vision. There is marked controversy on their pathogeneses, clinical features and particularly their management. Recently, advances in clinical research added anti-VEGF, corticosteroids and sustained-release implants to our armamentarium in the management of retinal vein occlusions [1]. Despite the existence of several therapeutic options, none is entirely satisfactory. Short-term effectiveness such as VA improvement may be significant, however, their long-term curative rates are still disappointing requiring expensive and repetitive treatments, for they only focus on the symptoms such as macular edema, not the disease. TCM has always been focusing on the diseases instead of the symptoms alone, so whether it may have some effectiveness on retinal vascular occlusive disorders is yet to be studied.

TCM is a unique system of theory, diagnosis and treatment tools, and is commonly used in Asian countries. Compared with western medicine, the TCM approach treats the function and dysfunction of living organisms in a more holistic way. However, the complexity of the chemical components and the actions in vivo often lead to great difficulties to elucidate the molecular mechanisms of TCM, which has been always the bottleneck of modern TCM study.

In this research, we studied TSA, which is an herbal monomer with a clear chemical structure, isolated from Danshen (Salvia miltiorrhiza). Danshen, a herbal medicine derived from the dried root of Salvia miltiorrhiza Bunge, is a hemorheologic agent that may have protective effect in patients with unstable angina [4] and has been used for cardiovascular disorders for hundreds of years in China and now is widely used in other countries as well. Danshen consists of a mixture of compounds, among which TSA represents the most biologically active ingredient [8]. Animal and cellular studies have shown various potential benefits of the agent, including neuroprotective effect in cerebral ischemia and reperfusion [9], antioxidant potential to prevent oxidation of low-density lipoproteins [10], reducing cellular damage by free radicals [11], protecting cardiomyocytes against oxidative stress-mediated apoptosis [12], and so on. Human studies also have demonstrated cardioprotective effects of TSA, including reduction of myocardial infarct size and decrease of myocardial consumption of oxygen [13]. TSA has drawn extensive attention because of its therapeutic efficacy in cardiovascular diseases, metabolic diseases as well as cancers [14]. As a multi-target drug, whether TSA may have protective effects on retinal vascular diseases has not been proved. Therefore, this study was designed to assess the safety and efficacy of TSA in treating RVO patients.

Here, we found that after 6 months SS injections, most patients in Treatment Group showed a good response with a significant reduction of CRT, RCT and an increase in VA. To date, initial VA is the most reliable prognostic factor of visual prognosis. Initial CRT can be useful for evaluating the severity of ME associated with RVO, and seems to be important toward the presentation of visual function after treatment, while initial RCT can reflect the status of retinal circulation. During the follow-up period, no one was lost and all required data were collected in this trial.

This prospective study had a number of potential limitations. The sample size was small, the investigators and patients were not masked. Considering the strength of the evidence, more rigorously designed trials are required for assessing the effects of SS injection before it can be recommended routinely.

5. Conclusion

In summary, SS injection was an effective and safe modality for treating RVO patients based on the comparison of mean BCVA and OCT images and FFA results between the two groups. SS injection appeared to be an effective and safe treatment option for RVO.

Acknowledgements

This work was supported by a grant from Shanghai First People's Hospital. The author was grateful to Professor Wu from Shanghai First People's Hospital for final edict of this manuscript.

References

[1] Querques, G., Triolo, G., Casalino, G., García-Arumí, J., Badal, J., Zapata, M., Boixadera, A., Castillo, V.M. and Bandello, F. (2013) Retinal Venous Occlusions: Diagnosis and Choice of Treatments. *Ophthalmic Research*, **49**, 215-222. http://dx.doi.org/10.1159/000346734

[2] Hahn, P. and Fekrat, S. (2012) Best Practices for Treatment of Retinal Vein Occlusion. *Current Opinion in Ophthalmology*, **23**, 175-181. http://dx.doi.org/10.1097/ICU.0b013e3283524148

[3] Cernak, M. and Struharova, K. (2012) Current Therapy for Retinal Vein Occlusion. *Bratisl Lek Listy*, **113**, 228-231. http://dx.doi.org/10.4149/BLL_2012_052

[4] Zhou, L., Zuo, Z. and Chow, M.S. (2005) Danshen: An Overview of Its Chemistry, Pharmacology, Pharmacokinetics, and Clinical Use. *The Journal of Clinical Pharmacology*, **45**, 1345-1359. http://dx.doi.org/10.1177/0091270005282630

[5] Chen, Y., Wu, X., Yu, S., Lin, X., Wu, J., Li, L., Zhao, J. and Zhao, Y. (2012 Neuroprotection of Tanshinone IIA against Cerebral Ischemia/Reperfusion Injury through Inhibition of Macrophage Migration Inhibitory Factor in Rats. *PLoS ONE*, **7**, e40165. http://dx.doi.org/10.1371/journal.pone.0040165

[6] Fu, J., Huang, H., Liu, J., Pi, R., Chen, J. and Liu, P. (2007) Tanshinone IIA Protects Cardiac Myocytes against Oxidative Stress-Triggered Damage and Apoptosis. *European Journal of Pharmacology*, **568**, 213-221. http://dx.doi.org/10.1016/j.ejphar.2007.04.031

[7] Park, O.K., Choi, J.H., Park, J.H., Kim, I.H., Yan, B.C., Ahn, J.H., Kwon, S.H., Lee, J.C., Kim, Y.S., Kim, M., Kang, I.J., Kim, J.D., Lee, Y.L. and Won, M.H. (2012) Comparison of Neuroprotective Effects of Five Major Lipophilic Diterpenoids from Danshen Extract against Experimentally Induced Transient Cerebral Ischemic Damage. *Fitoterapia*, **83**, 1666-1674. http://dx.doi.org/10.1016/j.fitote.2012.09.020

[8] Shang, Q.H., Xu, H. and Huang, L. (2012) Tanshinone IIA: A Promising Natural Cardioprotective Agent. *Evidence-Based Complementary and Alternative Medicine*, **2012**, Article ID: 716459. http://dx.doi.org/10.1155/2012/716459

[9] Chen, Y.L., Wu, X.M., Yu, S.S., Lin, X.M., Wu, J.X., Li, L., Zhao, J. and Zhao, Y. (2012) Neuroprotection of Tanshinone IIA against Cerebral Ischemia/Reperfusion Injury through Inhibition of Macrophage Migration Inhibitory Factor in Rats. *PLoS ONE*, **7**, e40165. http://dx.doi.org/10.1371/journal.pone.0040165

[10] Li, X.X., Xu, X., Wang, J.N., Yu, H., Wang, X., Yang, H.J., Xu, H.Y., Tang, S.H., Li, Y., Yang, L., Huang, L.Q., Wang, Y.H. and Yang, S.L. (2012) A System-Level Investigation into the Mechanisms of Chinese Traditional Medicine: Compound Danshen Formula for Cardiovascular Disease Treatment. *PLoS ONE*, **7**, e43918. http://dx.doi.org/10.1371/journal.pone.0043918

[11] Wang, A.-M., Sha, S.-H., Lesniak, W. and Schacht, J. (2003) Tanshinone (*Salviae miltiorrhizae* Extract) Preparations

Attenuate Aminoglycoside-Induced Free Radical Formation *in Vitro* and Ototoxicity *in Vivo*. *Antimicrobial Agents and Chemotherapy*, **47**, 1836-1841. http://dx.doi.org/10.1128/AAC.47.6.1836-1841.2003

[12] Zhang, M.-Q., Zheng, Y.-L., Chen, H., Tu, J.-F., Shen, Y., Guo, J.-P., Yang, X.-H., Yuan, S.-R., Chen, L.-Z., Chai, J.-J., Lu, J.-H. and Zhai, C.-L. (2013) Sodium Tanshinone IIA Sulfonate Protects Rat Myocardium against Ischemia-Reperfusion Injury via Activation of PI3K/Akt/FOXO3A/Bim Pathway. *Acta Pharmacologia Sinica*, **34**, 1386-1396. http://dx.doi.org/10.1038/aps.2013.91

[13] Tan, X.Y., Li, J.P., Wang, X.Y., Chen, N., Cai, B.Z., Wang, G., Shan, H.L., Dong, D.L., Liu, Y.J., Li, X.D., Yang, F., Li, X., Zhang, P., Li, X.Q. Yang, B.F. and Lu, Y.J. (2011) Tanshinone IIA Protects against Cardiac Hypertrophy via Inhibiting Calcineurin/Nfatc3 Pathway. *International Journal of Biological Sciences*, **7**, 383-389. http://dx.doi.org/10.7150/ijbs.7.383

[14] Xu, S. and Liu, P. (2013) Tanshinone II-A: New Perspectives for Old Remedies. *Expert Opinion on Therapeutic Patents*, **23**, 149-153. http://dx.doi.org/10.1517/13543776.2013.743995

miRNAs Expression and Role of Dicer on Podocyte Injury in PAN Nephrosis Rats

Chunqing Li[1,2], Wei Sun[2,3*], Haochang Du[1], Dong Zhou[3], Jihong Chen[3], Lu Zhang[3], Jiade Shao[3]

[1]Nephrology Department of Wuxi No. 3 Hospital, Wuxi, China
[2]Discipline of Chinese and Western Integrative Medicine, Nanjing University of Chinese Medicine, Nanjing, China
[3]Nephrology Department of Jiangsu Province Hospital of Traditional Chinese Medicine, Nanjing, China
Email: *jssunwei@163.com

Abstract

Objective: microRNAs (miRNAs) are regulatory RNAs that act as important players in diverse biologic and pathologic processes. Under circumstance as podocye-injury triggering proteinuria, which miRNAs are up-regulated or down-regulated? This experiment aims at detecting miRNAs changes in PAN nephrosis rats based on miRNA arrays and exploring the therapeutic targets of Leizhi capsule. Methods: Fifty male wistar rats were randomly divided into five groups, including control group, model group, leizhi capsule group, *Tripterygium glucosides* group, and valsartan group. PAN nephrosis models were made by jugular vein injection of PAN (100 mg/kg body weight, dissolve in physiological saline), while control group rats were made by jugular vein injection of physiological saline with equal volume. Other groups rats had been given medicines by irrigating stomach once a day for ten days. Blood and urine samples were collected, and renal tissues were processed after rats being euthanasised. The 24 h urinary protein excretion and blood biochemistry parameters were measured by routine methods. The glomerular morphology and podocyte ultrastructure were observed with light microscopy and transmission electron microscopy respectively. miRNA expression profile was detected by Exiqon miRNA Array. Real time RT-PCR analysis for mature miRNAs was used to validate differentially expressed miRNAs. Results: 1) In day 3 - 5, model rats had decreased urine volume, ascites, malnutrition and wight loss. From day 7 to day 10, the nephrotic syndromes were worst in model rats, but which had no skin edema. Some rats died in serious ascites, the mortality is 3/10. 2) miRNA array detection shows 106 miRNAs up regulated and 62 miRNAs down regulated in PAN nephrosis rats. Fold change (model vs. control group) varies from 1.8 to 7.0. For leizhi capsule group and model sample, there are 90 miRNAs differentially expressed, with 65 miRNAs up and 25 miRNAs down. The most important finding in our research is the discovery of the specific miRNAs related to PAN nephrosis (rno-miR23a, rno-miR-24, rno-miR-30c and rno-miR-300-3p), which have been validated by Real time RT-PCR anal-

---

*Corresponding author.

ysis. 3) Compared with control sample, immune fluorescence intensity of dicer, expression profile of nephrin, podocin and synaptopodin mRNA and protein decrease in PAN nephrosis rats. After treated with Leizhi Capsule, immune fluorescence intensity of the above molecules improved. Conclusion: 1) Characteristic miRNAs of PAN nephrosis were screening. Up-regulated miRNAs (rno-miR-23a, rno-miR-300-3p) may trigger podocyte injury and proteinuria, while down-regulated miRNAs (rno-miR-24, rno-miR-30c) may be protective factors by anti-apoptosis. 2) Dicer and these miRNAs (rno-miR-24, rno-miR-30c, rno-miR-23a) may be are probably key molecules therapeutic targets of Leizhi capsule.

Keywords

microRNAs, Podocyte Injury, Puromycin Aminonucleoside Nephrosis Model, Proteinuria, Leizhi Capsule

---

1. Introduction

microRNAs (miRNA) are a group of non-coding small RNA (approximately 22-nt) that are present in lower through higher organism and function to regulate gene expression by translation repression or transcript degradation of target genes. Dicer is a key enzyme in miRNA biosynthetic, by which pri-miRNAs are processed into approximately 22-nt mature microRNA [1] [2]. In addition, Dicer is involved in the immediate downstream effecter steps of this pathway, whereby it serves as an essential component of miRNA-containing catalytic enzyme complexes, such as the RNA-induced silencing complex. Thus, as a physical platform and a functional bridge, Dicer couples miRNA biogenesis to miRNA-mediated gene silence [3].

Proteinuria is a dangerous factor of chronic kidney disease (CKD). Podocyte injury is not only the key link of proteinuria, but also closely contacts with CKD progress. Some microRNAs may induce slit diaphragm (SD) molecules expression via triggering nephrin phosphorylation to reduce proteinuria [4]-[6]. As a key enzyme of miRNA biosynthesis, dicer probabaly have a role on proteinuria of CKD. Podocyte-selective deletion of dicer induces proteinuria and glomerulosclerosis [1] [7], also alter cytoskeletal dynamics and causes glomerular disease [1] [2] [8], leading to rapid glomerular and tubular injury [3] [9]. It is suggested that dicer and these miRNAs are probably key regulated targets. How dicer enzyme have effects on podocyte in PAN (puromycin aminonucleoside, PAN) nephrosis pathlogy? So the aim of our experiment is to explore how dicer has effects on podocyte apotosis and cytoskeleton.

2. Methods

Fifty male Wistar rats were divided into five groups, including: 1) control group, 2) PAN model group, 3) leizhi group, 4) *Tripterygium glucosides* (GTW) group, and 5) valsartan group.

PAN model rats were made by jugularly intravenous injecting with PAN (100 mg/kg) [10], while control group rats were made by intravenous injecting with physiological saline. After injection, all rats were feeding with clear water and food for ten days in metabolic cage.

By irrigation stomach once a day for ten days, all rats had been given medicines as follows:

1) Physiological saline (2 ml) for control group and model group;

2) *Tripterygium glucosides* (2 mg) dissolved in Erzhi (containing Ligustrum lucidum and Drought Ephraim grass) solusion (1 ml) for Leizhi group;

3) *Tripterygium glucosides* 1 mg/kg/d for *Tripterygium glucosides* group;

4) Triptolid 2 mg/200g/d for triptolid group ;

5) Valsartan valsartan 1.5 mg/200g/d for valsartan group.

Urine was collected on alternate day, and blood sample were gathered before and after experiment. After all rats being euthanasised, kidneys and livers were removed for Electron microscopy, Immunofluorescence stain and RT-PCR and western bloting.

miRNA Array analysis has been accomplished by Shanghai KangChen Biological engineering company. miRNA expression profile was detected by Exiqon miRNA Array, including: prepare the RNA Sample and

RNA Sample QC, miRNA labeling, miRNA array hybridization, miRNA array scanning and analysis. Real time RT-PCR analysis for mature miRNAs was used to validate 4 differentially expressed miRNAs between control and model group in microRNA microarray assays.

3. Results

PAN nephrosis rats were made successfully by jugular vein injection of PAN (100 mg/kg body weight). In day 5, model rats were in low spirits, with decreased urine volume, ascites, malnutrition and weight loss. From day 7 to day 10, proteinueia for 24 h were worst in PAN model rats, but without skin edema, see **Table 1**. Some rats died of serious ascites, the mortality is 30% (3/10).

Morphologic changes in light microscope include epithelial cells degeneration renal tubular and transparent cast, but there are no obvious changes in glomerulus and renal interstitial. Podocyte processes effacement was obvious in model groups sample in electronic microscope. See in **Figure 1**.

miRNA array detection shows 106 miRNA up regulated and 62 miRNA down regulated in PAN nephrosis rats. Fold change (model vs. control group) vary from 1.8 to 7.0. For leizhi capsule high-dose group and model sample, there are 90 miRNA differentially expressed, with 65 up and 25 down. see **Figure 2** and **Figure 3**.

The most important finding in our study is the discovery of the specific miRNA related to PAN nephrosis (rno-miR23a, rno-miR-24, rno-miR-30c and rno-miR-300-3p, which have been validated by Real time RT-PCR analysis. See **Table 2**.

Compared with control sample, Immune Fluorescence intensity of nephrin, podocin and synaptopodin reduced in model sample. See in **Figure 3**. In addition, apoptosised podocytes increase in PAN sample.

Table 1. Proteinuria for 24 h among each group.

Group	Dose mg·kg^{-1}	Pre-trial	3 d	9 d
NS	—	4.63 ± 1.82	4.43 ± 1.05	5.33 ± 1.69
PNS	—	5.29 ± 2.68	$73.45 \pm 68.76^{1)}$	$90.04 \pm 65.38^{1)}$
Leizhi	10	4.81 ± 3.77	$38.24 \pm 13.41^{2)}$	$28.23 \pm 15.26^{2)}$
GTW	10	6.82 ± 4.09	$54.68 \pm 25.32^{2) 3)}$	$33.23 \pm 14.14^{2)}$
Valsartan	7.5	5.47 ± 1.68	$44.46 \pm 17.66^{2)}$	$23.09 \pm 5.41^{2)}$

Compared with NS group, [1]representing $p < 0.05$, compared with PNS group, [2]representing $p < 0.05$, compared with Leizhi group, [3]representing $p < 0.05$.

Table 2. miRNAs expression by miRNA Array and realtime RT PCR. (a) miRNA expression (model versus NS). (b) miRNA expression (leizhi versus PAN).

(a)

miRNA	miRNA Array	Realtime RT PCR
rno-mir-24	0.32	0.312
rno-mir-30c	0.30	0.555
rno-mir-23a	3.23	2.472
rno-mir-300-3p	2.93	2.514

(b)

miRNA	miRNA Array	Realtime RT PCR
rno-mir-24	3.49	0.312
rno-mir-30c	2.32	0.555
rno-mir-23a	0.50	2.472
rno-mir-300-3p	0.53	2.514

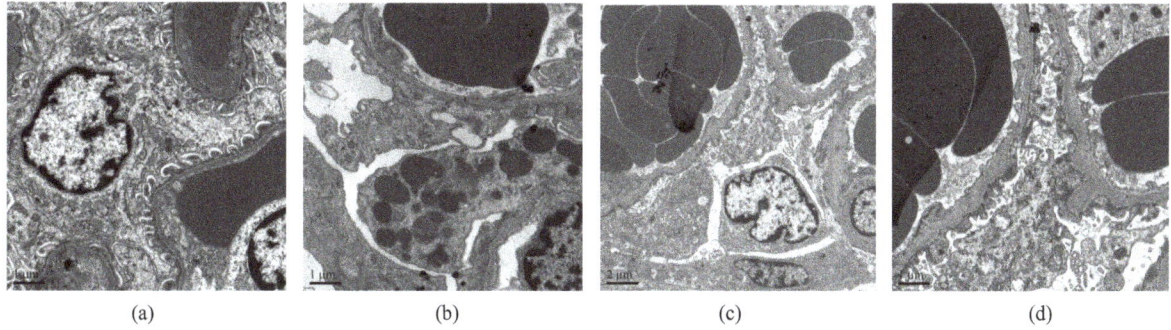

Figure 1. Change of foot process of glomerular podocyte in PAN rats. (a) NS, (b) PAN, (c) Leizhi, (d) GTW (8000×).

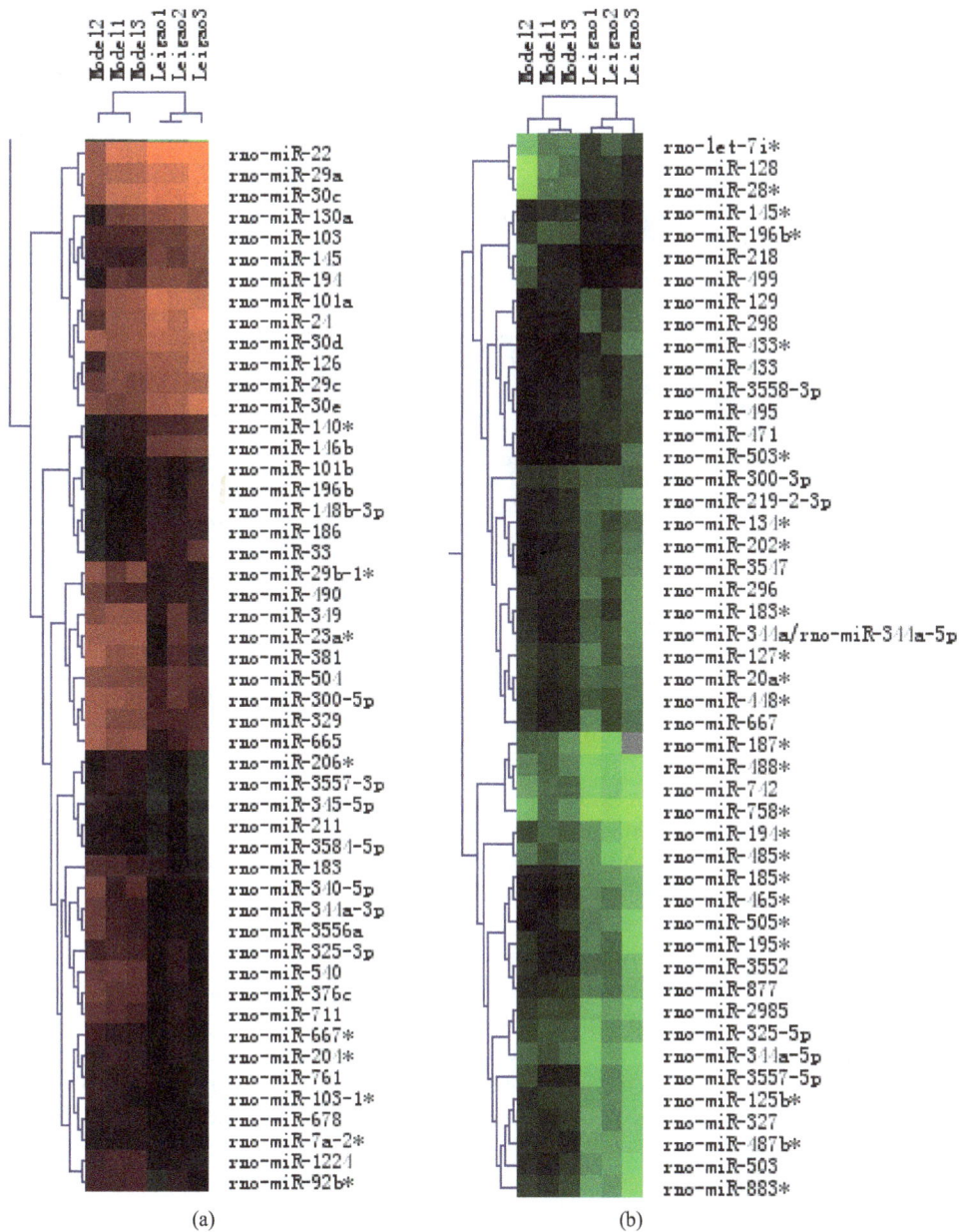

Figure 2. Differentially expressed miRNAs screening by miRNA Arrays. (a) Up-expressed miRNAs; (b) Down-expressed miRNAs.

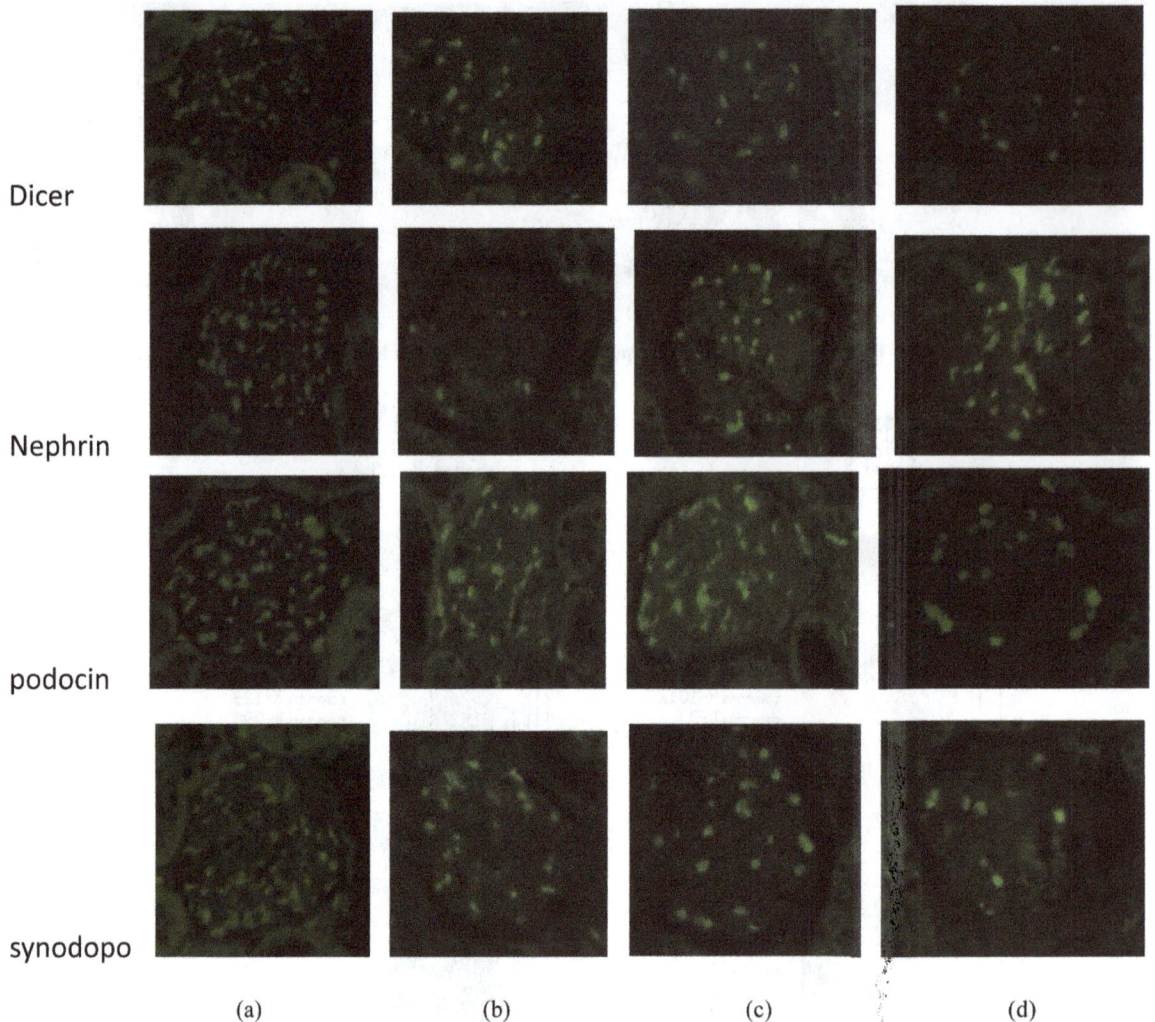

Figure 3. Immunoflunce of dicer, nephrin, podocin, and synodopotoptin in glomerular. (a) NS, (b) PAN, (c) Leizhi, (d) GTW.

4. Discussion

PAN nephrosis rats can be made successfully by jugular vein injection of PAN. PAN can selectively injury podocytes but not mesangium or endothelial cells in glomerular, inducing proteinuria, foot process effacement, and glomerular basement membrane abnormalities. So PAN nephrosis has been a classic podocyte-injury model.

Dicer is key to miRNA mature, which can mentain podocyte function and structure of SD in kidney. Our results show that dicer correlates well with proteinuria, but correlating negatively with nephrin and podocin. The most important finding in our study is the specific miRNA related to PAN nephrosis (rno-miR23a, rno-miR-24, rno-miR-30c and rno-miR-300-3p), which have been validated by Real time RT-PCR analysis. Up-regulated miRNAs (rno-miR-23a, rno-miR-300-3p) may trigger podocyte injury and proteinuria, while down-regulated miRNAs (rno-miR-24, rno-miR-30c) may be protective factors by anti-apoptosis. These miRNA may function corporately, because they located in the same chromosome [11] [12]. To explore dicer role in glomerular function, Harvey [8] *et al.* used a conditional *Dicer* allele to disrupt miRNA biogenesis in mouse podocytes. Mutant mice developed proteinuria and progressed rapidly to end-stage kidney disease. The pathology included foot process effacement, vacuolization, and hypertrophy with crescent formation. Their findings demonstrate a critical role for miRNA in glomerular function and suggest that podocyte may participate in the pathogenesis of kidney diseases. Shi [7] *et al.* inactivated dicer selectively in mouse podocytes. Mutant mice developed proteinuria 4 to 5 weeks after birth and died several weeks later, presumably from kidney failure. Multiple abnormalities including foot process effacement, irregular and split areas of the glomerular basement membrane, podocyte apoptosis and depletion, and glomerulosclerosis were observed. Four members of the mir-30 miRNA family were identified, known to be expressed and/or functional in podocytes. These results suggest functional roles for the mir-30 miRNA family in podocyte homeostasis and podocytopathies. Ho [9] *et al.* generated mice lacking functional miRNAs in the developing podocyte through podocyte-specific knockout of Dicer, Podocyte-specific loss of miRNAs resulted in significant proteinuria, rapid progression of marked glomerular and tubular injury, and death. Expression of the slit diaphragm proteins nephrin and podocin was decreased, and expression of the transcription factor WT1 remained unchanged. To identify miRNA-mRNA interactions that contribute to this phenotype, they profiled the glomerular expression of miRNAs; three miRNAs expressed in glomeruli were identified: mmu-miR-23b, mmu-miR-24, and mmu-miR-26a. These results suggest that miRNA function is dispensable for the initial development of glomeruli but is critical to maintain the glomerular filtration barrier. Connect to the database of miRNA Base [13] [14], target genes of miR-24, miR-23a and miR-30c correlate with phosphatase phosphatkinase and Protease C, suggesting these miRNA may participate in nephrin phosphorylation in podocyte homeostasis and podocyte injury.

Dicer can be down-regulated in PAN induced rats treated with *Tripterygium* preparation. Expression profile of nephrin, podocin and synaptopodin mRNA and protein decrease in samples treated with *Tripterygium wilfordii* Hook by triggering dicer-miRNA, which play the podocyte protection role by inhibiting podocyte apotosis. So these miRNAs (rno-miR-24, rno-miR-30c, rno-miR-23a) and dicer may be target moculars of leizhi capsule on treating proteinuria in PAN nephrosis. They may be are probably key molecules therapeutic targets.

From our work, we can conclude that characteristic miRNAs of PAN nephrosis were screening. Up-regulated miRNAs (rno-miR-23a, rno-miR-300-3p) may trigger podocyte injury and proteinuria, while down-regulated miRNAs (rno-miR-24, rno-miR-30c) may be protective factors by anti-apoptosis. Dicer and these miRNAs (rno-miR-24, rno-miR-30c, rno-miR-23a) may be are probably key molecules therapeutic targets of Leizhi capsule. But the fine mechanisms remain to be clarified by more researches.

Acknowledgements

miRNA Array analysis has been accomplished by Shanghai Kang Chen Biological engineering company.

Financial Support

The experiment is funded by Jiangsu province natural science fund (BK2009462) and the Priority Academic Program Development of Jiangsu Higher Education Institutions (PAPD).

Conflict of Interest Statement

The authors declare no conflicts of interest.

References

[1] Lee, R.C., Feinbaum, R.L. and Ambros, V. (1993) The *C. elegans* Heterochronic Gene lin-4 Encodes Small RNAs with Antisense Complementarity to lin-14. *Cell*, **75**, 843-854. http://dx.doi.org/10.1016/0092-8674(93)90529-Y

[2] Reinhart, B.J., Slack, F.J., Basson, M., *et al.* (2000) The 21-Nucleotide let-7 RNA Regulates Developmental Timing in *Caenorhabditis elegans. Nature*, **403**, 901-906. http://dx.doi.org/10.1038/35002607

[3] Muljo, S.A., Kanellopoulou, C. and Aravind, L. (2010) MicroRNA Targeting in Mammalian Genomes: Genes and Mechanisms. *Wiley Interdisciplinary Reviews: Systems Biology and Medicine*, **2**, 148-161. http://dx.doi.org/10.1002/wsbm.53

[4] Ohashi, T., Uchida, K., Asamiya, Y., *et al.* (2010) Phosphorylation Status of Nephrin in Human Membranous Nephropathy. *Clinical and Experimental Nephrology*, **14**, 51-55. http://dx.doi.org/10.1007/s10157-009-0241-z

[5] Welsh, G.I. and Saleem, M.A. (2010) Nephrin-Signature Molecule of the Glomerular Podocyte? *Journal of Pathology*, **220**, 328-337.

[6] Qin, X.S., Tsukaguchi, H., Shono, A., *et al.* (2009) Phosphorylation of Nephrin Triggers Its Internalization by Raft-Mediated Endocytosis. *Journal of the American Society of Nephrology*, **20**, 2534-2545. http://dx.doi.org/10.1681/ASN.2009010011

[7] Shi, S., Yu, L., Chiu, C., *et al.* (2008) Podocyte-Selective Deletion of Dicer Induces Proteinuria and Glomerulosclero-

sis. *Journal of the American Society of Nephrology*, **19**, 2159-2169. http://dx.doi.org/10.1681/ASN.2008030312

[8]   Harvey, S.J., Jarad, G., Cunningham, J., *et al.* (2008) Podocyte-Specific Deletion of Dicer Alters Cytoskeletal Dynamics and Causes Glomerular Disease. *Journal of the American Society of Nephrology*, **19**, 2150-2158.
       http://dx.doi.org/10.1681/ASN.2008020233

[9]   Ho, J., Ng, K.H., Rosen, S., *et al.* (2008) Podocyte-Specific Loss of Functional microRNAs Leads to Rapid Glomerular and Tubular Injury. *Journal of the American Society of Nephrology*, **19**, 2069-2075.
       http://dx.doi.org/10.1681/ASN.2008020162

[10]   Liu, L.H., Zhu, C.F. and Ou, L.Z. (2005) Optimization and Evaluation of Puromycin Amioenucleoside Nephropathy Model in Rats. *Fudan University Journal of Medical Sciences*, **32**, 488-492.

[11]   Chhabra, R., Dubey, R. and Saini, N. (2010) Cooperative and Individualistic Functions of the microRNAs in the miR-23a~27a~24-2 Cluster and Its Implication in Human Diseases. *Molecular Cancer*, **9**, 232.
       http://dx.doi.org/10.1186/1476-4598-9-232

[12]   Chhabra, R., Adlakha, Y.K., Hariharan, M., *et al.* (2009) Upregulation of miR-23a-27a-24-2 Cluster Induces Caspase-Dependent and -Independent Apoptosis in Human Embryonic Kidney Cells. *PLoS One*, **4**, e5848.
       http://dx.doi.org/10.1371/journal.pone.0005848

[13]   Griffiths-Jones, S. (2010) miRBase: microRNA Sequences and Annotation. *Current Protocols in Bioinformatics*, **12**, 12-19.

[14]   Griffiths-Jones, S., Grocock, R.J., van Dongen, S., *et al.* (2006) miRBase: microRNA Sequences, Targets and Gene Nomenclature. *Nucleic Acids Research*, **34**, D140-D144. http://dx.doi.org/10.1093/nar/gkj112

7

The Effect of Electroacupuncture on Neuronal Apoptosis and Related Functions in Rats with Acute Spinal Cord Injury

Liang Zhang[1], Changming Li[1], Renfu Quan[2*], Shangju Xie[1]

[1]Research Institute of Orthopedics, Zhejiang Chinese Medical University, Hangzhou, China
[2]Department of Orthopedics, Xiaoshan Traditional Chinese Medical Hospital, Hangzhou, China
Email: *quanrenfu@126.com

Academic Editor: Qingshan (Bill) Fu, Harvard Medical School, USA

Abstract

Objective: To investigate the effect and significance of electroacupuncture (EA) on neuronal apoptosis and hindlimb motor and bladder functional improvement in rats with acute spinal cord injury (SCI). *Methods*: Sixty healthy Sprague Dawley rats were randomly assigned to sham, model, EA, and EA control groups (n = 15 each). EA group rats received EA treatment at Zhibian and Shuidao acupoints seven times daily, whereas EA control group rats received EA at two points, 0.5 cm away from Zhibian and Shuidao, respectively. Histomorphological changes in spinal cord tissue were examined using hematoxylin-eosin staining. Neuronal apoptosis was detected by TUNEL assay. Bcl-2, Bax, and Bad protein levels were detected using immunohistochemistry. Additionally, hindlimb motor function, residual urine volume and maximum bladder capacity were measured. *Results*: HE staining revealed a morphologically and structurally intact spinal cord in the EA group, and the tissue contained scattered blood cells without edema. In the EA control group, there were small morphological defects in the spinal cord, and the tissue contained fewer blood cells with local edema. Compared with the EA control and model groups, Bax and Bad levels were significantly decreased in the EA group and Bcl-2 expression was increased ($P < 0.05$). After SCI, hindlimb function scores, residual urine volume, and maximum bladder capacity in rats of the EA group significantly differed from those of the EA control group ($P < 0.05$). *Conclusion*: EA may induce SCI-induced improvements in hindlimb motor and bladder functions by affecting neuronal apoptosis and relevant gene expression changes.

#Corresponding author.

Keywords

Electroacupuncture, Spinal Cord Injury, Neuronal Apoptosis, Molecular Mechanism

1. Introduction

Spinal cord injury (SCI) is a serious threat to human health. It often causes paraplegia and quadriplegia, leading to a series of serious complications and sequelae, such as urinary tract infection, respiratory tract infection, renal function impairment, and bedsores [1] [2]. SCI can substantially affect quality of life and family life situations, making it an urgent, worldwide problem to be addressed in the field of medicine. In recent years, there have been an increasing number of studies focused on the treatment, rehabilitation, and mechanisms of acute SCI. It is currently believed that mechanical injury to the spinal cord itself destroys its continuity and integrity. Following primary injury, the body initiates secondary injury to the spinal cord, leading to changes in the microenvironment, such as ischemia and hypoxia, inflammation, intracellular and extracellular calcium imbalance, excessive production of free radicals, excitatory amino acid changes, cytotoxic substances, and apoptosis, which are counterproductive to spinal cord functional recovery.

Electroacupuncture (EA) is an important part of traditional Chinese medicine, with a dual therapeutic effect of acupuncture and electrostimulation. EA stimulation at certain acupoints promotes Qi and blood circulation *via* meridian vessels to help regulate yin and yang and strengthen resistance to pathogenic factors. Previous acupuncture studies have focused on the analgesic, antispastic, and antidepressant effects [3]. Apoptosis is an important biological process, which involves a series of gene-regulated, initiative, cell death processes. Apoptosis exists in a number of diseases, such as Alzheimer's disease, Parkinson's disease, and traumatic injury [4] [5]. However, abnormal apoptosis can cause drastic deterioration in a variety of neurodegenerative diseases. Previous studies have documented the role of neuronal apoptosis and apoptotic gene expression in SCI [6]. In addition, Bcl-2 family proteins are key regulators of apoptosis, among which the proportion of Bcl-2, Bad, and Bax expression is the "molecular switch" to initiate apoptosis [7] [8]. It has been shown that down-regulation of Bcl-2 expression and up-regulation of Bax expression are non-conducive to the survival of hippocampal neurons [9]. A number of reports document that EA has a curative effect on neurodegenerative diseases, such as SCI [10] [11], although the underlying mechanisms remain unclear. The present study investigated the effect of EA treatment at Zhibian and Shuidao acupoints on neuronal apoptosis in rats with SCI. We further examined relevant changes in Bad, Bax and Bcl-2 expression to explore the possible molecular mechanisms of EA for promoting neuronal functional improvement after SCI.

2. Materials and Methods

2.1. Experimental Animals and Grouping

A total of 60 healthy, adult, male Sprague Dawley (SD) rats (220 - 250 g body weight) were purchased from the Experimental Animal Center of Xiamen University, Fujian Province, China (License No.: SYXK (Fujian) 2013-0006). After 1 week of adaptive feeding, the rats were randomly assigned to the sham, model, EA, and EA control groups (n = 15 each). Animals were sacrificed at 7 d post-surgery, and a 0.5-cm-long tissue sample was taken from above and below the injured spinal cord segment for further testing.

2.2. Reagents and Instruments

Bcl-2, Bax, and Bad were purchased from Bioworld (Louis Park, MN, USA). The TUNEL kit was purchased from Beijing Zhongshan Reagent Company (Beijing, China). Disposable Hwato acupuncture needles and an electroacupuncture device were purchased from Suzhou Medical Appliance Factory (Jiangsu Province, China). The fixative was prepared with 4% paraformaldehyde in phosphate-buffered saline (PBS).

2.3. Animal Model Establishment

An SD rat model with moderate SCI was established using a modified Allen's method [12] [13]. Rats were fasted for 8 h, and individual rats then underwent surgery in a random order. All groups were anesthetized via an intraperitoneal injection of 10% chloral hydrate (0.3 mL/100mg) and then fixed in a prone position. An approximately 2.5-cm-long, median, chest-back incision was aseptically made, through which the skin and subcutaneous tissues were dissected layer by layer to expose one vertebral body in the upper and lower positions, respectively. The T9-T10 spinous processes and complete vertebral plate were gouged to expose the 0.8-mm-wide spinal dura mater. A 10-g Kirschner wire was allowed to freely fall along a scaled catheter from a height of 60 mm, which hit a 4-mm-diameter, 2-mm-wide semicircle of thin, plastic material. The object was immediately removed, thereby inducing moderate injury to the posterior horn of the spinal cord. The surrounding tissues and skin were sutured layer by layer postoperatively using 4-0 silk. The entire surgery was performed at $37°C \pm 0.5°C$. Animals were intraperitoneally administered 800 million U/d penicillin postoperatively daily to prevent infection. Individuals were fed in separate cages at a room temperature of 20°C - 25°C and supplied with adequate food and water. The bladder was massaged twice daily using Crede's method [14] [15] to help void urine until the reestablishment of reflex bladder emptying. Specific criteria were assigned for the success of model establishment: following initial injury, the injured spinal cord segment showed bleeding and edema; the rat exhibited a tail-wagging reflex with retraction-like fluttering of both lower extremities and the body; and there was flaccid paralysis in both lower extremities upon return of consciousness after anesthesia.

2.4. Intervention Strategy

After successful model construction, the model and sham groups remained untreated. The EA group underwent EA treatment upon return of consciousness after anesthesia. The rat was fixed within a custom-made rat bag. Acupoints were chosen according to international standard acupoints developed by the World Health Organization. Zhibian (BL54) was located in the lower hip, *i.e.*, at the joint of outer and middle 1/3 intervals of the connection between the greater trochanter and sacral vertebra-coccygeal vertebra junction. Shuidao (ST28) was located in the abdomen, approximately 2 cm away from the third equal interval above the pubic symphysis on the midline between pubic symphysis and xiphosternal symphysis (divided into 13 equal parts) (**Figure 1**). Skin at the acupoints was prepared and disinfected. Stainless steel 0.25-mm-diameter acupuncture needles were used to punctuate the acupoints to 4 - 5 mm deep, followed by 1 min of twirling and 15 min of retaining. The ipsilateral Zhibian and Shuidao points were connected to a JL2B electrical pulse stimulator to form a loop, and 2/100 Hz frequency and 1 mA current were applied for 15 min of stimulation. The EA treatment alternated left and right daily. For the EA control group, treatment was performed as described for the EA group at two points 0.5 cm away for Zhibian and Shuidao, respectively.

2.5. Evaluation Indices and Methods

2.5.1. Behavioral and Motor Function Scoring

Following model establishment, the motor function in rats of different groups was scored using the Basso, Beattie, and Bresnahan locomotor rating scale (BBB scale). SCI rats were allowed free activity in an open space. Because of limited hindlimb mobility, the rat was unable to support its body, and the hindlimbs and buttocks dragged on the ground. Rats scoring >2 points were considered to be failed model establishment and were subsequently excluded from the experimental group. Rats were later supplemented to these groups. BBB scoring was performed prior to model establishment, as well as immediately and 7 d after model establishment to ex-

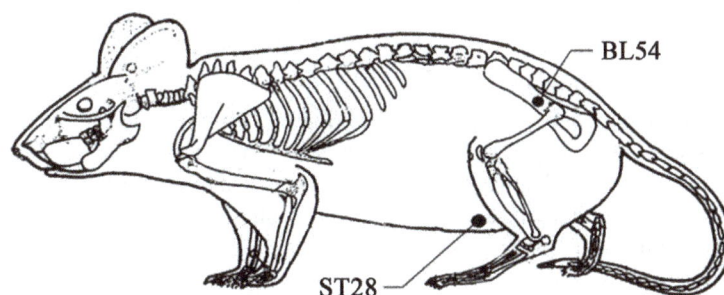

Figure 1. Schematic showing the Zhibian and Shuidao acupoints in the rat.

amine hindlimb motor functional recovery following acute SCI. Scoring criteria included the number of movable hindlimb joints, motor coordination, and fine motor joint function. Scores were divided into 21 grades. The higher the score, the better the recovery of motor function.

2.5.2. Residual Urine Volume Measurement

At 1 and 7 d post-surgery, residual urine volume was measured by manual expression of the bladder. When held in an upright position, rats often exhibited automatic micturition. After the rat supported itself and voided urine, forefingers of both hands were used to squeeze three times from the abdomen to the pelvis. During this process, pre-weighed absorbent papers were placed underneath. Following manual expression, the absorbent papers were weighed again. Increase in the weight of papers (g) was taken as the residual urine volume (mL), because the density of urine is close to that of water, $\rho \approx 1$.

2.5.3. Maximum Bladder Capacity Measurement

Maximum bladder capacity was measured at 1 and 7 d post-surgery. The rat was fixed in a supine position on a custom-made board. Iodophor was used to disinfect the external urethral orifice and anus. Two catheters were filled with sterile saline to remove the contained gas prior to use. Following lubrication with paraffin oil, one sterilized F3 urinary catheter was slowly inserted into the urethra and bladder (4.0 - 5.0 cm depth) via the external urethral orifice. The second F3 catheter was then lubricated with paraffin oil and slowly inserted along the end of the first catheter to the deeper depth. Crede's method was used to void urine. Once the residual urine was completely voided from the bladder through the catheter, sterile saline was slowly injected into the bladder perfusion catheter with a 1-mL syringe. The other discharger catheter placed on the rat board was subjected to close observation, and perfusion was stopped when liquid overflowed. The total volume of injected saline solution was recorded as the bladder's maximum functional capacity.

2.5.4. Spinal Cord Tissue Sampling

At 7 d after model establishment, the rats were anesthetized via intraperitoneal injection with 10% chloral hydrate (0.3 mL/100g). After thoracotomy, intubation was performed from the left ventricle to the aorta, and the right atrial appendage was then cut. The tissue was perfused with 150 mL 9% normal saline and then fixed with 250 mL 40 g/L paraformaldehyde. After 2 h, a 0.5-cm-long spinal cord tissue was taken from above and below the injured segment, respectively. The specimens were fixed in the same fixative for another 24 h, followed by conventional paraffin embedding. Serial sections (~6 μm thick) were prepared for hematoxylin-eosin (HE) staining, terminal deoxyribonucleotidyl transferase-mediated dUTP nick-end labeling (TUNEL) assay, and immunohistochemical (IHC) analysis.

2.5.5. HE Staining

HE staining was performed on three tissue sections randomly selected from each rat in different groups. After dewaxing, the sections were rinsed with double-distilled water for 1 min and stained with hematoxylin for 10 min. Excess dye was removed with double-distilled water, and specimens were immersed in 1% hydrochloric alcohol for 1 min of color separation (to avoid over-separation). Following treatment with an alkaline pro-blue solution, the sections were rinsed with flowing water and then counterstained with eosin for 2 min, dehydrated with graded ethanol (50%, 70%, 80%, 90%, and 100%), clarified using xylene, and mounted with neutral gum. Changes in the structure and morphology of spinal cord tissues were examined under an Olympus optical microscope.

2.5.6. TUNEL Detection of Apoptotic Cells

Three tissue sections from each rat were dewaxed and digested with proteinase K (0.02% mass fraction) for 30 min. The sections were fixed in 40 g/L paraformaldehyde and then incubated with drops of horseradish peroxidase at 37°C for 30 min. Finally, diaminobenzine (DAB) was used for coloration, followed by counterstaining with lighter hematoxylin, dehydration, and mounting. The number of positive cells was quantified, and the apoptotic index (AI) = number of apoptotic nuclei/total number of nuclei.

2.5.7. IHC Staining

Three tissue sections from each rat were used to detect Bcl-2, Bad, and Bax expression with an SP kit following the manufacturer's instructions. After conventional dewaxing, the sections were processed with 3% hydrogen peroxide, followed by high-temperature restoration and serum blocking. The sections were incubated with drops of primary antibody (dilution factor 1:150) at 4°C overnight. The negative control was prepared with PBS substituting the primary antibody. On the following day, secondary antibody was dropped onto the sections and incubated for 20 min, followed by incubation with strept avidin-biotin complex (SABC) at 37°C for 20 min. Thereafter, DAB was added for coloration and the color development background was examined by microscopy. Between the above steps, sections were rinsed three times with 0.01 mol/L PBS for 5 min each. Finally, the sections were dehydrated with gradient alcohol, clarified with xylene, and mounted with neutral resin. Morphological changes in spinal cord tissue were examined under a light microscope.

2.6. Statistical Analysis

Data are presented as mean ± standard deviation ($\bar{x}$ ± s). For normally distributed data with equal variances, comparison of group means was performed using one-way analysis of variance with the LSD and SNK methods. For normally distributed data with unequal variances, the Tamhane T2 and Dunnett T3 methods were used for variance test and pairwise comparison. Data that did not follow a normal distribution were analyzed using the rank-sum test. Statistical analysis was performed using SPSS13.0 (SPSS, Chicago, IL, USA).

3. Results

3.1. Behavioral Observations and BBB Scores

Prior to surgery, all groups had normal BBB scores. Immediately post-surgery, only the sham group had a BBC score of 21, whereas the remaining three groups had the same BBC score of 0, indicating successful model establishment. Compared with the model group, the EA and EA control groups had no significant difference in BBC score immediately or 1 d post-surgery ($P > 0.05$). However, BBC scores were significantly greater in the latter two groups than in the model group at 3 and 7 d post-surgery ($P < 0.05$). Compared with the EA control group, the EA group had significantly increased BBC scores at 7 d post-surgery ($P < 0.05$) (**Table 1**).

3.2. Residual Urine Volume

Residual urine volume was measured in rats at 1 d post-surgery and remeasured after 7 d of treatment. Compared with the model group, the EA and EA control groups had no significant difference in residual urine volume at 1 d post-surgery ($P > 0.05$). However, the residual urine volume of rats was significantly less in the EA group compared with the model group at 7 d post-surgery ($P < 0.05$). The decrease in residual urine volume of the EA group was more significant when compared with the EA control group at 7 d post-surgery ($P < 0.05$) (**Table 2**).

3.3. Maximum Bladder Capacity

Maximum bladder capacity was measured in rats at 1 d post-surgery and remeasured after 7 d of treatment. There was no significant difference in maximum bladder capacity of rats in the EA and EA control groups compared with the model group at 1 d post-surgery ($P > 0.05$). However, maximum bladder capacity was significantly less in the EA group compared with the model group at 7 d post-surgery ($P < 0.05$). The decrease in maximum bladder capacity was more significant in the EA group compared with the EA control group at 7 d post-surgery ($P < 0.05$) (**Table 3**).

Table 1. Comparison of BBB scores at different time points after spinal cord injury in different groups of rats ($\bar{x}$ ± s).

Group	BBB score			
	Immediately post-surgery	1 d post-surgery	3 d post-surgery	7 d post-surgery
Model	0 ± 0	0.6 ± 0.52	1.9 ± 0.74	3.9 ± 1.20
EA	0 ± 0	0.7 ± 0.53	2.9 ± 1.10■■	7.5 ± 1.58■■◆◆
EA control	0 ± 0	0.8 ± 0.52	2.7 ± 0.95■■	5.3 ± 1.95■■
Sham	21 ± 0	21 ± 0	21 ± 0	21 ± 0

Note: EA, electroacupuncture; 3 and 7 d post-surgery, compared with the model group, ■■$P < 0.05$; and 7 d post-surgery, compared with the EA control group, ◆◆$P < 0.05$.

Table 2. Comparison of residual urine volume at different time points after spinal cord injury in different groups of rats ($\bar{x} \pm s$).

Group	Number of rats	Residual urine volume (mL)	
		1 d post-surgery	7 d post-surgery
Model	15	2.02 ± 0.20	1.41 ± 0.07
EA	15	1.99 ± 0.15	1.14 ± 0.09■■◆◆
EA control	15	2.00 ± 0.16	1.23 ± 0.06■■

Note: EA, electroacupuncture; 7 d post-surgery, compared with the model group, ■■$P < 0.05$; and 7 d post-surgery, compared with the EA control group, ◆◆$P < 0.05$.

Table 3. Comparison of maximum bladder capacity at different time points after spinal cord injury in different groups of rats ($\bar{x} \pm s$).

Group	Number of rats	Maximum bladder capacity (mL)	
		1 d post-surgery	7 d post-surgery
Sham	15	0.93 ± 0.06	0.94 ± 0.09
Model	15	3.16 ± 0.14	1.67 ± 0.07■■
EA	15	2.95 ± 0.11	2.79 ± 0.12■■◆◆
EA control	15	2.89 ± 0.13	2.65 ± 0.11■■

Note: EA, electroacupuncture; 7 d post-surgery, compared with the model group, ■■$P < 0.05$; and compared with the EA control group, ◆◆$P < 0.05$.

3.4. HE Staining

Light microscopy revealed histological changes in rat spinal cord tissue specimens of different groups. In the sham group (**Figure 2(A)**), the spinal cord displayed intact morphology and structure; gray matter neurons exhibited normal morphology and uniform distribution, with normal cell membrane, nucleus, and interstitial spaces; and white matter fibers were evenly distributed, with intact myelin sheath in an orderly arrangement.

In the model group (**Figure 2(B)**), the spinal cord appeared incomplete with defects of nerve tissue; the tissue presented with severe bleeding in the presence of a large number of blood cells; tissue was loose and had edema, while cells exhibited vacuolar degeneration with some karyopyknosis; nerve fibers were dissolved and missing; there was a decreased number of gray matter neurons, with neuronal swelling, karyorrhexis; the extracellular matrix exhibited a vacuolated pattern; and white matter fibers were decreased, unevenly distributed, and demyelinated, showing incomplete morphology with mutual integration.

In the EA group (**Figure 2(C)**), the morphology and structure of the spinal cord were generally intact, and the tissue contained scattered blood cells without edema; gray matter neurons exhibited normal morphology and vacuolar degeneration was alleviated; vacuolar degeneration still existed in some cells and the nuclei showed no significant pyknosis; and white matter fibers were evenly distributed and appeared morphologically intact without demyelination.

In the EA control group (**Figure 2(D)**), the spinal cord had a small amount of defects and the tissue contained fewer blood cells, with local edema; there were slightly less gray matter neurons, some of which still presented with vacuolar degeneration and karyopyknosis; and white matter fibers were slightly decreased and unevenly distributed, some of which were demyelinated (**Figure 2**).

3.5. TUNEL Data

TUNEL data showed that apoptosis was widely present in the spinal cord tissues. The number of TUNEL-positive cells was significantly increased in the model group. By comparison, EA treatment substantially reduced the number of TUNEL-positive cells ($P < 0.01$). The reduction in TUNEL-positive cell number was significant in the EA group compared with the EA control group ($P < 0.05$), indicating that EA treatment at Zhibian and Shuidao significantly reduced neuronal apoptosis in the spinal cord after injury (**Table 4, Figure 3**).

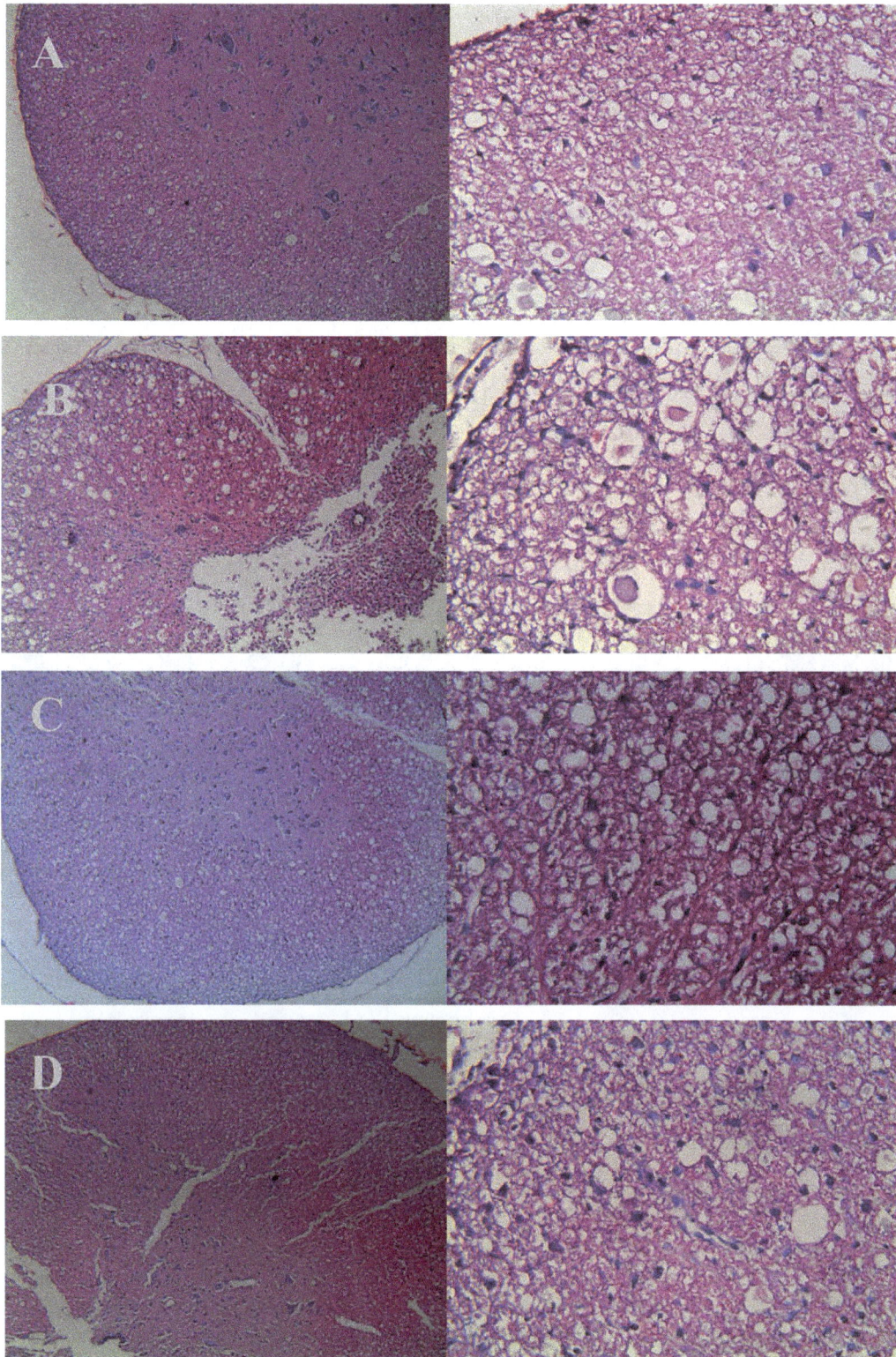

Figure 2. Microscopic observations of HE staining in injured spinal cord tissue specimens from rats of different groups at 7 d post-surgery (left, ×100, and right, ×400 for each group). (A) Sham group; (B) Model group; (C) Electroacupuncture (EA) group; and (D) EA control group. After spinal cord injury, the spinal cord showed incomplete morphology, with nervous tissue defects. After EA treatment, the spinal cord displayed intact morphology and structure, significantly better than those in the model and EA control groups.

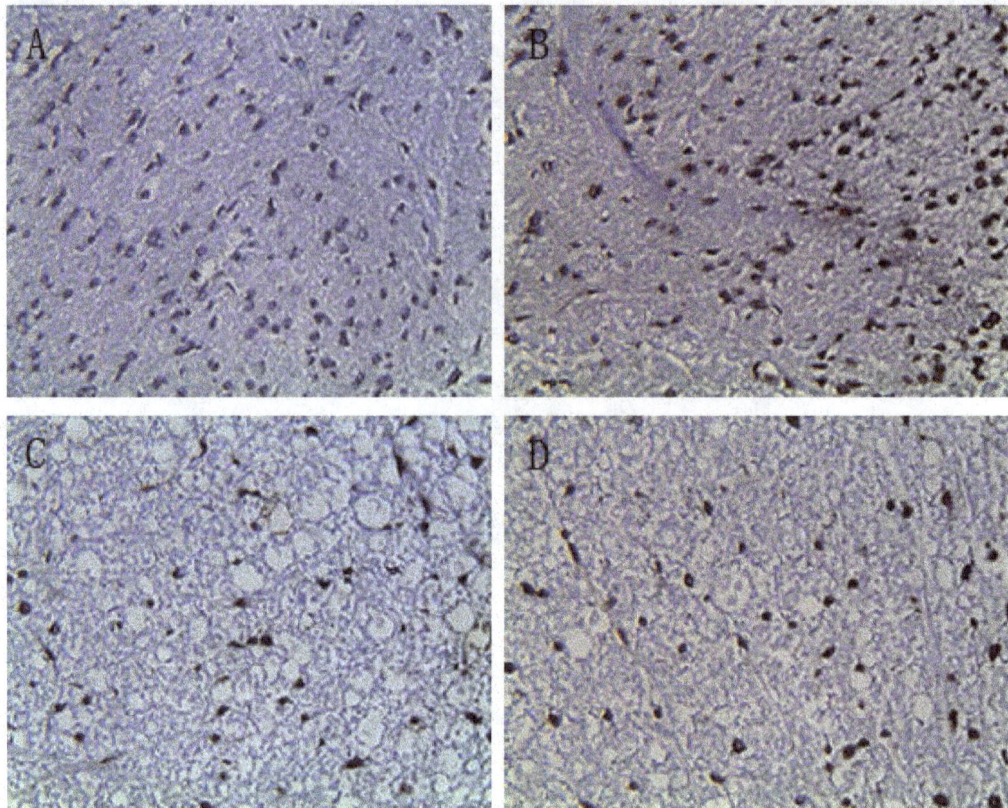

Figure 3. Microscopic observations of TUNEL staining in injured spinal cord tissue specimens from rats of different groups at 7 d post-surgery (×100). (A) Sham group; (B) Model group; (C) Electroacupuncture (EA) group; and (D) EA control group. After spinal cord injury, spinal cord neurons showed different degrees of apoptosis, as well as proliferating gliocytes. The EA group had fewer apoptotic neurons, indicating that EA treatment inhibited apoptosis and promoted spinal cord injury repair. There were more apoptotic neurons in the spinal cord tissue of the EA control group, indicating that EA treatment at Zhibian and Shuidao acupoints was more effective.

Table 4. The results of TUNEL assay on injured spinal cord tissue at 7 d post-surgery in different groups of rats ($\overline{x} \pm s$).

Group	Number of rats	Apoptotic index
Sham	15	0.161 ± 0.11
Model	15	0.953 ± 0.02
EA	15	$0.691 \pm 0.06^{\star\star\blacklozenge\blacklozenge}$
EA control	15	$0.838 \pm 0.04^{\bullet\bullet}$

Note: EA, electroacupuncture; compared with the model group, $^{\star\star}P < 0.05$, $^{\bullet\bullet}P < 0.05$; and compared with the EA control group, $^{\blacklozenge\blacklozenge}P < 0.05$.

3.6. IHC Staining

Positive IHC staining presented as a brown color. At 7 d after SCI, the number of Bcl-2-positive cells significantly decreased, but the number of Bax- and Bad-positive cells increased. After Zhibian and Shuidao EA treatment, the number of Bcl-2-positive cells significantly increased, while the number of Bax- and Bad-positive cells significantly decreased. These quantitative changes were statistically significant between the EA and EA control groups ($P < 0.05$), indicating that EA treatment at both acupoints and non-acupoints promoted Bcl-2 expression and inhibited Bax and Bad expression, but the regulatory effect was more significant in the EA group (**Table 5**, **Figure 4**).

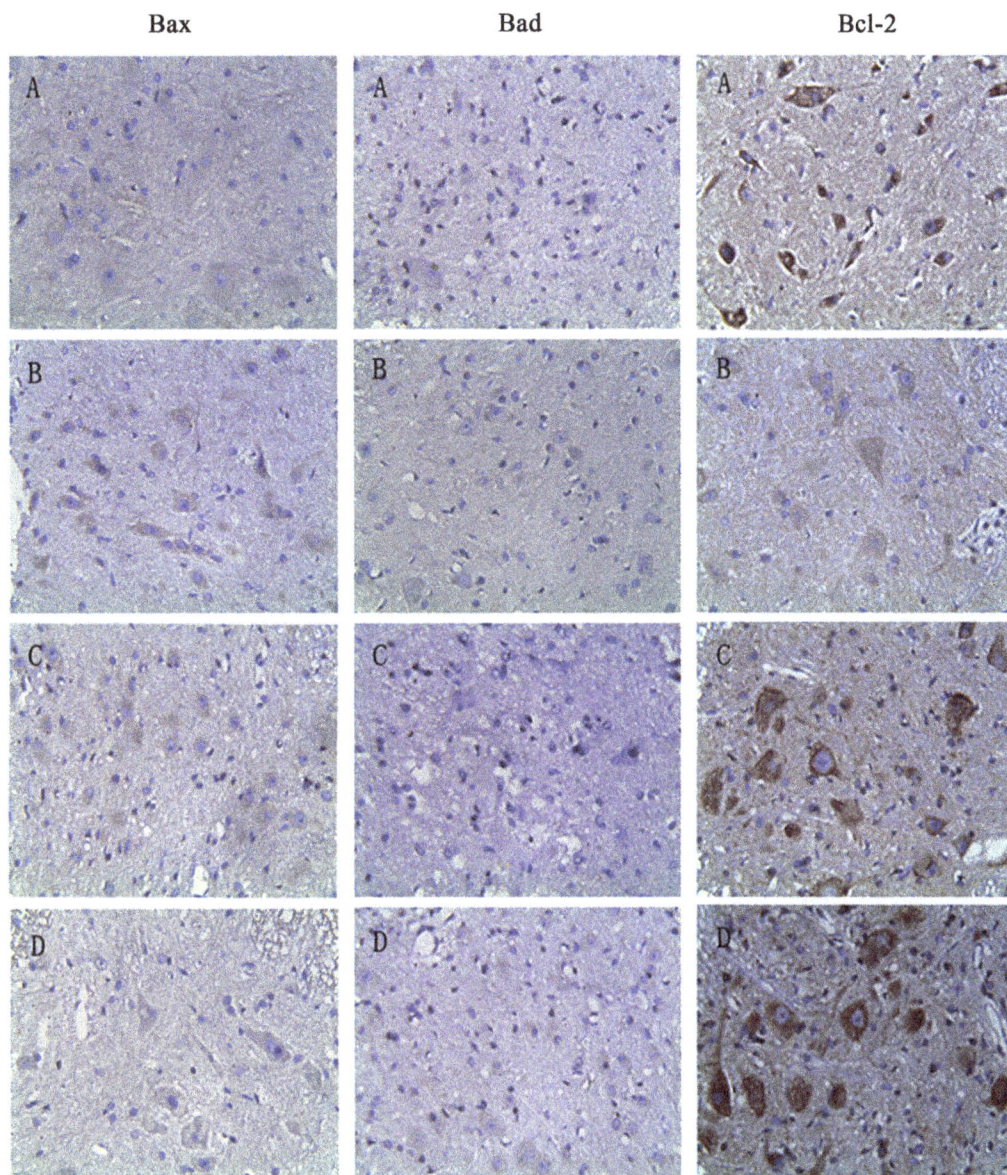

Figure 4. Microscopic observations of Bad, Bax, and Bcl-2 expression in injured spinal cord tissue specimens from rats of different groups at 7 d post-surgery (×100). (A) Sham group; (B) Model group; (C) Electroacupuncture (EA) group; and (D) EA control group. After spinal cord injury, Bad and Bax expression increased, while Bcl-2 expression decreased. EA treatment significantly promoted Bcl-2 expression, but inhibited Bad and Bax expression.

Table 5. The results of immunohistochemical analysis of Bax, Bad, and Bcl-2 in injured spinal cord tissue at 7 d post-surgery in different groups of rats ($\bar{x} \pm s$).

Group	Bad	Bax	Bcl-2
Sham	0.06895 ± 0.012	0.027039 ± 0.004	0.187429 ± 0.006
Model	0.128251 ± 0.021	0.150294 ± 0.003	0.103892 ± 0.014
EA	0.054116 ± 0.009★★■■	0.078775 ± 0.007★★■■	0.173388 ± 0.004★★■■
EA control	0.071302 ± 0.004●●	0.117657 ± 0.018●●	0.145866 ± 0.005●●

Note: EA, electroacupuncture; compared with the model group, ★★$P < 0.01$, ●●$P < 0.05$; and compared with EA control group, ■■$P < 0.05$.

4. Discussion

Presently, SCI is characterized by high mortality, high disability rate, difficult rehabilitation, longer course, and high cost of treatment. SCI prevention, treatment, and rehabilitation have attracted increasing attention in the field of medicine and there is a great need for a simple and efficient means of treatment for this disease. Acupuncture is well known for its simple operation. It is also free of toxic side effects, has a low price, and has proven efficacy. Research shows that acupuncture plays a positive role in neurodegenerative diseases. It can stimulate the release of substances from the central nervous system, such as endorphins, calcitonin gene-related peptides, and neuropeptide Y [16] [17]. Additionally, acupuncture regulates enzyme activity to maintain neuronal self-protective mechanisms [18]. Moreover, it can promote proliferation and differentiation of endogenous neural stem cells in the central nervous system [19]. The present study found that motor nerve function in rats after EA treatment was significantly better than in the model and EA control groups. Additionally, bladder capacity tended to stabilize, with no significant trend towards a decrease in the EA group. These results indicated that the early application of EA stimulation promoted restoration of motor function in rats. However, the protective mechanism of EA for SCI and relevant complications is still unclear. Further studies are needed to better understand the role EA plays in neuronal apoptosis.

Traumatic brain injury, SCI, and stroke are all associated with the occurrence of apoptosis [20]. Crowe *et al.* [21] first found that the occurrence of apoptosis after SCI caused motor and sensory dysfunction. There is a sequential process of primary and secondary injuries after SCI, and the ultimate extent of the injury is mainly determined by secondary injury initiated by a variety of factors. Apoptosis is an important secondary injury factor that mainly involves the death receptor pathway and mitochondrial signaling pathway. The mitochondrial signaling pathway is the primary pathway for disease development and progression, whereas the Bcl-2 family plays a key role in regulating the execution phase of apoptosis. Common apoptotic genes include Bcl-2, Bax, Bcl-xl, and Bad, among which Bax and Bcl-2 are antagonistic to each other, whereby the Bcl-2/Bax ratio determines the extent of apoptosis [22]. The anti-apoptotic factor Bcl-2 is mainly localized in the mitochondrial outer membrane, endoplasmic reticulum, and nuclear membrane. When cells receive apoptotic stimuli, Bcl-2 and Bcl-xL form heterodimers with the anti-apoptotic protein of the Bcl-2 family through the BH3 domain. This mechanism maintains the localization of pro-apoptotic proteins within the cell and protects cells from undergoing the apoptosis process. Bax and Bad are both pro-apoptotic genes. Increased Bax expression initiates apoptosis possibly through two mechanisms: on one hand, Bax forms a heterodimer with Bcl-2, thereby inhibiting the anti-apoptotic effects of Bcl-2. On the other hand, Bax itself forms a heterodimer to exert a pro-apoptotic effect. Bad is normally localized in the cytoplasm, and when cells are subject to apoptotic stimuli, Bad rapidly dephosphorylates and migrates to the mitochondria, thereby inducing apoptosis [23].

In the present study, a large number of apoptotic neurons were present in spinal cord tissue of the model and treatment groups after SCI. Following EA treatment for 7 d, the number of apoptotic cells in the EA group significantly decreased compared with the model and EA control groups. Additionally, Bcl-2 expression was relatively low after SCI, but significantly increased after 7 d of EA treatment compared with the model and EA control groups. These results coincided with previous studies [24] [25] and showed that Bax and Bad expression substantially increased after SCI, but decreased after EA intervention. As the key anti-apoptotic and pro-apoptotic factors, increased Bcl-2 expression and drastically reduced Bax and Bad expression may be related to positive and negative regulation of Bcl-2 and Bax. After EA stimulation, Bcl-2 competitively binds to the Bax protein to form a stable Bax/Bcl-2 heterodimer, counteracting Bax/Bax-induced apoptosis. Bad can bind to Bcl-2 and Bcl-xl to form heterodimers. However, after EA stimulation, p-Bad can bind to the chaperone protein 14-3-3 and thus interfere with the binding of Bad to Bcl-2 and Bcl-xl, further inhibiting apoptosis. Therefore, mutual regulation of Bcl-2, Bax, and Bad proteins can inhibit neuronal apoptosis after SCI, whereas EA treatment promotes Bcl-2 expression and reduces Bax and Bad expression. This may be one of the reasons why EA inhibits injured spinal cord apoptosis and promotes spinal cord repair.

5. Conclusion

In conclusion, this study demonstrated that EA treatment at the Zhibian and Shuidao acupoints significantly improved relevant functions after SCI. One of the possible mechanisms is that EA treatment inhibits expression of pro-apoptotic genes Bax and Bad, but promotes expression of anti-apoptotic gene Bcl-2. However, the occurrence of apoptosis is a complex regulatory process. It includes three stages of gene regulation, signal transduction, and apoptotic execution, respectively, ultimately eliminating unnecessary or abnormal cells. Activation of the signal transduction pathway during the early stages of apoptosis is a necessary precondition for the occurrence of apoptosis and has been increasingly used in studies of neurological diseases in recent years. Nevertheless, further studies are needed to determine the exact mechanism underlying the promotion of spinal cord injury repair by EA treatment.

Acknowledgements

This study was supported by the Zhejiang Chinese Medical Science Research Foundation (No. 2008CB067).

References

[1]   Xia, L.P., Fan, F., Tang, A.L. and Ye, W.Q. (2014) Effects of Electroacupuncture Combined with Bladder Training on the Bladder Function of Patients with Neurogenic Bladder after Spinal Cord Injury. *International Journal of Clinical and Experimental Medicine*, **7**, 1344-1348.

[2]   Fischer, M.J., Krishnamoorthi, V.R., Smith, B.M., Evans, C.T., St Andre, J.R., Ganesh, S., *et al.* (2012) Prevalence of Chronic Kidney Disease in Patients with Spinal Cord Injuries/Disorders. *American Journal of Nephrology*, **36**, 542-548. http://dx.doi.org/10.1159/000345460

[3]   Xing, G.G., Liu, F.Y., Qu, X.X., Han, J.S. and Wan, Y. (2007) Long-Term Synaptic Plasticity in the Spinal Dorsal Horn and Its Modulation by Electroacupuncture in Rats with Neuropathic Pain. *Experimental Neurology*, **208**, 323-332. http://dx.doi.org/10.1016/j.expneurol.2007.09.004

[4]   Hwang, L., Choi, I.Y., Kim, S.E., Ko, I.G., Shin, M.S., Kim, C.J., *et al.* (2013) Dexmedetomidine Ameliorates Intracerebral Hemorrhage-Induced Memory Impairment by Inhibiting Apoptosis Andenhancing Brain-Derived Neurotrophic Factor Expression in the Rat Hippocampus. *International Journal of Molecular Medicine*, **31**, 1047-1056.

[5]   Sung, Y.H., Kim, S.C., Hong, H.P., Park, C.Y., Shin, M.S., Kim, C.J., *et al.* (2012) Treadmill Exercise Ameliorates Dopaminergic Neuronal Loss through Suppressing Microglial Activation in Parkinson's Disease Mice. *Life Sciences*, **91**, 1309-1316. http://dx.doi.org/10.1016/j.lfs.2012.10.003

[6]   Okuno, S., Saito, A., Hayashi, T. and Chan, P.H. (2004) The c-Jun N-Terminal Protein Kinase Signaling Pathway Mediates Bax Activation and Subsequent Neuronal Apoptosis through Interaction with Bim after Transient Focal Cerebral Ischemia. *Journal of Neuroscience*, **24**, 7879-7887. http://dx.doi.org/10.1523/JNEUROSCI.1745-04.2004

[7]   Chen, M.H., Ren, Q.X., Yang, W.F., Chen, X.L., Lu, C. and Sun, J. (2013) Influences of HIF-1α on Bax/Bcl-2 and VEGF Expressions in Rats with Spinal Cord Injury. *International Journal of Clinical and Experimental Pathology*, **6**, 2312-2322.

[8]   Li, Y., Gu, J., Liu, Y., Long, H., Wang, G., Yin, G., *et al.* (2013) iNOS Participates in Apoptosis of Spinal Cord Neurons via p-BAD Dephosphorylation Following Ischemia/Reperfusion (I/R) Injury in Rat Spinal Cord. *Neuroscience Letters*, **545**, 117-122. http://dx.doi.org/10.1016/j.neulet.2013.04.043

[9]   Sun, W., Winseck, A., Vinsant, S., Park, O.H., Kim, H. and Oppenheim, R.W. (2004) Programmed Cell Death of Adult-Generated Hippocampal Neurons Is Mediated by the Proapoptotic Gene Bax. *Journal of Neuroscience*, **24**, 11205-11213. http://dx.doi.org/10.1523/JNEUROSCI.1436-04.2004

[10]   Norrbrink, C. and Lundeberg, T. (2011) Acupuncture and Massage Therapy for Neuropathic Pain Following Spinal Cord Injury: An Exploratory Study. *Acupuncture in Medicine*, **29**, 108-115. http://dx.doi.org/10.1136/aim.2010.003269

[11]   Pei, J., Sun, L., Chen, R., Zhu, T., Qian, Y. and Yuan, D. (2001) The Effect of Electro-Acupuncture on Motor Function Recovery in Patients with Acute Cerebral Infarction: A Randomly Controlled Trial. *Journal of Traditional Chinese Medicine*, **21**, 270-272.

[12]   Lin, H.S., Ji, Z.S., Zheng, L.H., Guo, G.Q., Chen, B., Zhang, G.W. and Wu, H. (2012) Effect of Methylprednisolone on the Activities of Caspase-3, -6, -8 and -9 in Rabbits with Acute Spinal Cord Injury. *Experimental and Therapeutic Medicine*, **4**, 49-54.

[13]   Zhou, Y., Liu, X.H., Qu, S.D., Yang, J., Wang, Z.W., Gao, C.J., *et al.* (2013) Hyperbaric Oxygen Intervention on Expression of Hypoxia-Inducible Factor-1α and Vascular Endothelial Growth Factor in Spinal Cord Injury Models in Rats. *Chinese Medical Journal* (*English*), **126**, 3897-3903.

[14]   Rajan, R.K., Juler, G. and Eltorai, I.M. (2000) Sigmoid Colon Rupture Secondary to Credé's Method in a Patient with Spinal Cord Injury. *The Journal of Spinal Cord Medicine*, **23**, 90-91.

[15]   Nomura, S., Ishido, T., Teranishi, J. and Makiyama, K. (2000) Long-Term Analysis of Suprapubic Cystostomy Drainage in Patients with Neurogenic Bladder. *Urologia Internationalis*, **65**, 185-189. http://dx.doi.org/10.1159/000064873

[16]   Feng, X.D., Yang, S.L., Liu, J., Huang, J., Peng, J., Lin, J.M., *et al.* (2013) Electroacupuncture Ameliorates Cognitive

Impairment through Inhibition of NF-κB-Mediated Neuronal Cell Apoptosis in Cerebral Ischemia-Reperfusion Injured Rats. *Molecular Medicine Reports*, **7**, 1516-1522.

[17] Lee, B., Sur, B., Shim, J., Hahm, D.H. and Lee, H. (2014) Acupuncture Stimulation Improves Scopolamine-Induced Cognitive Impairment via Activation of Cholinergic System and Regulation of BDNF and CREB Expressions in Rats. *BMC Complementary and Alternative Medicine*, **14**, 338.

[18] Cha, M.H., Bai, S.J., Lee, K.H., Cho, Z.H., Kim, Y.B., Lee, H.J., *et al.* (2010) Acute Electroacupuncture Inhibits Nitric oxide Synthase Expression in the Spinal Cord of Neuropathic Rats. *Neurological Research*, **32**, 96-100. http://dx.doi.org/10.1179/016164109X12537002794363

[19] Liu, Z., Ding, Y. and Zeng, Y.S. (2011) A New Combined Therapeutic Strategy of Governor Vessel Electro-Acupuncture and Adult Stem Cell Transplantation Promotes the Recovery of Injured Spinal Cord. *Current Medicinal Chemistry*, **18**, 5165-5171. http://dx.doi.org/10.2174/092986711797636144

[20] Kim, D.H., Ko, I.G., Kim, B.K., Kim, T.W., Kim, S.E., Shin, M.S., *et al.* (2010) Treadmill Exercise Inhibits Traumatic Brain Injury-Induced Hippocampal Apoptosis. *Physiology & Behavior*, **101**, 660-665. http://dx.doi.org/10.1016/j.physbeh.2010.09.021

[21] Crowe, M.J., Bresnahan, J.C., Shuman, S.L., Masters, J.N. and Beattie, M.S. (1997) Apoptosis and Delayed Degeneration after Spinal Cord Injury in Rats and Monkeys. *Nature Medicine*, **3**, 73-76.

[22] Hou, Q., Cymbalyuk, E., Hsu, S.C., Xu, M. and Hsu, Y.T. (2003) Apoptosis Modulatory Activities of Transiently Expressed Bcl-2: Roles in Cytochrome *c* Release and Bax Regulation. *Apoptosis*, **8**, 617-629. http://dx.doi.org/10.1023/A:1026187526113

[23] Zhang, X.H., Chen, S.Y., Tang, L., Shen, Y.Z., Luo, L., Xu, C.W., *et al.* (2013) Myricetin Induces Apoptosis in HepG2 Cells through Akt/p70S6K/Bad Signaling and Mitochondrial Apoptotic Pathway. *Anti-Cancer Agents in Medicinal Chemistry*, **13**, 1575-1581. http://dx.doi.org/10.2174/18715206136661311251123059

[24] Bleicken, S., Wagner, C. and Garcia-Saez, A.J. (2013) Mechanistic Differences in the Membrane Activity of Bax and Bcl-xL Correlate with Their Opposing Roles in Apoptosis. *Biophysical Journal*, **104**, 421-431. http://dx.doi.org/10.1016/j.bpj.2012.12.010

[25] Wang, T., Liu, C.Z., Yu, J.C., Jiang, W. and Han, J.X. (2009) Acupuncture Protected Cerebral Multi-Infarction Rats from Memory Impairment by Regulating the Expression of Apoptosis Related Genes Bcl-2 and Bax in Hippocampus. *Physiology & Behavior*, **96**, 155-161. http://dx.doi.org/10.1016/j.physbeh.2008.09.024

8

Molecular Identification of Chinese Materia Medica and Its Adulterants Using ITS2 and *psbA-trnH* Barcodes: A Case Study on Rhizoma Menispermi

Pei Yang[1*], Xiwen Li[1,2*], Hong Zhou[1], Hao Hu[3], Hui Zhang[4], Wei Sun[2], Yitao Wang[3], Hui Yao[1#]

[1]Institute of Medicinal Plant Development, Chinese Academy of Medical Sciences and Peking Union Medical College, Beijing, China
[2]Institute of Chinese Materia Medica, China Academy of Chinese Medical Sciences, Beijing, China
[3]State Key Laboratory of Quality Research in Chinese Medicine, Institute of Chinese Medical Sciences, University of Macau, Macau, China
[4]Development Center of Traditional Chinese Medicine and Bioengineering, Changchun University of Chinese Medicine, Changchun, China
Email: [#]scauyaoh@sina.com

Abstract

Rhizoma Menispermi, derived from the rhizoma of *Menispermum dauricum* DC., is one of the most popular Chinese medicines. However Rhizoma Menispermi is often illegally mixed with other species in the herbal market, including *Aristolochia mollissimae* Hance, which is toxic to the kidneys and potentially carcinogenic. The use of DNA barcoding to authenticate herbs has improved the management and safety of traditional medicines. In this paper, 49 samples belonging to five species, including 34 samples of *M. dauricum*, from different locations and herb markets in China were collected and identified using DNA barcoding. The sequences of all 34 samples of Rhizoma Menispermi are highly consistent, with only one site variation in internal transcribed spacer 2 (ITS2) of nuclear ribosomal DNA and no variations in the *psbA-trnH* region. The intra-specific genetic distance is much smaller than inter-specific one. Phylogenetic analysis shows that both sequences allow the successful identification of all species. Nearest distance and BLAST1 methods for the ITS2 and *psbA-trnH* regions indicate 100% identification efficiency. Our research shows that DNA barcoding can effectively distinguish Rhizoma Menispermi from its adulterants from both commercial and original samples, which provides a new and reliable way to monitor com-

---

[*]These two authors contributed equally to this work.
[#]Corresponding author.

mercial herbs and to manage the modern medicine market.

Keywords

Rhizoma Menispermi, *Menispermum dauricum* DC., ITS2, *psbA-trnH*, Identification, Adulterants

---

1. Introduction

Rhizoma Menispermi (Beidougen) is a commonly used traditional Chinese herbal medicine recorded in Chinese Pharmacopoeia as an analgesic and antipyretic drug. Rhizoma Menispermi is derived from the rhizoma of the plant *Menispermum dauricum* DC. (Menispermaceae), which is widely distributed in North China. Recent studies have shown that the alkaloids from *M. dauricum* have various bioactivities, which include anti-arrhythmic and anti-tumor effects [1]. Zhao *et al.* stated that the phenolic alkaloids in the rhizome of *M. dauricum* could protect against brain ischemia injury [2]. In addition, the water-soluble polysaccharides extracted from Rhizoma Menispermi significantly inhibit cell proliferation and DNA synthesis in human ovarian carcinoma SKOV3 cells [3]. Rhizoma Menispermi has become a focus of research because of its newly discovered medicinal properties.

Medication safety is currently a research hot spot, which has become necessary with the increase in market demand for medicinal plants. The rhizome of *Aristolochia mollissimae* Hance (Aristolochiaceae), an adulterant of Rhizoma Menispermi, shows profound nephrotoxicity and carcinogenicity [4]. Radix et Rhizoma Sophorae Tonkinensis (Shandougen), the root and the rhizome of *Sophora tonkinensis* Gagnep., is the most common adulterant in the herb market. Several studies have explored traditional methods to distinguish these two medicinal species [5]. In China, *M. dauricum* is the only species in the genus *Menispermum*; however, medicinal plants in the same family, such as *Stephania tetrandra* S. Moore and *Cocculus orbiculatus* (L.) DC, are commonly interchanged because of their similar morphological characteristics. An accurate identification of these medicinal plants is essential to ensuring the purity and safety of medicines for consumers.

The traditional identification of herbal medicines is mainly based on the morphological characteristics of the source plants, microscopic observations, and the physical form or chemical compositions. These parameters are subjective and can be affected by the external environment, leading to inaccurate classification of herbal authenticity. DNA barcoding has emerged as a cost-effective standard for species identification and has brought a renaissance to the study of taxonomy [6]. DNA barcoding has been proven highly effective in identifying medicinal herbs with high accuracy and reproducibility. The internal transcribed spacer 2 (ITS2) of nuclear ribosomal DNA has been validated as a novel DNA barcode to identify medicinal plant species [7] and is now recommended as the universal DNA barcode for plants [8]. In addition, the China Plant Barcode of Life Group [9] has confirmed that ITS/ITS2 should be incorporated into the core barcode set for seed plants. The chloroplast intergenic spacer, *psbA-trnH*, has been suggested as a candidate barcode sequence after a large-scale study found high variability and efficiency of detection across a broad range of flowering plants [10]. This region is one of the most variable non-coding regions of the plastid genome in angiosperms [11]. In this study, the ITS2 and *psbA-trnH* regions were used to distinguish Rhizoma Menispermi from its adulterants. The extraction of DNA from different tissues of herb species may be hampered by different chemical compositions and growing environments. Leaves and other fresh tissues are generally used in published literatures, whereas roots, which have high polysaccharides and polyphenols content, are rarely used. In this study, *M. dauricum* rhizomas were used to verify the use of DNA barcoding in the identification of *M. dauricum* and its adulterants. Commercial materials were included to evaluate the prospective application of the DNA barcoding method in monitoring crude drugs in the market.

2. Material and Method

2.1. Taxon Sampling

Forty-nine samples of various herbal species were collected from different locations and markets in China (**Table 1**). A total of 4 original plant samples and 30 rhizoma samples of *M. dauricum* were collected from main

Table 1. Detailed information of experimental samples in this study.

Taxon	Sampling part	Voucher No.	Location	GenBank Accession NO.	
				ITS2	*psbA-trnH*
Menispermum dauricum	Rhizoma	YC0146MT01	Chengde, Hebei	KC902480	KC902468
M. dauricum	Rhizoma	YC0146MT02	Chengde, Hebei	KC902481	/
M. dauricum	Leaf	YC0146MT03	Songfengshan, Heilongjiang	KC902482	KC902460
M. dauricum	Rhizoma	YC0146MT04	Songfengshan, Heilongjiang	KC902483	KC902467
M. dauricum	Rhizoma	YC0146MT05	Songfengshan, Heilongjiang	KC902484	KC902466
M. dauricum	Leaf	YC0146MT06	Chifeng, Inner Mongolia	KC902485	KC902465
M. dauricum	Rhizoma	YC0146MT07	Xiaoxinganling, Heilongjiang	KC902486	KC902464
M. dauricum	Rhizoma	YC0146MT08	Fushun, Liaoning	KC902487	KC902463
M. dauricum	Rhizoma	YC0146MT09	Wangqing, Jilin	KC902488	KC902459
M. dauricum	Rhizoma	YC0146MT10	Wangqing, Jilin	KC902489	/
M. dauricum	Rhizoma	YC0146MT11	Fengcheng, Liaoning	KC902490	KC902462
M. dauricum	Rhizoma	YC0146MT12	Fengcheng, Liaoning	KC902491	KC902461
M. dauricum	Leaf	YC0146MT13	Yichun, Heilongjiang	KC902492	KC902458
M. dauricum	Rhizoma	YC0146MT14	Fushun, Liaoning	KC902493	KC902476
M. dauricum	Rhizoma	YC0146MT15	Xiaoxinganling, Heilongjiang	KC902494	KC902475
M. dauricum	Rhizoma	YC0146MT16	Chifeng, Inner Mongolia	KC902495	KC902474
M. dauricum	Rhizoma	YC0146MT18	Qingdao, Shandong	KC902496	KC902473
M. dauricum	Rhizoma	YC0146MT19	Qingdao, Shandong	KC902497	KC902472
M. dauricum	Rhizoma	YC0146MT20	Shangluo, Shaanxi	KC902498	KC902471
M. dauricum	Rhizoma	YC0146MT21	Shangluo, Shaanxi	KC902499	KC902470
M. dauricum	Rhizoma	YC0146MT22	Ziyang, Sichuan	KC902500	KC902469
M. dauricum	Rhizoma	YC0146MT23	Anguo Medicine Market, Hebei	KC902501	KC902479
M. dauricum	Rhizoma	YC0146MT25	Bozhou Medicine Market, Anhui	KC902502	KC902477
M. dauricum	Rhizoma	YC0146MT26	Bozhou Medicine Market, Anhui	KC902503	/
M. dauricum	Rhizoma	YC0146MT28	Drug Store I, Beijing	KC902504	/
M. dauricum	Rhizoma	YC0146MT29	Drug Store I, Beijing	KC902505	/
M. dauricum	Rhizoma	YC0146MT31	Drug Store II, Beijing	KC902506	KC902457
M. dauricum	Rhizoma	YC0146MT32	Drug Store II, Beijing	KC902507	KC902456
M. dauricum	Rhizoma	YC0146MT33	Drug Store III, Beijing	KC902508	KC902455
M. dauricum	Rhizoma	YC0146MT34	Drug Store III, Beijing	KC902509	/
M. dauricum	Rhizoma	YC0146MT35	Drug Store IV, Beijing	KC902510	KC902454
M. dauricum	Rhizoma	YC0146MT36	Drug Store IV, Beijing	KC902511	KC902453
M. dauricum	Rhizoma	YC0146MT37	Drug Store V, Beijing	KC902512	/
M. dauricum	Leaf	PS0345MT01	IMPLAD, Beijing	GQ434390	/

Continued

Sophora tonkinensis	Root	YC0104MT01	Drug Store II, Beijing	KC902514	KC902515
So. tonkinensis	Root	YC0104MT02	Drug Store III, Beijing	KJ766117	KJ766122
So. tonkinensis	Root	YC0104MT03	Tianlin County, Guangxi	KJ766116	KJ766123
So. tonkinensis	Root	YC0104MT04	Meilin County, Guangxi	KJ766118	KJ766124
So. tonkinensis	Leaf	PS0228MT01	Nanning, Guangxi	GQ434351	GQ434960
Aristolochia mollissima	Leaf	YC0514MT01	Nanyang, Henan	KJ766113	KJ766119
A. mollissima	Leaf	YC0514MT02	Nanyang, Henan	KJ766114	KJ766120
A. mollissima	Leaf	YC0514MT03	South China Botanical Garden, Guangdong	KJ766115	KJ766121
Stephania tetrandra	Leaf	PS0348MT01	Danfeng, Shaanxi	/	GQ434988
St. tetrandra	Leaf	PS0348MT02	Xuancheng, Anhui	/	GQ434989
St. tetrandra	Root	YC0200MT01	Anguo Medicine Market, Hebei	/	KJ766125
St. tetrandra	Root	YC0200MT02	Anguo Medicine Market, Hebei	/	KJ766126
Cocculus orbiculatus	Leaf	PS0353MT02	Xuancheng, Anhui	GQ434395	GQ434990
C. orbiculatus	Leaf	PS0353MT03	Chengdu, Sichuan	GQ434396	GQ434991
C. orbiculatus	Leaf	PS0353MT04	Putian, Fujian	GQ434397	GQ434992

"/" means the sample failed to obtain the sequence.

producing areas and different drug stores and markets. Additional 15 samples of species, which were often confused as *M. dauricum*, were also obtained. All samples were identified by Professor Yulin Lin of Institute of Medicinal Plant Development (IMPLAD), Chinese Academy of Medical Sciences, Peking Union Medical College. The samples were deposited in the herbarium of the institute.

2.2. DNA Extraction, Amplification and Sequencing

The surface of the rhizoma samples was first wiped with 75% ethanol, and the outer epidermis was scraped off. Approximately 40 mg for rhizoma samples and 20 mg for the leaves were used to extract genomic DNA using Bioteke DNA Exaction Kit (Bioteke Co., Beijing). For the rhizome samples, 1% PVP (Polyvinylpyrrolidone) was mixed before they were crushed. Then the crushed samples with lysate were heated to 56°C by water bath for 8 h - 12 h. The succeeding steps were consistent with those used for the leaf samples. The primers and Polymerase Chain Reaction (PCR) conditions were previously described [7] [12]. All amplified products were bi-directionally sequenced. Data analysis was conducted according to the methods used in previous study [8].

2.3. Sequence Alignment, Genetic Analysis and Species Identification

Intra- and inter-specific genetic distances were computed with MEGA 5.0 [13] on the basis of the Kimura 2-Parameter (K2P) model. The sequence lengths and GC contents are listed in **Table 2**. Phylogenetic trees were constructed according to ITS2 and *psbA-trnH* regions with the use of the neighbor-joining (NJ) method, with 1000 bootstraps, in MEGA 5.0. Finally, BLAST1 and Nearest Distance methods were applied to species identification, as described in previous studies [7] [14].

3. Results

3.1. PCR, Sequencing Efficiency and Sequence Characteristics

Most genomic DNA samples showed smearing on agarose gel electrophoresis, which indicated DNA degradation. However, most of the samples were successfully amplified except the ITS2 sequence of *S. tetrandra*, suggesting that amplification of both ITS2 and *psbA-trnH* was not affected by the degradation of genomic DNA.

Table 2. Sequence characteristics of ITS2 and *psbA-trnH* of *M. dauricum* and its adulterants.

	ITS2	*psbA-trnH*
Amplification efficiency of *M. dauricum* (%)	100	100
Sequencing efficiency of *M. dauricum* (%)	100	76.5
Length of *M. dauricum* (bp)	203	315
Amplification efficiency of all taxa (%)	91.8	100
Sequencing efficiency of all taxa (%)	91.8	83.7
Length of all taxa (bp)	181 - 277	215 - 656
Aligned length (bp)	331	743
GC content range in *M. dauricum* (%)	52.7	24.4
GC content range (mean) in all taxa (%)	49.3 - 74.4 (62.8)	23.6 - 41.4 (26.6)
Number (and %) of variable sites in all taxa	163 (49.2)	319 (42.9)

The amplification efficiency of *psbA-trnH* was 100%, whereas the sequencing efficiency of *psbA-trnH* was 76.5% (**Table 2**). We failed to obtain the ITS2 sequence for *S. tetrandra* by using the universal ITS2 primer pairs described by Chen *et al.* [6]. However, the *psbA-trnH* region was obtained from all the samples of this species.

The sequence length of ITS2 in *M. dauricum* was 203 bp, with only one variable site observed in 34 sequences. The result of inter-specific sequence alignment showed that the length of ITS2 was 331 bp with 163 bp variable sites (49.2%). The sequence length of *psbA-trnH* in all *M. dauricum* samples was 315 bp, which indicated high consistency. The length of *psbA-trnH* sequences alignment was 743 bp with high variability (42.9%) across taxa. The GC contents of ITS2 and *psbA-trnH* of *M. dauricum* were 52.7% and 24.4%, which averaged 62.8% and 26.6%, respectively across all taxa (**Table 2**). One of the adulterants, *A. mollissima*, had the highest GC content with 74.4% in the ITS2 locus.

3.2. Intra- and Inter-Specific Genetic Distances and Species Identification

The intra- and inter-specific K2P distances of ITS2 and *psbA-trnH* of *M. dauricum* and its adulterants are presented in **Table 3**. All the experimental samples of *M. dauricum* were highly conserved in ITS2 and *psbA-trnH* regions. The maximum intra-specific distance (0.005 in ITS2) was due to a single C-A variation at the 82 bp site. The inter-specific K2P distances of the two sequences were expectedly higher, with an average of 0.457 and 0.428 for ITS2 and *psbA-trnH* respectively. NJ trees indicated that both sequences allowed the successful identification of all species; with each separate species grouped into distinct clades (**Figure 1** and **Figure 2**). All the sequences were examined by the Nearest Distance and BLAST1 methods. The successful identification rates of the two regions were 100% with the two methods.

4. Discussion

Fresh leaves have been traditionally used as the raw material for DNA barcoding. Currently, DNA barcoding is used to identify traditional Chinese medicines derived from other source tissues such as Rhizoma et Radix Notopterygii [15], Radix Gentianae Macrophyllae [16], Herba Ephedrae [17], and Flos Lonicerae Japonicae [18]. Chiou *et al.* [19] described that DNA extracted from various medicinal tissues and processed materials was usually degraded and even contaminated by microorganisms. For root and rhizome medicinal materials, the accumulation of secondary metabolites, such as polysaccharides and polyphenols, can affect the quantity and purity of the extracted DNA and the success of downstream applications, including PCR. The general approaches to improve the quality and quantity of DNA extracted from medicinal parts include extending the water bath time to 8 h - 12 h at 56°C, increasing the amount of the sample, and simultaneously increasing the use of beta-mercaptoethanol and PVP. In addition, extracting the crushed samples by buffer for two to three times [20] will help to remove the polysaccharides and polyphenols in the medicinal parts of crude drugs. In this study, 36 rhizoma samples were collected, including 16 dried and long-stored rhizoma samples of commercial materials, and successfully

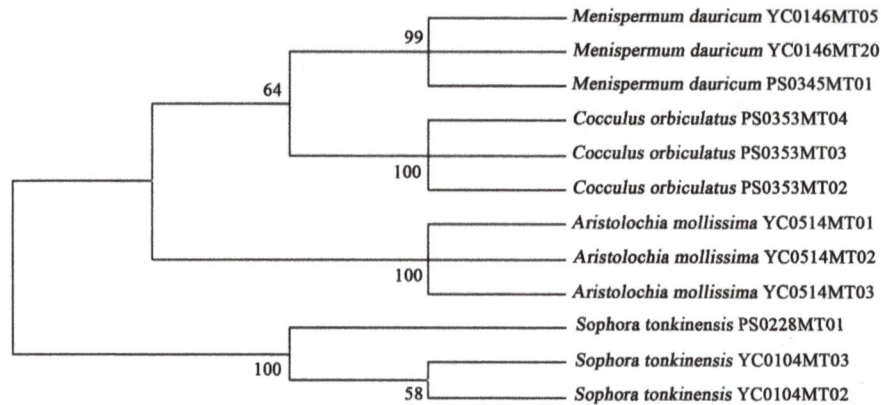

Figure 1. Phylogenetic tree of Rhizoma Menispermi and its adulterants constructed with the representative ITS2 sequences using NJ method. The bootstrap scores (1000 replicates) are shown (≥50%) for each branch.

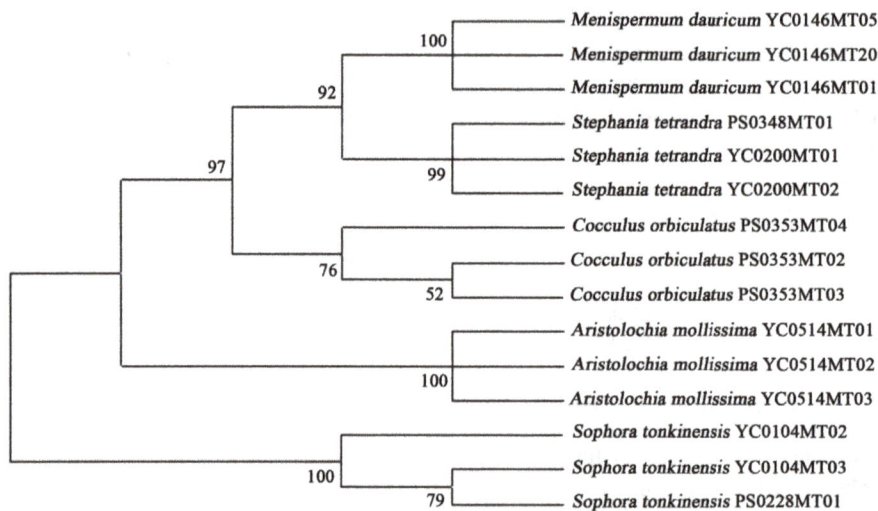

Figure 2. Phylogenetic tree of Rhizoma Menispermi and its adulterants constructed with the representative *psbA-trnH* sequences using NJ method. The bootstrap scores (1000 replicates) are shown (≥50%) for each branch.

Table 3. The K2P genetic distances of ITS2 and *psbA-trnH* sequences of Rhizoma Menispermi and its adulterants.

K2P genetic distances	Range of genetic distances (mean)	
	ITS2	*psbA-trnH*
Intra-specific distances of *M. dauricum*	0 - 0.005 (0.000)	0 (0.000)
Inter-specific distances between Rhizoma Menispermi and its adulterants	0.035 - 0.509 (0.457)	0.033 - 0.624 (0.428)

amplified by PCR. The result showed that the primers used were universal, and the ITS2 and *psbA-trnH* loci were easy to amplify. Wiping with 75% ethanol and scraping the outer epidermis helped prevent the risk of soil fungal contamination to a certain extent. No fungal sequence interference was observed during the experiments. Xu *et al.* [21] verified the operability of ITS2 locus between *S. tonkinensis* and its adulterants, including *M. dauricum*, using sequences downloaded from GenBank and several plant materials. DNA barcoding could identify fresh original plant samples of *S. tonkinensis* and its adulterants. However, no medicinal material samples were included. In this study, we focused on testing the applicability of DNA barcoding to distinguish medicinal materials.

New technology contributes to the success of identification methods. In the 2010 edition of *Chinese Pharmacopoeia*, allele-specific diagnostic PCR was recorded as a new method of identifying *Zaocys dhumnades* (Cantor). DNA barcoding technology uses universal primers and the same PCR reaction conditions across samples to construct a reference database. These factors increase the value of such a method in practical applications. The Food and Drug Administration approved DNA barcoding for seafood identification [22]. In the contemporary medicine market, this technology will help stop the spread of fake and adulterant materials with similar appearance to true medicines. Kool *et al.* [23] used root samples sold by herbalists in Marrakech, Morocco, to determine the applicability of DNA barcoding to modern drug markets. The results of their study showed that *rpoC*1, *psbA-trnH*, and ITS had high sequencing success rates, and combining all three loci allowed the identification of the majority of the market samples up to the genus level. DNA barcoding was used to successfully detect substitution and contamination in herbal products in North America [24]. These two previous studies indicated that DNA barcoding can be applied to the identification of commercial herbs. In the current study, we collected 16 commercial medicinal materials, including Rhizoma Menispermi, Radix et Rhizome Sophorae Tonkinensis, and Radix Stephaniae Tetrandrae. DNA is expected to show increasing degradation with an increase in storage time in dried commercial root drugs. We show that all the commercial materials were effectively identified, and the results were consistent with the information indicated on the medicinal drug labels. Sequence conservation in commercial medicinal materials and original samples from a single species indicated that DNA barcoding can consistently identify commercialized medicinal plants.

The *psbA-trnH* region is among the most variable non-coding regions in the chloroplast genome, and this variation means that this intergenic spacer can offer high levels of species discrimination [11]. However, Chase *et al.* [25] stated that a high rate of insertion/deletion may hamper application to barcoding. Agarose gel electrophoresis demonstrated that both ITS2 and *psbA-trnH* had high amplification efficiency. However, the sequencing efficiency of *psbA-trnH* sequences was almost 10% lower than that of the ITS2 sequences, even if bidirectional sequencing was used. This result was likely due to poly-A and poly-T structures in the *psbA-trnH* intergenic spacer. When a continuous repeated A or T structure emerges, the quality of the followed sequence will decrease, so the determination of the complete intergenic spacer is limited. The sequencing efficiency caused a 23.5% decline compared with the amplification efficiency in *M. dauricum*. In all samples used in this study, we also observed continuous repeated nucleotide structures belonging to Menispermaceae and *S. tonkinensis* (Leguminosae).

DNA barcoding technology has contributed to the development of taxonomy [6] and authentication, especially in traditional Chinese herbal medicine. A stable and accurate method is urgently needed for the circulation and standard management of traditional Chinese herbal medicines. This study is the first to use DNA barcoding to authenticate Rhizoma Menispermi (particularly commercial variants) and its adulterants. The stability and accuracy of the two regions (ITS2 and *psbA-trnH*) were examined. The intra-specific genetic distances and sequence alignment indicated that *M. dauricum* from different production areas had few variable sites in ITS2 and *psbA-trnH* sequences. The existence of multiple copies of the ITS2 region in plants may affect the stability of the obtained sequences. However, Song *et al.* [26] showed that despite multiple intra-genomic variants, the use of the major variants alone was sufficient for phylogenetic construction and species determination in most cases. The ITS2 sequences of *M. dauricum* were highly consistent; intra-specific variations were nearly absent. Multi-copies of ITS2 did not affect sequence amplification, sequencing, and analysis in *M. dauricum*. The high conservation of the ITS2 region was also discovered in *Panax ginseng* and *Panax quinquefolius* [27].

5. Conclusion

In conclusion, both ITS2 and *psbA-trnH* can be successfully amplified from commercial and natural samples of the important traditional Chinese medicine, Rhizoma Menispermi and its adulterants. As a result, accurate species identification and validation of product authenticity are facilitated. Compared with the ITS2 regions, the *psbA-trnH* sequence should not be the first choice for the DNA barcoding of Menispermaceae species on the basis of high poly-N structures and reduced sequencing efficiency. However, in consideration of the results for *S. tetrandra*, *psbA-trnH* can still be used as a complementary barcode for ITS2 in species identification.

Acknowledgements

We thank Dr. Jingyuan Song from Institute of Medicinal Plant Development, Chinese Academy of Medical

Sciences for revising an earlier version of this manuscript. This work was supported by the Program for Changjiang Scholars and Innovative Research Team (No. IRT1150), and National Natural Science Foundation of China (No. 81073001, 81373922).

References

[1]   Shan, B.E., Ren, F.Z., Liang, W.J., Zhang, J., Li, Q.X. and Zeng, Y.P. (2006) Isolation and Purification of Antitumor Component in Rhizoma Menispermi and Analysis of Its Activity. *Carcinogenesis, Teratogenesis & Mutagenesis*, **3**, No. 007.

[2]   Zhao, B., Chen, Y., Sun, X., Zhou, M., Ding, J., Zhan, J.J. and Guo, L.J. (2012) Phenolic Alkaloids from *Menispermum dauricum* Rhizome Protect against Brain Ischemia Injury via Regulation of GLT-1, EAAC1 and ROS Generation. *Molecules*, **17**, 2725-2737. http://dx.doi.org/10.3390/molecules17032725

[3]   Lin, M., Xia, B., Yang, M., Gao, S., Huo, Y. and Lou, G. (2013) Characterization and Antitumor Activities of a Polysaccharide from the Rhizoma of *Menispermum dauricum*. *International Journal of Biological Macromolecules*, **53**, 72-76. http://dx.doi.org/10.1016/j.ijbiomac.2012.11.012

[4]   Hoang, M.L., Chen, C.H., Sidorenko, V.S., He, J., Dickman, K.G., Yun, B.H., Moriya, M., Niknafs, N., Douville, C., Karchin, R., Turesky, R.J., Pu, Y.S., Vogelstein, B. and Papadopoulos, N. (2013) Mutational Signature of Aristolochic Acid Exposure as Revealed by Whole-Exome Sequencing. *Science Translational Medicine*, **5**, 197ra102.

[5]   Chen, H. (2010) The Difference and the Reasonable Application of *Menispermum dauricum* and *Sophorae tonkinensis*. *Chinese Medicine Modern Distance Education of China*, **8**, 60-61.

[6]   Miller, S.E. (2007) DNA Barcoding and the Renaissance of Taxonomy. *Proceedings of the National Academy of Sciences of the United States of America*, **104**, 4775-4776. http://dx.doi.org/10.1073/pnas.0700466104

[7]   Chen, S.L., Yao, H., Han, J.P., Liu, C., Song, J.Y., Shi, L.C., Zhu, Y.J., Ma, X.Y., Gao, T., Pang, X.H., Luo, K., Li, Y., Li, X.W., Jia, X.C., Lin, Y.L. and Leon, C. (2010) Validation of the ITS2 Region as a Novel DNA Barcode for Identifying Medicinal Plant Species. *PLoS One*, **5**, e8613. http://dx.doi.org/10.1371/journal.pone.0008613

[8]   Yao, H., Song, J., Liu, C., Luo, K., Han, J.P., Li, Y., Pang, X.H., Xu, H.X., Zhu, Y.J., Xiao, P.G. and Chen, S.L. (2010) Use of ITS2 Region as the Universal DNA Barcode for Plants and Animals. *PLoS One*, **5**, 13102. http://dx.doi.org/10.1371/journal.pone.0013102

[9]   Li, D.Z., Gao, L.M., Li, H.T., Wang, H., Ge, X.J., Liu, J.Q., Chen, Z.D., Zhou, S.L., Chen, S.L., Yang, J.B., Fu, C.X., Zeng, C.X., Yan, H.F., Zhu, Y.J., Sun, Y.S., Chen, S.Y., Zhao, L., Wang, K., Yang, T. and Duan, G.W. (2011) Comparative Analysis of a Large Dataset Indicates That Internal Transcribed Spacer (ITS) Should Be Incorporated into the Core Barcode for Seed Plants. *Proceedings of the National Academy of Sciences of the United States of America*, **108**, 19641-19646. http://dx.doi.org/10.1073/pnas.1104551108

[10] Kress, W.J., Wurdack, K.J., Zimmer, E.A., Weigt, L.A. and Janzen, D.H. (2005) Use of DNA Barcodes to Identify Flowering Plants. *Proceedings of the National Academy of Sciences of the United States of America*, **102**, 8369-8374. http://dx.doi.org/10.1073/pnas.0503123102

[11] Shaw, J., Lickey, E.B., Schilling, E.E. and Small, R.L. (2007) Comparison of Whole Chloroplast Genome Sequences to Choose Noncoding Regions for Phylogenetic Studies in Angiosperms: The Tortoise and the Hare III. *American Journal of Botany*, **94**, 275-288. http://dx.doi.org/10.3732/ajb.94.3.275

[12] White, T.J. (1990) Amplification and Direct Sequencing of Fungal Ribosomal RNA Genes for Phylogenetics. In: *PCR Protocols, a Guide to Methods and Applications*, 315-322.

[13] Tamura, K., Peterson, D., Peterson, N., Stecher, G., Nei, M. and Kumar, S. (2011) MEGA5: Molecular Evolutionary Genetics Analysis Using Maximum Likelihood, Evolutionary Distance, and Maximum Parsimony Methods. *Molecular Biology and Evolution*, **28**, 2731-2739. http://dx.doi.org/10.1093/molbev/msr121

[14] Ross, H.A., Murugan, S. and Li, W.L. (2008) Testing the Reliability of Genetic Methods of Species Identification via Simulation. *Systematic Biology*, **57**, 216-230. http://dx.doi.org/10.1080/10635150802032990

[15] Xin, T.Y., Yao, H., Luo, K., Xiang, L., Ma, X.C., Han, J.P., Lin, Y.L., Song, J.Y. and Chen, S.L. (2012) Stability and Accuracy of the Identification of Notopterygii Rhizoma et Radix Using the ITS/ITS2 Barcodes. *Yao Xue Xue Bao*, **47**, 1098-1105.

[16] Luo, K., Ma, P., Yao, H., Xin, T.Y., Hu, Y., Zhen, S.H., Huang, L.F., Liu, J. and Song, J.Y. (2012) Identification of Gentianae Macrophyllae Radix Using the ITS2 Barcodes. *Yao Xue Xue Bao*, **47**, 1710-1717.

[17] Pang, X.H., Song, J.Y., Xu, H.B. and Yao, H. (2012) Using ITS2 Barcode to Identify Ephedraeherba. *China Journal of Chinese Materia Medica*, **37**, 1118-1121.

[18] Hou, D.Y., Song, J.Y., Shi, L.C., Ma, X.C., Xin, T.Y., Han, J.P., Xiao, W., Sun, Z.Y., Cheng, R.Y. and Yao, H. (2013) Stability and Accuracy Assessment of Identification of Traditional Chinese Materia Medica Using DNA Barcoding: A

Case Study on Flos Lonicerae Japonicae. *BioMed Research International*, **2013**, Article ID: 549037.

[19] Chiou, S.J., Yen, J.H., Fang, C.L., Chen, H.L. and Lin, T.Y. (2007) Authentication of Medicinal Herbs Using PCR-Amplified ITS2 with Specific Primers. *Planta Medica*, **73**, 1421-1426. http://dx.doi.org/10.1055/s-2007-990227

[20] Li, J.L., Wang, S., Yu, J., Wang, L. and Zhou, S.L. (2013) A Modified CTAB Protocol for Plant DNA Extraction. *Chinese Bulletin of Botany*, **48**, 72-78. http://dx.doi.org/10.3724/SP.J.1259.2013.00072

[21] Xu, X.L., Shi, L.C., Song, J.Y., Han, J.P., Yao, H., Chen, S.L., *et al.* (2012) Molecular Identification of Sophorae Tonkinensis Radix et Rhizoma Original Plant and Its Adulterants Based on ITS2 DNA Barcode. *World Science and Technology/Modernization of Traditional Chinese Medicine and Materia Medica*, **14**, 1147-1152.

[22] Yancy, H.F., Zemlak, T.S., Mason, J.A., Washington, J.D., Tenge, B.J. and Nguen, N.T. (2008) Potential Use of DNA Barcodes in Regulatory Science: Applications of the Regulatory Fish Encyclopedia. *Journal of Food Protection*, **71**, 210-217.

[23] Kool, A., Boer, H.J., Kruger, A., Rydberg, A., Abbad, A., Bjork, L. and Martin, G. (2012) Molecular Identification of Commercialized Medicinal Plants in Southern Morocco. *PLoS One*, **7**, e39459. http://dx.doi.org/10.1371/journal.pone.0039459

[24] Newmaster, S.G., Grguric, M., Shanmughanandhan, D., Ramalingam, S. and Ragupathy, S. (2013) DNA Barcoding Detects Contamination and Substitution in North American Herbal Products. *BMC Medicine*, **11**, 222. http://dx.doi.org/10.1186/1741-7015-11-222

[25] Chase, M.W., Cowan, R.S., Hollingsworth, P.M., Berg van den, C., Madrinan, S., Petersen, G. and Seberg, O. (2007) A Proposal for a Standardised Protocol to Barcode All Land Plants. *Taxon*, **56**, 295-299.

[26] Song, J.Y., Shi, L.C., Li, D.Z., Sun, Y.Z., Niu, Y.Y., Chen, Z.D., Luo, H.M., Pang, X.H., Sun, Z.Y., Liu, C., Lv, A.P., Deng, Y.P., Larson-Rabin, Z., Wilkinson, M. and Chen, S.L. (2012) Extensive Pyrosequencing Reveals Frequent Intra-Genomic Variations of Internal Transcribed Spacer Regions of Nuclear Ribosomal DNA. *PLoS One*, **7**, e43971. http://dx.doi.org/10.1371/journal.pone.0043971

[27] Chen, X.C., Liao, B.S., Song, J.Y., Pang, X.H., Han, J.P. and Chen, S.L. (2013) A Fast SNP Identification and Analysis of Intraspecific Variation in the Medicinal Panax Species Based on DNA Barcoding. *Gene*, **530**, 39-43. http://dx.doi.org/10.1016/j.gene.2013.07.097

9

The Protective Effect of Compound Danshen Dripping Pills on Oxidative Stress after Retinal Ischemia/Reperfusion Injury in Rats

Bingwen Lu, Xingwei Wu*

Ophthalmology Department, Shanghai First People's Hospital, Shanghai, China
Email: *704487389@qq.com

Abstract

Objective: To investigate the effect of Compound Danshen Dripping Pills (CDDP) on oxidative stress after ischemia/reperfusion (I/R) injury in the rat retina. Methods: Adult male SD rats were randomly divided into 3 groups: sham (group A), I/R (group B), and I/R plus CDDP (group C). Retinal ischemia/reperfusion injury (RIRI) was introduced by increasing the intraocular pressure (IOP) to 110 mmHg for 60 min via cannulation into the anterior chamber. Right after the insult, CDDP was administered intragastrically (450 mg/kg/d) for 7 days. The levels of malondialdehyde (MDA), the activities of superoxide dismutase (SOD), glutathione peroxidase (GSH-Px), and catalase (CAT) in the retinal tissues were determined on d1 and d7 after the ischemic insult. Results: Following ischemia, the MDA levels in group B and group C were significantly higher than those in group A ($p < 0.01$). CDDP significantly lowered MDA levels in group C when compared with group B ($p < 0.01$). The activities of SOD, GSH-Px and CAT were higher in group A than in group B and group C ($p < 0.01$). CDDP could increase the activities of SOD, GSH-Px and CAT remarkably in group C when compared with group B ($p < 0.01$). Conclusion: CDDP can protect the retina from I/R injury through reducing oxidative stress, and thus may be a promising method for the treatment of ischemic retinal disorders.

Keywords

Compound Danshen Dripping Pills (CDDP), Retinal Ischemia/Reperfusion Injury (RIRI), Oxidative Stress, Rats

1. Introduction

Ischemia/reperfusion (I/R) occurs in many clinical conditions and can seriously impair the affected organ or tis-

---

*Corresponding author.

sues [1]. Retinal ischemia/reperfusion injury (RIRI) is a common cause of visual impairment and blindness. Central retinal artery occlusion (CRAO), central retinal vein occlusion (CRVO), branch retinal artery occlusion (BRAO), branch retinal vein occlusion (BRVO), acute glaucoma, diabetic retinopathy, and age-related macular degeneration (AMD) are all associated with retinal ischemia [2]. The retina is highly dependent on its oxygen supply, while restoration of blood flow after ischemia paradoxically initiates more serious tissue injury and cell death, leading to an irreversible impairment of retinal function [2]. Therefore, the management of RIRI is crucial.

Compound Danshen Dripping Pills (CDDP) is a Chinese patent medicine, developed on the basis of Traditional Chinese Medicine (TCM) theory and modern preparation technologies. It is widely used in the prevention and treatment of coronary arteriosclerosis, angina pectoris, hyperlipidemia, and other cardiovascular diseases in China [3]. This new drug compound mainly consists of salvia miltiorrhiza and panax notoginseng [4]. In the past few decades, CDDP has been demonstrated to have antioxidant, anti-inflammatory properties, and it can also protect endothelial function, inhibit platelet adhesion as well as improve microcirculation [5]-[8]. Because of its characters of multi-components, multi-effects, and multi-targets, CDDP went through phase II clinical research in USA in 2010 [9]. Although many studies have provided evidences that CDDP is I/R protective in cardiovascular disorders, its potential protective effects in ameliorating retina ischemic disorders have received little attention. Thus, we hypothesized that CDDP could have some therapeutic efficacy on RIRI. In our previous study, we have already demonstrated that CDDP can exert protective effects on the retina under ischemic conditions through examining resultant ERG and histological findings [10].

I/R-induced oxidative stress is thought to be the direct cause of retinal injury. MDA, a degraded product of lipid peroxidation, produces cytotoxicity by reacting with the amino of nucleic acid [11], whereas SOD, GSH-Px and CAT are major scavengers of reactive oxygen species (ROS), which are known to trigger apoptosis and are massively generated during I/R [12]. Previous study showed that changes of MDA levels and SOD activities were indicators for lipid peroxidation degrees and therefore reflected the severity of tissue damage [13]. Therefore, in the present study, in order to elucidate whether CDDP exerts protective effects on the retinal under ischemic conditions against oxidative stress, we examined the MDA level and the activities of SOD, GSH-Px, and CAT in the retina tissues.

2. Materials and Methods

2.1. Research Objects and Grouping

Fifty-four adult male SD rats, weighing from 200 to 350 g, were provided by Joinn Laboratories (Suzhou). The animal care strictly conformed to the Association for Research in Vision and Ophthalmology Statement for the Use of Animals in Ophthalmology and Vision Research. The animals were housed under controlled conditions: a 12-hour light/dark cycle; a temperature of 20°C to 26°C, and humidity in the range of 40% to 70%. The animals had free access to standard food and drinking water.

Rats were randomly divided into three groups: sham (group A) (n = 18), I/R (group B) (n = 18), and I/R plus CDDP (group C) (n = 18).

2.2. Experiment Medicine

CDDP was provided by Tasly Pharmaceutical Co., Ltd. (Tianjin, China). The CDDP was dissolved in a certain amount of water to a certain concentration of per milliliter of drug solution. Group C was treated with drug solution at a dose of 450 mg/kg/d for seven days. Meanwhile, Group A and Group B were treated with the same volume of 0.9% saline solution.

2.3. Experiment Methods

2.3.1. Establishment of RIRI Model in Rats

Animals were anesthetized intraperitoneally with 1% pentobarbital sodium (0.7 ml/100g). Body temperature was maintained at 36.5°C - 37°C using a heated blanket. For corneal analgesia, one drop of 0.4% oxybuprocaine hydrochloride was used. Pupillary dilation was achieved with 0.5% tropicamide and 0.5% phenylephrine.

Retinal ischemia was induced by increasing the IOP in the right eye to 110 mmHg for 60 min. After dilation of the pupil, the anterior chamber of the right eye (only the right eye was used experimentally) was cannulated with a 30-gauge needle connected to a physiological saline bag. The IOP was raised to 110 mmHg by keeping the bag at 150 cm above the eye. Retinal ischemia was confirmed when there was whitening of the iris and loss of the red reflex of the retina. After 60 min of ischemia, the needle was removed and the IOP was returned to normal pressure. For the sham group, the procedure was performed without elevating the saline bag.

2.3.2. Determination of the Levels of MDA and Activities of SOD, GSH-Px, and CAT

The levels of MDA and the activities of SOD, GSH-Px, and CAT were determined in each retina 1 day and 7 days after the ischemic insult.

The retina samples were prepared as a 10% homogenate in 0.9% saline using a homogenizer on ice according to their respective weight. Then, the homogenate was centrifuged at 3500 rpm for 15 min, and the supernatant was collected and diluted.

MDA levels were determined using the double heating method. Briefly, 2.5 ml of thiobarbituric acid (TBA) means thiobarbituric acid solution (100 g/L) was added to 0.5 mL of homogenate in each centrifuge tube, and the tubes were placed in boiling water for 15 min. After cooling with flowing water, the tubes were centrifuged at 1000 rpm for 10 min, 2 mL of the supernatant was added to 1 mL of the TBA solution (6.7 g/L), and the tube was placed in boiling water for another 15 min. After cooling, the amount of thiobarbituric acid-reactive species was measured at 532 nm. The MDA concentration was calculated from the absorbance coefficient of the MDA-TBA complex.

SOD activity was determined through the inhibition of nitrotetrazolium blue (NTB) reduction by the xanthine/xanthine oxidase system as a superoxide generator. The activity was assessed in the supernatant after the addition of 1.0 mL of ethanol/chloroform (5/3, v/v) to the same volume of sample and centrifugation for 15 min at 3000 rpm. The production of formazan was determined at 560 nm. One unit of SOD activity was defined as the amount of protein that inhibited the rate of NTB reduction by 50%.

GSH-Px activity was measured by the method of Paglia and Valentine. The enzymatic reaction in the tube that contained reduced nicotinamide adenine dinucleotide phosphate, reduced glutathione, sodium azide, and glutathione reductase was initiated by the addition of H_2O_2, and the change in absorbance at 340 nm was monitored by spectrophotometry. The data are expressed as U/g of protein.

CAT activity was measured by the method of Cohen. The principle of the assay was based on the determination of the rate constant (s-1, k) of H_2O_2 decomposition. The rate constant of the enzyme was determined by measuring the absorbance change per minute. The data are expressed as k/g of protein.

2.4. Statistical Methods

Data were represented as the mean ± SEM. To determine the significance of differences, analysis of variance (ANOVA) were carried out using SPSS 18.0 software. P values less than 0.05 were considered statistically significant in this study.

3. Results

3.1. Effects of CDDP on the MDA Level and Activities of SOD, GSH-Px, and CAT on d1 after RIRI

To estimate the anti-oxidative effect of CDDP, the MDA level and the activities of SOD, GSH-Px, and CAT of the retina tissue were measured on d1 after I/R injury. As a marker of lipid peroxidation, the MDA level in the retina tissues of group B was remarkably higher than that in group A ($p < 0.01$). CDDP significantly inhibited MDA production in the retina tissue after RIRI when compared with group B ($p < 0.01$). Data are shown in **Figure 1(a)**.

SOD, GSH-Px, and CAT are pivotal enzymes scavenging ROS in vivo. The activities of SOD, GSH-Px, and CAT were greatly reduced in group B than in goup A after I/R injury ($p < 0.01$). Compared with group B, CDDP could significantly increase the activities SOD, GSH-Px, and CAT ($p < 0.01$). Data are shown in **Figures 1(b)-(d)**, respectively.

3.2. Effects of CDDP on the MDA Level and Activities of SOD, GSH-Px, and CAT on d7 after RIRI

Seven days after RIRI, the MDA level in the group B was lower than those of day 1. However, compared with

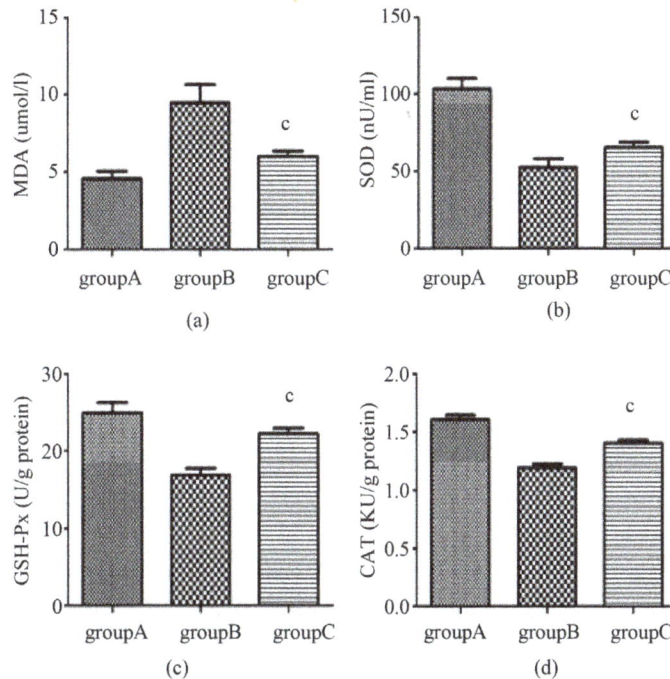

Figure 1. Effects of CDDP on MDA levels and the activities of SOD, GSH-Px and CAT on the retina tissue from I/R-induced retinal injury on d1. Data are expressed as mean ± SD and are representative of 3 experiments (n = 9). ^{c}p < 0.01 vs. group B with group C.

group C, the MDA levels were still significantly higher in group B (p < 0.01). Data are shown in **Figure 2(a)**. The activities of SOD, GSH-Px, and CAT were higher than those of d1. Compared with group C, the activities were still significantly lower in the group B (p < 0.01). Data are shown in **Figures 2(b)-(d)**, respectively.

4. Discussion

The present study was performed to evaluate the protective effects of CDDP against oxidative stress on the retina following RIRI in the rats. We found that CDDP improved the oxidative parameters of the retinal tissue in the I/R model, which suggested that CDDP might be a potential choice for the treatment of RIRI-related eye diseases.

A number of ocular diseases have been associated with retinal ischemia reperfusion injury, including retinal vascular occlusion, acute glaucoma, diabetic retinopathy, and retinopathy of prematurity [14]. Oxygen-free radicals [15], endogenous excitatory amino acids [16], calcium imbalances [17], and nitric oxide [18] [19], are involved in the pathogenesis of I/R injury. The exact mechanism of RIRI is complicated, mediated by a variety of factors, which makes it a hot pot problem around the world. Accordingly, finding a way to reduce or prevent RIRI, thus reduce visual impairment is of great importance.

Oxygen is crucial for life and metabolic processes, however, reactive metabolites of oxygen can be toxic to cells [20] [21]. Particularly, the sudden reintroduction of oxygen into tissues during reperfusion may exacerbate the cellular damage secondary to ischemia. ROS is considered to be a critical mediator of ischemia reperfusion injury. The generation of excess ROS can affect subcellular structures and functions, resulting in mitochondrial dysfunction, lipid peroxidation of polyunsaturated fatty acids in membranes, and alterations in protein or DNA structure [21]-[23].

Abundant studies of retinal tissue have shown that oxidative stress was an fundamental factor in cellular damage during IR injury. MDA is a naturally occurring product of lipid peroxidation, a process in which unsaturated fatty acids are oxidized to form radicals [24]. The level of MDA is currently used to assess oxidative tissue damage after I/R injury [24]. Free radicals produced in living organisms can be scavenged by intrinsic antioxidant enzymes, including SOD, CAT, and GSH-Px, thus, the activities of these enzymes may reflect the anti-

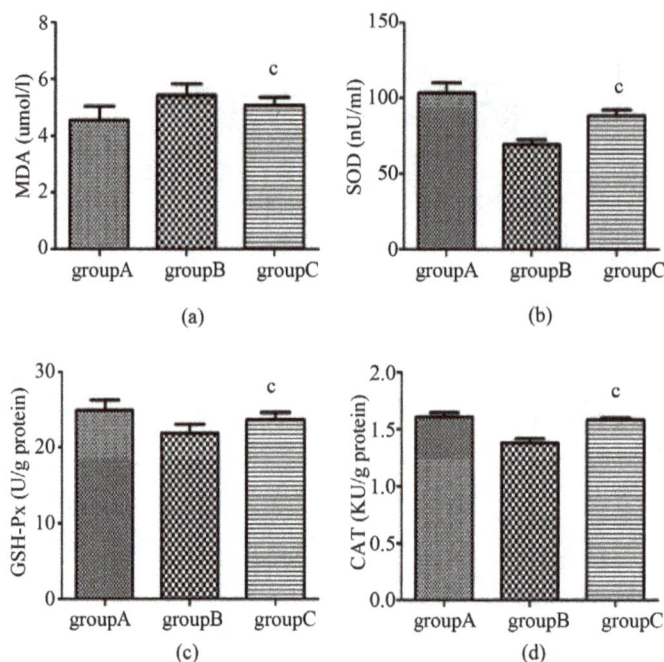

Figure 2. Effects of CDDP on MDA levels and the activities of SOD, GSH-Px and CAT on the retina tissue from I/R-induced retinal injury on d7. Data are expressed as mean ± SD and are representative of 3 experiments (n = 9). [c]p < 0.01 vs. group B with group C.

oxidative ability of the body [25]-[27].

Therefore, the aim of this study is to investigate the protective effects of CDDP against oxidative stress on the retina following RIRI in the rats through examining the MDA level and the activities of SOD, GSH-Px, and CAT in the retina tissues.

In the present study, we examined the changes in the levels of MDA, SOD, CAT, and GSH-Px, to elucidate the mechanism by which CDDP protects retinal cell injuries from oxidative stress. The results of d1 and d7 after RIRI have shown that I/R injury resulted in a significant increase in the MDA levels and decrease in the activities of SOD, CAT, and GSH-Px in the retina. However, CDDP could significantly decrease the MDA level and enhance the antioxidant enzyme activity in retinal tissue, implying that CDDP ameliorated the injury. The anti-oxidative stress effect of CDDP may be part of its protective mechanisms in RIRI.

CDDP is a new drug compound preparation in treating cardiovascular diseases. The chemical analysis of CDDP reported previously shows that the main ingredients are salvia miltiorrhiza and panax notoginseng [4]. One pill of CDDP (obtained from Tasly Pharmaceutical, Tianjin, China) contains 9 mg of salvia miltiorrhiza and 1.76 mg of panax notoginseng. Salvia miltiorrhiza could improve cardiac function through improving antioxidant activity [5], and through preventing cardiomyocyte apoptosis [6]. Panax notoginseng could protect against myocardial damage and decrease lipid peroxidation [7]. With the combination of multiple components, CDDP hits multiple targets, and exerts the synergistic therapeutic effects. CDDP has been reported to be effective in the prevention of tissue damage in the heart and brain after IR injury, whereas there are few studies on the protective effect of CDDP against retinal damage caused by I/R, which is commonly seen in clinical practice. Thus, our studies investigated the protective effect and the underlying mechanisms.

In this study, the dose of CDDP chosen was the high-dose (450 mg/kg/d) used in the Li *et al.* study [28]. Our previous study demonstrated that the high-dose CDDP (450 mg/kg/d) could exert protective effects on the retina under ischemic conditions through examining resultant ERG and histological findings [10]. Those positive results provided proof for the use of the dosage of CDDP.

However, it should be noted that the anti-oxidative stress effect may not be the sole protective mechanism of CDDP. Various other mechanisms, such as anti-inflammatory and anti-apoptosis activities, could also play a role in the observed protective effects of CDDP during I/R injury. Further investigations should be carried out to clarify this.

5. Conclusion

In conclusion, the present study demonstrates that CDDP is effective at protecting the retina during I/R injury. CDDP protected the retina from IR injury, possibly via a mechanism involving the regulation of oxidative parameters.

Acknowledgements

This work was supported by a grant from Shanghai First People's Hospital. The author was grateful to Professor Wu from Shanghai First People's Hospital for final edict of this manuscript.

References

[1]   Grace, P.A. (1994) Ischemia-Reperfusion Injury. *British Journal of Surgery*, **81**, 637-647. http://dx.doi.org/10.1002/bjs.1800810504

[2]   Osborne, N.N., Casson, R.J., Wood, J.P., Chidlow, G., Graham, M. and Melena, J. (2004) Retinal Ishchemia: Mechanisms of Damage and Potential Therapeutic Strategies. *Progress in Retinal and Eye Research*, **23**, 91-147. http://dx.doi.org/10.1016/j.preteyeres.2003.12.001

[3]   Jia, Y., Huang, F., Zhang, S. and Leung, S.W. (2012) Is Danshen (*Salvia miltiorrhiza*) Dripping Pill More Effective than Isosorbide Dinitrate in Treating Angina Pectoris? A Systematic Review of Randomized Controlled Trials. *International Journal of Cardiology*, **157**, 330-340. http://dx.doi.org/10.1016/j.ijcard.2010.12.073

[4]   Zheng, X.H., Zhao, X.F., Zhao, X., Wang, S.X., Wei, Y.M. and Zheng, J.B. (2007) Determination of the Main Bioactive Metabolites of *Radix Salvia miltiorrhizae* in Compound Danshen Dripping Pills and the Tissue Distribution of Danshensu in Rabbit by SPE-HPLC-MS^n. *Journal of Separation Science*, **30**, 851-857. http://dx.doi.org/10.1002/jssc.200600287

[5]   Wang, S.B., Tian, S., Yang, F., Yang, H.G., Yang, X.Y. and Du, G.H. (2009) Cardioprotective Effect of Salvianolic Acid A on Isoproterenol-Induced Myocardial Infarction in Rats. *European Journal of Pharmacology*, **615**, 125-132. http://dx.doi.org/10.1016/j.ejphar.2009.04.061

[6]   Li, M., Zhao, M.Q., Kumar Durairajan, S.S., Xie, L.X., Zhang, H.X., Kum, W.F., Goto, S. and Liao, F.L. (2008) Protective Effect of Tetramethylpyrazine and Salvianolic Acid B on Apoptosis of Rat Cerebral Microvascular Endothelial Cell Under High Shear Stress. *Clinical Hemorheology and Microcirculation*, **38**, 177-187.

[7]   Ruan, J.Q., Leong, W.I., Yan, R. and Wang, Y.T. (2010) Characterization of Metabolism and *in Vitro* Permeability Study of Notoginsenoside R1 from Radix Notoginseng. *Journal of Agricultural and Food Chemistry*, **58**, 5770-5776. http://dx.doi.org/10.1021/jf1005885

[8]   Yuan, R.Y. and Li, G.P. (2009) Multi-Target Effects of Compound Danshen Dripping Pills in Prevention and Treatment of Cardiovascular Diseases. *Chinese Journal of New Drugs*, **18**, 377-380.

[9]   Anonymous (2010) Compound Danshen Dripping Pills Passed Phase II Clinical Trials by FDA. *China Journal of Pharmaceutical Economics*, **4**, 94.

[10] Lu, B.-W. and Wu, X.-W. (2014) Protective Effects of Compound Danshen Dripping Pills on Retinal Ischemia-Reperfusion Injury in Rats. *Recent Advances in Ophthalmology*, **34**, 1030-1034.

[11] Banin, E., Berenshtein, E., Kitrossky, N., Pe'er, J. and Chevion, M. (2000) Gallium-Desferrioxamine Protects the Cat Retina against Injury after Ischemia and Reperfusion. *Free Radical Biology and Medicine*, **28**, 315-323. http://dx.doi.org/10.1016/S0891-5849(99)00227-0

[12] Anderson, R.E., Maude, M.B. and Neilsen, J.C. (1985) Effect of Lipid Peroxidation on Rhodopsin Regeneration. *Experimental Eye Research*, **4**, 65-71. http://dx.doi.org/10.3109/02713688508999969

[13] Xie, Z., Wu, X., Gong, Y., Song, Y., Qiu, Q. and Li, C. (2007) Intraperitoneal Injection of Ginkgo Biloba Extract Enhances Antioxidation Ability of Retina and Protects Photoreceptors after Light-Induced Retinal Damage in Rats. *Current Eye Research*, **32**, 471-479. http://dx.doi.org/10.1080/02713680701257621

[14] Shibuki, H., Katai, N., Yodoi, J., Uchida, K. and Yoshimura, N. (2000) Lipid Peroxidation and Peroxynitrite in Retinal Ischemia-Reperfusion Injury. *Investigative Ophthalmology Visual Science*, **41**, 3607-3614.

[15] Kwon, Y.H., Rickman, D.W., Baruah, S., Zimmerman, M.B., Kim, C.S., Boldt, H.C., Russell, S.R. and Hayreh, S.S. (2005) Vitreous and Retinal Amino Acid Concentrations in Experimental Central Retinal Artery Occlusion in the Primate. *Eye* (*London*), **19**, 455-463. http://dx.doi.org/10.1038/sj.eye.6701546

[16] Pannicke, T., Uckermann, O., Iandiev, I., Biedermann, B., Wiedemann, P., Perlman, I., Reichenbach, A. and Bring-

mann, A. (2005) Altered Membrane Physiology in Müller Glial Cells after Transient Ischemia of the Rat Retina. *Glia*, **50**, 1-11. http://dx.doi.org/10.1002/glia.20151

[17]   Toriu, N., Akaike, A., Yasuyoshi, H., Zhang, S., Kashii, S., Honda, Y., Shimazawa, M. and Hara, H. (2000) Lomerizine, a Ca^{2+} Channel Blocker, Reduces Glutamate-Induced Neurotoxicity and ischemia/Reperfusion Damage in Rat Retina. *Experimental Eye Research*, **70**, 475-484. http://dx.doi.org/10.1006/exer.1999.0809

[18]   Yoneda, S., Tanihara, H., Kido, N., Honda, Y., Goto, W., Hara, H. and Miyawaki, N. (2001) Interleukin-1Beta Mediates Ischemic Injury in the Rat Retina. *Experimental Eye Research*, **73**, 661-667. http://dx.doi.org/10.1006/exer.2001.1072

[19]   Sanchez, R.N., Chan, C.K., Garg, S., Kwong, J.M., Wong, M.J., Sadun, A.A. and Lam, T.T. (2003) Interleukin-6 in Retinal Ischemia Reperfusion Injury in Rats. *Investigative Ophthalmology Visual Science*, **44**, 4006-4011. http://dx.doi.org/10.1167/iovs.03-0040

[20]   Di Mascio, P., Murphy, M.E. and Sies, H. (1991) Antioxidant Defense Systems: The Role of Carotenoids, Tocopherols, and Thiols. *The American Journal of Clinical Nutrition*, **53**, 194S-200S.

[21]   Marnett, L.J. (2000) Oxyradicals and DNA Damage. *Carcinogenesis*, **21**, 361-370. http://dx.doi.org/10.1093/carcin/21.3.361

[22]   Szabo, M.E., Droy-Lefaix, M.T., Doly, M., Carré, C. and Braquet, P. (1991) Ischemia and Reperfusion-Induced Histologic Changes in the Rat Retina. Eemonstration of a Free Radical-Mediated Mechanism. *Investigative Ophthalmology Visual Science*, **32**, 1471-1478.

[23]   Nayak, M.S., Kita, M. and Marmor, M.F. (1993) Protection of Rabbit Retina from Ischemic Injury by Superoxide Dismutase and Catalase. *Investigative Ophthalmology Visual Science*, **34**, 2018-2022.

[24]   Del Rio, D., Stewart, A.J. and Pellegrini, N. (2005) A Review of Recent Studies on Malondialdehyde as Toxic Molecule and Biological Marker of Oxidative Stress. *Nutrition, Metabolism Cardiovascular Diseases*, **15**, 316-328. http://dx.doi.org/10.1016/j.numecd.2005.05.003

[25]   Chance, B., Sies, H. and Boveris, A. (1979) Hydroperoxide Metabolism in Mammalian Organs. *Physiological Reviews*, **59**, 527-605.

[26]   Crack, P.J., Taylor, J.M., de Haan, J.B., Kola, I., Hertzog, P. and Iannello, R.C. (2003) Glutathione Peroxidase-1 Contributes to the Neuroprotection Seen in the Superoxide Dismutase-1 Transgenic Mouse in Response to Ischemia/Reperfusion Injury. *Journal of Cerebral Blood Flow Metabolism*, **23**, 19-22. http://dx.doi.org/10.1097/00004647-200301000-00002

[27]   Liochev, S.I. and Fridovich, I. (2002) Superoxide and Nitric Oxide: Consequences of Varying Rates of Production and Consumption: A Theoretical Treatment. *Free Radical Biology Medicine*, **33**, 137-141. http://dx.doi.org/10.1016/S0891-5849(02)00864-X

[28]   Li, Y.M., Liu, X.Q., Chen, H.Q., Chen, X.A. and Liu, L.Y. (2010) Effect of Fufang danshen diwan on Atherosclerosis and the Level of TAFI in Rats. *Chinese Journal of Gerontology*, **29**, 280-281.

10

Introduction on the Emotion-Will Overcoming Therapy (EWOT): A Novel Alternative Approach of Psychological Treatment from Chinese Medicine

Hui Zhang[1], Xiangeng Zhang[1*], Xiaoli Liang[1], Han Lai[2], Jin Gao[1], Qin Liu[1], Hongyan Wang[1]

[1]The School of Nursing, Chengdu University of TCM, Chengdu, China
[2]The School of Foreign Language, Chengdu University of TCM, Chengdu, China
Email: *jeffery.h.zhang@gmail.com

Abstract

Emotional disorders and mental illnesses constitute a significant part of diseases. In Chinese medicine, emotional disorders and mental illnesses are classified as emotion-will (*Qing Zhi*) disorders. Emotion-will, *i.e.* seven emotions (*Qi Qing*: happiness, anger, anxiety, pensiveness, sorrow, fear, and fright) and five wills (*Wu Zhi*: happiness, anger, thinking, sorrow, and fear), play a basic role in the onset, progress and prognosis of almost all diseases, not only the mental illnesses. The emotion-will overcoming therapy (EWOT) is defined as a psychological approach that a therapist employs single or multiple emotions to overcome and eliminate patients' abnormal morbid emotions and to heal mind-body disorders derived from the abnormality. EWOT lays a foundation for the philosophical foundation of Chinese medicine, *i.e.* *Yin* and *Yang*, and five elements, which is believed to be the most commonly utilized and effective modality in dealing with mental illnesses. This essay covers the origin and development, underlying mechanism, clinical application, basic researches of emotion-will system and EWOT and the comparison with conventional therapies. Thus, EWOT could draw more attention in the field of psychology and spread in clinical practice.

Keywords

CM Psychology, Emotion-Will Overcoming Therapy, Psychology, Seven Emotions, Five Wills

---

*Corresponding author.

1. Introduction

The theory of emotion and will refers to the seven emotions (*Qi Qing*: happiness, anger, worry, thinking, sorrow, fear, and fright) and five wills (*Wu Zhi*: happiness, anger, thinking, sorrow, and fear) [1]. Hereby, "will" means normal emotional activities and "emotion" means hyperactive activities. In Chinese medicine, emotion-will plays a basic role in the onset, progress, and prognosis of almost all diseases, not only the psychological and psychiatric disorders. The emotion-will overcoming therapy (EWOT) derived from the philosophical foundation of Chinese medicine, *i.e. Yin* and *Yang*, and five elements, is believed to be the most effective modality in dealing with mental illness.

For thousands years, medical experts have been exploring the importance of emotion-will and efficacy of EWOT in medical records since the establishment of Chinese medicine theoretic and therapeutic structure in *Yellow Emperor's Inner Classic* (*Huang Di Nei Jing*) [2]. At present, Chinese medicine practitioners still frequently utilize EWOT in treating depression, anxiety, phobia, etc. and nursing chronic diseases such as apoplexy sequelae, cancer, diabetes, irritable bowel movement and so on [3]-[6]. From the 1980s on, Chinese researchers have been trying to translate this emotion-will with very Chinese characteristic in conventional psychological language. Some promising results have been made. For instance, relationships and similarities among EWOT and cognitive and behavior therapy (CBT) [7], positive psychology therapy [8], and Morita therapy (MT) [9] [10] have been discussed. But, regrettably the emotion-will system and EWOT have not been introduced to the Chinese medicine practitioners and psychology therapists outside China except for rare literature with rough description [11] [12]. Comparing with the prosperous spread of acupuncture and herbal medicine, two major therapy approaches in Chinese medicine, EWOT is, however, a brand-new option and promising method dealing with mental illness [4] [13] [14]. This essay covers the origin and development, underlying mechanism, clinical application, basic researches of emotion-ill system and EWOT and the comparison with conventional therapies.

2. Origin and Development of Emotion-Will and EWOT

Records on emotion-will date back to *The Book of Rites* (*Li Ji*, 51-21 A.D.), in which *happiness, anger, sorrow, fear, love, hate, and desire*, the seven emotional reactions human beings have [15]. It is in *Yellow Emperor's Inner Classic that* the theoretic foundation is established. This book elaborates the relationship between emotion-will and organs, the pathogenesis of illness resulting from extreme emotions, and the treatment of emotional disorders, leading to a sound foundation for the development of the emotion-will theory.

The relationship is constructed on the model of five organ and five wills and emotions linked by the five elements theory, that are, liver-anger, heart-happiness, lungs-grief, spleen-pensiveness, kidneys-fear (**Figure 1**).

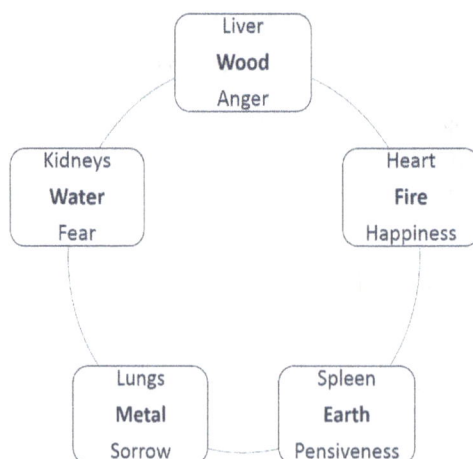

Figure 1. Organ-will pattern in understanding the correlation between five will and five organs in Chinese medicine and Chinese medicine psychology. A will and an organ, e.g. anger and liver are closely related because they have attributes of the element wood. Wood is featured by bending and straightening and likes orderly reaching. Anger drives the *Qi* circulation. Liver is the organ that governs free flow of *Qi*. Based on the attribute similarity of liver, anger-wood, organ-will pattern is established and so does happiness-heart, pensiveness-spleen, sorrow-lungs, and fear-kidneys by an extension of this logic.

This principle is considered as the foundation of emotion-will therapy in the treatment of emotional disorders and mental illnesses followed by later Chinese medicine practitioners supplementing and developing it. There are three representative advancements. First, Dr. Wuze Chen (1131-1189 A.D.) clarified the seven emotions, *i.e.* *Qi Qing*: happiness, anger, worry, thinking, sorrow, fear, and fright and differentiated the connotations of the Seven Emotions and five wills. Second, Congzheng Zhang (1156-1228 A.D.) recorded plenty of medical cases covering the utilization of EWOT in treating emotion-will disorders. Third, Wan Su Liu innovated a new understanding of extreme emotions, that is, a hyperactive emotion which gives rise to internal fire and accordingly injuries the related organ. In the 1980s, Prof. Miqu Wang and his peers believed in the modernization and systematization of the emotion-will theory. Thus Chinese medicine psychology (CMP), a new discipline, emerged, which bases on the philosophic essences of Chinese medicine and borrows the structure from current conventional psychology [16]. Still, in Chinese medicine psychology EWOT is a major approach.

3. Mechanism of EWOT

3.1. Five Elements

EWOT is defined as a psychological approach in which a therapist employs single or multiple emotions to overcome or eliminate patients' morbid emotions and to heal mind-body disorder derived from the abnormality. Speaking of the mechanism, pathogenesis and phatho-mechanism are the fundamental contents. From the perspective of pathogenesis, extreme performance of the five emotions engenders illness. When the will-emotion or psychological reaction manifests within the limits of rational range, it is the reflection of the normal function of internal organs *i.e.* "five will". A normal will benefit the *Qi* transformation or the function of intern organs, health, and longevity. Once an emotion-will presents abnormally (insufficiently and excessively), most excessively, it results in diverse illness, *i.e.* "Seven Emotion".

As for the patho-mechanism (*Bing Ji*), the injury of organs from the abnormality of emotion-will corresponds with the principle of the five elements, that is, hyper-anger harms liver, hyper happiness harms heart, hyper-pensiveness harms spleen, hyper-sorrow harms lungs, and hyper-fear harms kidneys (**Figure 2**). It is the abnormality of emotion-will that arouses the disorder of *Qi* circulation which is believed to be the primary reason for all diseases. According to *Yellow Emperor's Inner Classic*, anger drives *Qi* upward, happiness causes *Qi* to slacken, sorrow dissipates *Qi*, fear drives *Qi* downward, pensiveness causes *Qi* to bind, fright causes disruption of *Qi* (**Figure 3**). In terms of the treatment of emotion-will disorder, its theoretic foundation is laid on the over

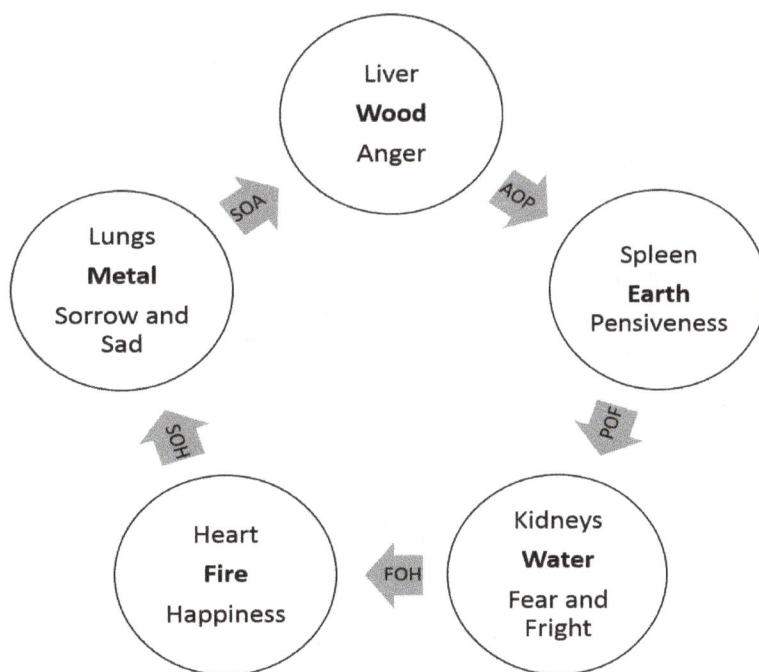

Figure 2. Emotion-will overcoming therapy (EWOT) model based on five elements.

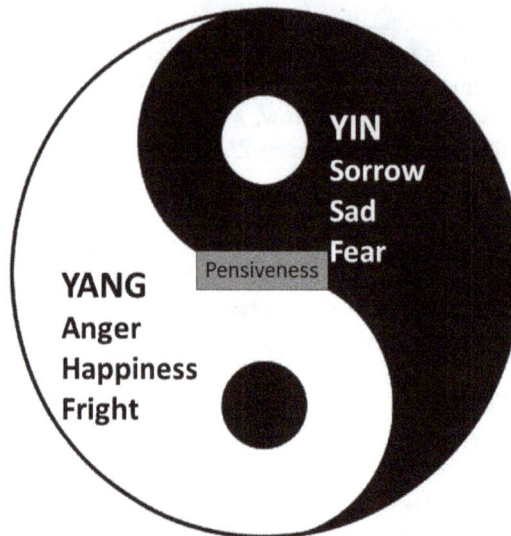

Figure 3. Emotion-will overcoming therapy (EWOT) model based on *Yin* and *Yang*. *Yin* can overcome hyperactive *Yang* and *vice versa*. Thus clinically, patient with emotional abnormalities of *Yang* (happiness, anger, and fright), are treated with emotions of *Yin* (sorrow, sad, and fear), while patient with emotional abnormalities of *Yin* (sorrow, sad, and fear), are treated with emotions of *Yang* (happiness, anger, and fright). In this way, the imbalance of *Yin* and *Yang* is restored, which indicates a mental illness is healed.

coming relationship among the five elements. It is constituted from five techniques: 1) sorrow overcomes the anger (SOA), 2) fear overcomes the happiness (FOH), 3) anger overcomes the pensiveness (AOP), 4) happiness overcomes the sorrow and sadness (HOSS), and 5) pensiveness overcomes the fear and fright (POFF) (**Figure 2**).

SOA: Sorrow attributes to the element metal and anger to the element wood. Because metal retrains wood, rational anger (one of the five wills) can overcome/neutralize hyperactive anger (one of the seven emotions).

FOH: Fear attributes to the element water and happiness to the element fire. Because water retrains fire, rational fear (one of the five wills) can overcome/neutralize hyperactive happiness (one of the seven emotions).

AOP: Anger attributes to the element wood and pensiveness to the element earth. Because wood retrains earth, rational anger (one of the five wills) can overcome/neutralize hyperactive pensiveness (one of the seven emotions).

HOSS: Happiness attributes to the element fire and sorrow to the element metal. Because fire retrains metal, rational happiness (one of the five wills) can overcome/neutralize hyperactive sorrow and sadness (two emotions of the seven emotions).

POFF: Pensiveness attributes to the element earth and fear to the element water. Because earth retrains water, rational pensiveness (one of the five wills) can overcome/neutralize hyperactive fear and fright (two emotions of the seven emotions).

SOA: Sorrow attributes to the element metal and anger to the element wood. Because metal retrains wood, rational anger (one of the five wills) can overcome hyperactive anger (one of the seven emotions).

FOH: Fear attributes to the element water and happiness to the element fire. Because water retrains fire, rational fear can overcome/neutralize hyperactive happiness.

AOP: Anger attributes to the element wood and pensiveness to the element earth. Because wood retrains earth, rational anger can overcome/neutralize hyperactive pensiveness.

HOSS: Happiness attributes to the element fire and sorrow to the element metal. Because fire retrains metal, rational happiness can overcome/neutralize hyperactive sorrow and sadness.

POFF: Pensiveness attributes to the element earth and fear to the element water. Because earth retrains water, rational pensiveness can overcome hyperactive fear and fright.

3.2. Role of *Yin* and *Yang*

Besides the Five Elements, *Yin* and *Yang* serves as another philosophical foundation in every aspects of Chinese medicine, from pathogenesis to treatment. Diverse discussions on the role the *Yin* and *Yang* plays can be found in *Yellow Emperor's Inner Classic*. For instance, when *Yang* is excessive, happiness presents; when *Yin* is excessive, anger presents (*Plain Questions, On Manipulating Needles* (*Su Wen, Xing Zhen*)). According to the attributes of *Yin* and *Yang*, Seven Emotions are categorized into two groups. First, happiness, anger, and fright attribute to *Yang* because the three emotions promote the circulation of *Qi* and blood. Second, sorrow, sad, and fear to *Yin*, which slow down the circulation. Pensiveness is a unique and neutralized emotion with both *Yin* and *Yang*'s qualities. As *Yin* can overcome hyperactive *Yang* and *vice versa*. Thus clinically, patient with emotional abnormalities of *Yang* (happiness, anger, fright), are treated with emotions of *Yin* (sorrow, sad, fear), while patient with emotional abnormalities of *Yin* (sorrow, sad, fear), are treated with emotions of *Yang* (happiness, anger, fright). In this way, the dis-balance of *Yin* and *Yang* is restored which is to say a mental illness is healed (**Figure 3**).

4. Clinical and Basic Research on EWOT

EWOT is regarded as a major clinical non-drug intervention in Chinese medicine psychology. For thousands years, a large amount of medical cases have been kept. Wang *et al.* [17] analyzed 196 ancient cases of disorders induced by seven emotion and found that EWOT was the most commonly applied approach. Yang *et al.* [18] analyzed 122 cases and found similar results as Wang's report. Meanwhile, other Chinese medicine psychology therapies were also applied such as suggestion therapy, stimulation therapy, behavior conduction therapy, etc., which were less frequently used than EWOT. Liu [19] (2009) treated 12 college students suffering phobia only with the technique of POF, resulting in satisfactory outcome. Clinically, EWOT is not only used to treat emotional disorders or mental illness, but also to treat and nurse other diseases e.g. menopause syndrome, irritable bowel syndrome, cardiovascular illnesses [20]-[22]. Ye *et al.* [23] found EWOT could alleviate anxiety and depression of stroke patients and enhanced their enthusiasm and initiative to take part in rehabilitation. Chen [24] reported a positive role EWOT played in the treatment of asthma, supported by the improved quality of life.

Current researches on the foundation are concentrated upon the sorting and editing ancient literature and experiments on the exploration of how the seven emotions impairs organ. Liu *et al.* [25] found the experimental evidence that prenatal fear derived from earthquake mimic could cause developmental insufficiency manifested as slower growth and poorer behavior performances. The finding is a convincing support for the understanding of EWOT. Zhang *et al.* [26] found that maternal fear negatively affected physical and nervous system development of the fetus, with specific alterations in neuro-hormones and gene expression. Interestingly, JKSQW (*Jin Kui Shen Qi Wan*) a preventative Chinese herbal formula reduced these negative outcomes which proved that the kidneys' function was disturbed by fear from another angel. Although plenty of clinical reports on EWOT are available, unfortunately, there are no reports available on fundamental researches of the underlying mechanism of the five techniques in EWOT.

5. EWOT and Conventional Psychology

EWOT plays an essential role in Chinese medicine psychology. It has a distinctive feature of Chinese culture. Recently, researchers have paid attention to the comparative study for it with conventional western psychology therapies. Yan *et al.* [27] found the application of EWOT in the treatment of emotional disorders and mental illnesses was in accordance with some therapies in conventional psychology, for instance, supportive therapy, behavior therapy, cognitive therapy, etc. Huang [8] believed that the technique HOS is pretty similar to positive psychology created by Martin E. P. Seligam. Positive psychology interventions (PPIs) is a promising approach to increase happiness and well-being, that is, treatment methods or intentional activities that aim to cultivate positive feelings, behaviors, or cognitions [28]. With intervention of HOS, approaches making a patient happier e.g. joyful music, conversation, favorite foods, reading and so on are employed to overcome the sorrow the patient encounters. Clinical cases on the treatment of depression and anxiety have been frequently reported [18] [29]. Sufficient evidence shows that PPI is an effective approach to treat depression, anxiety, and other psychological and psychiatric illness [30] [31].

Chen *et al.* [10] believed EWOT might share the same cultural origin with Morita Therapy and the skills of the two systems were similar. But differences existed between the procedures and appetencies. Morita therapy was regarded as the extension of EWOT in Chinese medicine psychology. The goals of Morita therapy are the recognition of facts, obedience to nature, focus on the present, the increase of spontaneous activities, the decrease of self-focused preoccupation, the elimination of indulgence in moods and emotions, the withholding of value judgments, the reduction of intellectualizing, the cessation of escape into a sick role, and the cultivation of a humble mind [32] [33]. The goal deeply rooted in Chinese Buddhism, Taoism and Confucianism [34].

Researchers compared EWOT with behavior therapy. Similarities were found in theoretic foundation and intervention intention, but the procedures, general protocol, and appetency were different [7] [12]. Taking HOS as example, behaviors such as jumping, dancing, howling, playing drum produce joyful emotion, which can decrease the disorders resulting from extreme sorrow or sadness. HOS is very similar with the positive reinforcement in behavior therapy. Positive reinforcement is applied to encourage and reward normal behaviors thus to suppress and replace bad behaviors [35].

6. Conclusion

In conclusion, EWOT is a unique therapeutic approach based on the emotion-will theory in Chinese medicine. Even though the conventional psychological modalities hold predominant status in China, it still requires localized adjustment to become more suitable for Chinese people. Although greatly influenced by western models, contemporary Chinese approaches to counseling reflect the philosophical traditions, cultural history, and indigenous help-seeking practices of a rapid modernizing society [36]. EWOT, rooted in Chinese culture and philosophy, ought to be more suitable without too big obstacles. Owing to the advantages of demanding simple environment, few disturbances, convenience, and compatibility with other Chinese medicine approaches, esp. acupuncture, EWOT is believed to have a promising prosperity and high value in dealing with psychological illness [37]. Disadvantages are unavoidable. Systemic therapeutic protocol has not been established. Lack of standards and effective evaluations remain a primary obstacle impeding the popularization and developing of EWOT. Our team and colleagues are trying to eliminate the obstacles in the following aspects: 1) designing rational trails and experiments to validate the efficacy and provide evidence for clinical use; 2) standardizing operation protocols; 3) developing assessment tools; 4) introducing EWOT abroad and studying it from cross-cultural perspective. We have strong faith in the bright future of this ancient, but new psychological therapy.

Acknowledgements

This study was under the support of National Science Funds of China (NSFC) with the Grant No. 81373710 and Science and Technology Development Fund of Chengdu University of TCM with the Grant No. (ZRMS-201348).

Conflict of Interests

The authors declare no conflict of interests.

References

[1]   Shi, L. and Zhang, C. (2012) Spirituality in Traditional Chinese Medicine. *Pastoral Psychology*, **61**, 959-974. http://dx.doi.org/10.1007/s11089-012-0480-x

[2]   Longhurst, J.C. (2010) Defining Meridians: A Modern Basis of Understanding. *Journal of Acupuncture and Meridian Studies*, **3**, 67-74. http://dx.doi.org/10.1016/S2005-2901(10)60014-3

[3]   Dobos, G. and Tao, I. (2011) The Model of Western Integrative Medicine: The Role of Chinese Medicine. *Chinese Journal of Integrative Medicine*, **17**, 11-20. http://dx.doi.org/10.1007/s11655-011-0601-x

[4]   Pilkington, K. (2010) Anxiety, Depression and Acupuncture: A Review of the Clinical Research. *Autonomic Neuroscience: Basic and Clinical*, **157**, 91-95. http://dx.doi.org/10.1016/j.autneu.2010.04.002

[5]   Wang, J., Li, Y., Ni, C., Zhang, H., Li, L. and Wang, Q. (2011) Cognition Research and Constitutional Classification in Chinese Medicine. *The American Journal of Chinese Medicine*, **39**, 651-660. http://dx.doi.org/10.1142/S0192415X11009093

[6]   Xutian, S., Zhang, J. and Louise, W. (2009) New Exploration and Understanding of Traditional Chinese Medicine. *The*

American Journal of Chinese Medicine, **37**, 411-426. http://dx.doi.org/10.1142/S0192415X09006941

[7] Chen, R., Bi, Y., Qin. Z. and Yang, Y.Q. (2006) Research on Relationship between Behavior Therapy and Three Psychotherapy of TCM. *J. Yunnan Univ. Tradit. Chin. Med.*, **29**, 10-12, 21. (In Chinese)

[8] Huang, Z.B. (2009) Compared Positive Psychotherapy and Emotional Counterbalance Therapy. *Chin. Med. Modern Distance Educ. China*, **7**, 84-85. (In Chinese)

[9] Aung, S.K. (1996) Medical Acupuncture and the Management of Psychosomatic Illness. *Acupuncture in Medicine*, **14**, 84-88. http://dx.doi.org/10.1136/aim.14.2.84

[10] Chen, R., Qin, Z., Zhao, Z.Y., Yang, Y.Q., Chu, G.W., Yang, W.D. and Chen, P. (2004) The Research to the Relationship between the Therapy of Mutual Promotion and Restraint between the Five Elements and the Sentian Therapy. *Chin. Arch. Tradit. Chin. Med.*, **22**, 1218-1219. (In Chinese)

[11] Chan, C., Ying Ho, P.S. and Chow, E. (2002) A Body-Mind-Spirit Model in Health: An Eastern Approach. *Social Work in Health Care*, **34**, 261-282. http://dx.doi.org/10.1300/J010v34n03_02

[12] Lin, K.M. (1981) Traditional Chinese Medical Beliefs and Their Relevance for Mental Illness and Psychiatry. *Normal and Abnormal Behavior in Chinese Culture*, **2**, 95-111. http://dx.doi.org/10.1007/978-94-017-4986-2_6

[13] Sarris, J., Panossian, A., Schweitzer, I., Stough, C. and Scholey, A. (2011) Herbal Medicine for Depression, Anxiety and Insomnia: A Review of Psychopharmacology and Clinical Evidence. *European Neuropsychopharmacology*, **21**, 841-860. http://dx.doi.org/10.1016/j.euroneuro.2011.04.002

[14] Tou, W.I., Chang, S.S., Lee, C.C. and Chen, C.Y.C. (2013) Drug Design for Neuropathic Pain Regulation from Traditional Chinese Medicine. *Scientific Reports*, **3**, 844. http://dx.doi.org/10.1038/srep00844

[15] Ma, Y.X. (2010) The Chinese Medicine Sentiment Will Theory Source and Course Searches Analysis. *Chinese Archives of Traditional Chinese Medicine*, **28**, 1838-1840. (In Chinese)

[16] Wang, X., Sun, H., Zhang, A., Sun, W., Wang, P. and Wang, Z. (2011) Potential Role of Metabolomics Approaches in the Area of Traditional Chinese Medicine: As Pillars of the Bridge between Chinese and Western Medicine. *Journal of Pharmaceutical and Biomedical Analysis*, **55**, 859-868. http://dx.doi.org/10.1016/j.jpba.2011.01.042

[17] Wang, M.Q., Zou, Y.Z., Zheng, Q., Chen, C. and Tang, C.H. (2006) Analysis of 196 Cases in *Ming Yi Lei An* about Morbidity Construction and Male and Female Characteristics of Seven Modes of Emotion Injury. *Modern J. Integrat. Tradit. Chin. West. Med.*, **15**, 983-984. (In Chinese)

[18] Yang, S.M., Gong, X.H. and Hui, L.J. (2008) Discussion about Chinese Medical Therapeutics on Depression Insomnia. *Lishizhen Medicine and Materia Medica Research*, **19**, 639-640. (In Chinese)

[19] Liu, Q. (2009) Clinical Use of Pensiveness Overcoming Fear. *J. Hubei Univ. Chin. Med.*, **11**, 52-53. (In Chinese)

[20] Kronenberg, F. and Fugh-Berman, A. (2002) Complementary and Alternative Medicine for Menopausal Symptoms: A Review of Randomized, Controlled Trials. *Annals of Internal Medicine*, **137**, 805-813. http://dx.doi.org/10.7326/0003-4819-137-10-200211190-00009

[21] Nedrow, A., Miller, J., Walker, M., Nygren, P., Huffman, L.H. and Nelson, H.D. (2006) Complementary and Alternative Therapies for the Management of Menopause-Related Symptoms: A Systematic Evidence Review. *Archives of Internal Medicine*, **166**, 1453-1465. http://dx.doi.org/10.1001/archinte.166.14.1453

[22] Zhang, H., Zhang, X.G., Liang, X.L., Wang, H.Y. and Liu, Y. (2014) Advance of Chinese Medicine Emotion Nursing. *Chinese Journal of Convalescent Medicine*, **23**, 208-209. (In Chinese)

[23] Ye, L.X., Chen, X.L. and Jiang, Y.X. (2012) Impact of Emotion-Will Therapy on the Anxiety of Stroke Patients. *Chin. J. Guangming Chin. Med.*, **27**, 2462-2463. (In Chinese)

[24] Chen, X.L. (2012) Impact of Emotion-Will Therapy on the QoL of Bronchial Asthma. *Chinese Journal of Modern Drug.* **6**, 118-119. (In Chinese)

[25] Liu, Q., Zhang, X.G., Liang, Q.F., Li, F.Y., Gao, J., Liang, X.L. and Yang, Y.Q. (2012) Expounding and Proving Favorable Environment and Earthquake Environment Model from SD Rat Offspring's Weight and Length. *J. Liaoning Univ. Tradit. Chin. Med*, **14**, 82-84. (In Chinese)

[26] Zhang, X.G., Zhang, H., Tan, R., Peng, J.C., Liang, X.L., Liu, Q., Wang, M.Q. and Yu, X.P. (2012) Mechanism of Earthquake Simulation as a Prenatal Stressor Retarding Rat Offspring Development and Chinese Medicine Correcting the Retardation: Hormones and Gene-Expression Alteration. *Evidence-Based Complementary and Alternative Medicine*, **2012**, Article ID: 670362. http://dx.doi.org/10.1155/2012/670362

[27] Yan, S.X., Zou, Y.Z., Cui, J.F. and Cao, Y.J. (2008) A Study of 122 Cases Analysis with Psychotherapy of Traditional Chinese Medicine. *Lishizhen Medicine and Materia Medica Research*, **19**, 1471-1474. (In Chinese)

[28] Sin, N.L. and Lyubomirsky, S. (2009) Enhancing Well-Being and Alleviating Depressive Symptoms with Positive Psychology Interventions: A Practice-Friendly Meta-Analysis. *Journal of Clinical Psychology*, **65**, 467-487. http://dx.doi.org/10.1002/jclp.20593

[29] Sun, Y. (2012) Approach of Application Classical Prescription in Treating Double Heart Disease. *Tianjin Journal of Traditional Chinese Medicine*, **29**, 361-362.

[30] Manicavasagar, V., Horswood, D., Burckhardt, R., Lum, A., Hadzi-Pavlovic, D. and Parker, G. (2014) Feasibility and Effectiveness of a Web-Based Positive Psychology Program for Youth Mental Health: Randomized Controlled Trial. *Journal of Medical Internet Research*, **16**, e140. http://dx.doi.org/10.2196/jmir.3176

[31] Schrank, B., Brownell, T., Tylee, A. and Slade, M. (2014) Positive Psychology: An Approach to Supporting Recovery in Mental Illness. *East Asian Arch Psychiatry*, **24**, 95-103.

[32] Hwang, K.K. and Chang, J. (2009) Self-Cultivation Culturally Sensitive Psychotherapies in Confucian Societies. *The Counseling Psychologist*, **37**, 1010-1032. http://dx.doi.org/10.1177/0011000009339976

[33] Gaudiano, B.A. (2009) Öst's (2008) Methodological Comparison of Clinical Trials of Acceptance and Commitment Therapy Versus Cognitive Behavior Therapy: Matching Apples with Oranges? *Behaviour Research and Therapy*, **47**, 1066-1070. http://dx.doi.org/10.1016/j.brat.2009.07.020

[34] Qian, M., Smith, C.W., Chen, Z. and Xia, G. (2001) Psychotherapy in China: A Review of Its History and Contemporary Directions. *International Journal of Mental Health*, **30**, 49-68.

[35] Kanter, J.W., Rusch, L.C., Busch, A.M. and Sedivy, S.K. (2009) Validation of the Behavioral Activation for Depression Scale (BADS) in a Community Sample with Elevated Depressive Symptoms. *Journal of Behavior Therapy and Experimental Psychiatry*, **31**, 36-42. http://dx.doi.org/10.1007/s10862-008-9088-y

[36] Chang, D.F., Tong, H., Shi, Q. and Zeng, Q. (2005) Letting a Hundred Flowers Bloom: Counseling and Psychotherapy in the People's Republic of China. *J. Mental Health Counseling*, **27**, 104-116.

[37] Gao, Z. (2013) The Strengths and Weaknesses of the Analysis of Emotion Therapy Clinical Applications. *Inner Mongolia J. Chin. Med.*, **32**, 140-141. (In Chinese)

11

Quantitative Estimation of Gallic Acid as Biomarker in Lipitame Tablets by HPTLC Densitometry for Diabetic Dyslipidemia

Sheeraz Siddiqui[1], Khan Usmanghani[1,2], Aqib Zahoor[2], Zeeshan Ahmed Sheikh[2], Saleha Suleman Khan[2]

[1]Faculty of Eastern Medicine, Hamdard University, Karachi, Pakistan
[2]Research and Development Department, Herbion Pakistan (Pvt.) Limited, Karachi, Pakistan
Email: ugk_2005@yahoo.com

Abstract

Lipitame is a poly herbal formulation comprised of *Terminalia arjuna*, *Terminalia belerica*, *Commiphora mukul* and *Phyllanthus emblica*. The formulation is investigated for its analysis evaluation. Biomarkers of three herbs such as *Terminalia arjuna*, *Terminalia belerica*, and *Phyllanthus emblica* have been already cited to contain gallic acid, which was qualitatively and quantitatively estimated. In the present study rapid and inexpensive qualification methods for the quality control of *Terminalia arjuna*, *Terminalia belerica*, *Commiphora mukul* and *Phyllanthus emblica* on thin layer chromatography (TLC) were developed and validated. The solvent system used was toluene:ethyl acetate:formic acid:methanol (12:9:4:0.5). The scanning of plate was performed linearly at 273 nm (absorption) by use of a TLC Scanner III CAMAG with a deuterium source, and the area of spots corresponding to Gallic acid standard was integrated. It was found that gallic acid has been found in the Lipitame tablets on HPTLC densitometry assessment compared with authentic gallic acid reference standard.

Keywords

Lipitame, Tablets, Quantitative Estimation, Densitometry, Diabetic Dyslipidemia

1. Introduction

Inadequately controlled hyperglycemia has been cited as a primary cause of diabetic complications. Increased serum levels of lipids in diabetics (as observed by high levels of triglycerides, total cholesterol and LDL-cholesterol) are partially responsible for and further exacerbate the damaging effects of diabetic hyperglycemia. Because there has been no effective and inexpensive therapeutic option to control glycemic or lipidemic levels in diabetic patients; these patients often suffer severe complications, including nephropathy, retinopathy, neuropathy and atherosclerosis. Although improved glycemic control can reduce the incidence and progression of diabetic complications, implementation and monitoring of glycemic control are arduous and expensive. Many diabetic complications are believed to occur through the oxidative action of glucose. In particular, the high oxidant activity in diabetics coupled with dyslipidemia can lead to the formation of advanced glycation endproducts (AGEs). The presence of AGEs is associated with the formation of arterial atheromas and ultimately, to the development of atherosclerosis. These complications can be mitigated in part by certain antioxidants, including superoxide dismutase, catalase and gluathione. Blocking the oxidative action of glucose responsible for diabetic vascular dysfunction has been validated as one approach to reduce the occurrence of diabetic complications. For example, aldose reductase inhibitors have been shown to prevent or reduce different components of vascular dysfunction, cataract formation, neuropathy and nephropathy in animal model. Furthermore, antioxidants (such as vitamin E, vitamin C and alpha lipoic acid) and antiplatelet agents (such as aspirin and ticlopidine) are being tested to determine their efficacy against the progression of certain diabetic complications, such as non-proliferative diabetic retinopathy.

Although some strides have been made to control glycemic levels and the associated oxidant activity in diabetics, little progress has been made to address the underlying problem of diabetic dyslipidemia. By lowering levels of triglycerides, total cholesterol and LDL-cholesterol in diabetics, development or progression of atherosclerosis and other diabetic complications could be slowed or eradicated. Advantageously, such therapy could be combined with hypoglycemic medications to synergistically treat diabetic patients. Therefore, it is of great importance for the long-term quality of life for diabetic patients that therapeutic options can be made available to treat diabetic dyslipidemia.

The present study is directed to a polyherbal formulation Lipitame comprised of *Terminalia arjuna*, *Terminalia belerica*, *Commiphora mukul* and *Phyllanthus emblica* or a mixture of the active ingredients that have been extracted from such herbs. The herbal compositions of the present invention are effective for the treatment of conditions involving atherosclerosis, stress and anxiety, for use in cardioprotection, cardio-toning, and hyperlipidemia. The medicinal herbal composition such as *Terminalia arjuna* (Roxb.) Wight & Arn., *Terminalia belerica* (Gaertn.) Roxb., *Commiphora mukul* (*Hook ex Stock*) Linn. and *Phyllanthus emblica* Linn. have been used in 10% - 15% by weight of selection of herbal drugs for hyperlipidemia to formulate the dosage which is in tablet form. The Unani herbal drugs have been cited for ethnobotanaical and scientific evidences and are selected for hyperlipidemia after thorough Qarabadini and published literature from electronic journals.

2. Material and Methods

2.1. Formula of Tablet Lipitame (Unani Medicine)

The Unani medicine based tablets "Lipitame" has the following ingredients: *Terminalia arjuna* Bark (Arjun) powder, 1000 gm; *Commiphora mukul* gum resin (muqil), 1300 gm; *Terminalia chebula* (epicarp, harh) powder, 500 gm; *Phyllanthus emblica* fruit (amla) powder, 500 gm.

2.2. Manufacturing Process

All herbs are purchased from the local market then cleaned and examined for their impurities and adulteration. The herbs are weighted according to the formulation and three drugs respectively; **Terminalia chebula, Phyllanthus emblica** and **Terminalia arjuna** are powdered through grinding machine and passed through the sieve no 50. The powder is further checked for its homogenous consistency. **Commiphora mukul** is soaked in water for a night and then boiled along with continuous stirring. After boiling and cooling the solution of *Commiphora mukul* is filtered and the impurities are separated. This cooled filter solution of **Commiphora mukul** is mixed with the powdered drug to develop the granules for tablet making by passing through the sieve no 80. The granules are mixed with binder gum acacia for half hour thoroughly in a mixer.

The granules are dried at 35°C for a day in oven and then these granules were used to make the compressed tablets weighing each 1 gm on average and they were stored in air tight plastic jars. After the above testing the tablets are then send for blister allo-allo foil. Each blister contains ten tablets. Three blisters are put in a box for

30 days dosage (recommended dose 1 tablet at bedtime with plane water).

2.3. Testing Specification

The tablets are checked for disintegration time which is 15 minutes for Lipitame. Hardness of tablets are checked which is 6 kg. Friability test under limit *i.e.* 0.5%. Moisture test is 3%.

2.4. Indications

Primary hyperlipidemia and mixed dyslipidemia, hypertriglyceridemia.

2.5. Dosage and Administration

Recommended dose for Lipitame is one tablet (1 gm) at bedtime with plane water.

2.6. Dosage Form and Packaging

Tablet: 1 gm, 30 tablets (10 × 3 unit dose).

2.7. Contraindication

Active liver and renal diseases, pregnancy, nursing mothers.

2.8. Adverse Effects

Mostly tolerated but in certain cases mild constipation, dry mouth and mild hypotension with headache.

3. Quantitative Estimation of Gallic Acid in Lipitame Tablet by HPTLC Densitometry

Lipitame tablets consist of *Phyllanthus emblica*, *Terminalia chebula*, *Commiphora mukul* and *Terminalia arjuna*. On literature citation it has been found that all the three drugs contains gallic acids where as *Commiphora mukul* elaborate no gallic acid.

Equipment: CAMAG Scanner III, CAMAG Linomat 5 or Equivalent

TLC Plates: HPTLC silica gel G60F$_{254}$

Solvent system:Toluene:Ethyl acetate:Formic acid:Methanol

12:9:4:0.5

Wave length: 273 nm

3.1. Standard Preparation

Prepare standard solution containing known concentration (0.4 mg/ml) by dissolving 4 mg standard of gallic acid monohydrate in 10 ml of methanol.

3.2. Sample Preparation

Weigh about 2.5 g of tablet powder (note exact weight) in to 100 ml of conical flask. Add 30 ml of methanol heat to boil on water bath for 15 minute filter the solution in 250 ml round bottomed flask. Repeat extraction of the remaining residue of tablet powder four times more using 30 × 4 ml portions (5 times in total) as mention above. Collect methanol soluble fraction into the same round-bottomed flask. Evaporate the methanol under vacuum. Dissolve the dry residue in 5 ml of methanol and transfer quantitatively into a 10 ml volumetric flask. Bring the solution's volume to the mark with methanol.

3.3. Procedure

3.3.1. TLC Preparation

a) Perform analysis on 10 × 10 cm HPTLC silica gel G60F$_{254}$ plates with fluorescent indicator.

b) Before start the analysis, HPTLC plate cleans by predevelopment with methanol by ascending method. (Note:

immerse HPTLC Plate in a CAMAG glass chamber (20 × 20 cm), contains 30 ml methanol as solvent system cover the chamber with glass lid and wait to develop the plate to the top with methanol. After complete development, remove the plate from TLC glass chamber and dry it in an oven at 105°C for 5 min.)

3.3.2. Application Procedure

a) Apply three spots of 10 μl (in the form of band) of standard preparation along with three spots of 10 μl of sample preparation as the bands on the same plate by means of a CAMAG Linomat 5 (automated spray-on applicator equipped with a 100 μl syringe and operated with the settings band length 6 mm, distance between bands 14 mm, distance from the plate side edge 15 mm, and distance from the bottom of the plate 15 mm).
b) After sample application, dry the plate in hot air oven at 105°C for 5 min.

3.3.3. TLC Development

a) Develop the plate by immersing sample HPTLC Plate in a CAMAG glass chamber (20 × 20 cm) contained the solvent system (Toluene:Ethyl acetate:Formic acid:Methanol (12:9:4:0.5)), wait to develop the plate to the distance of 8 to 9 cm (see **Figure 1**).
b) After complete development, allow the plate to dry by keeping in fume cupboard for 10 minutes and then keep in hot air oven for 5 min at 105°C.

3.3.4. TLC Scanning

a) Scan the plate in the densitometer by linear scanning at 273 nm (absorption) by use of a TLC Scanner III CAMAG with a deuterium source, and integrate the area of the spots of the sample (see **Figure 2**) and corresponding to gallic acid standard (see **Figure 3**).

Calculate the amount of gallic acid in mg per 10 ml in Lipitame tablet by following formula.

3.4. Content of Gallic Acid

$$\frac{A_{SMP} \times W_{STD} \times f \times \text{Dilution of Smp} \times \text{Application vol. of Smp} \times P \times 0.5}{A_{STD} \times \text{Dilution of Std} \times W_{SMP} \times \text{Application of vol. Std} \times 100}$$

A_{SMP} = Avg. Area of Sample;
A_{STD} = Avg. Area of Standard;
W_{STD} = Weight of Standard, mg;
W_{SMP} = Weight of Sample, g;
Dilution of Smp = Dilution of Sample, ml;
Dilution of Std = Dilution of Standard, ml;
P = Percent Purity of Standard;
f (0.904) = conversion factor of gallic acid monohydrate in gallic acid.
Note: quantity of gallic acid in Lipitame tablet should be NLT 2.72 mg/tablet.

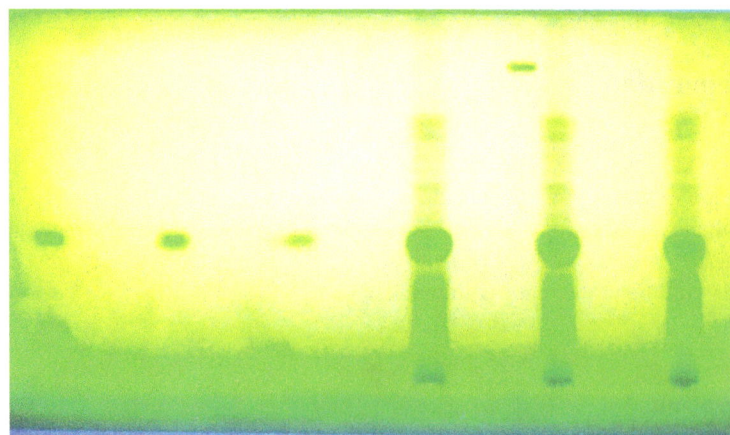

Figure 1. TLC image of gallic acid analysis in Lipitame tablet.

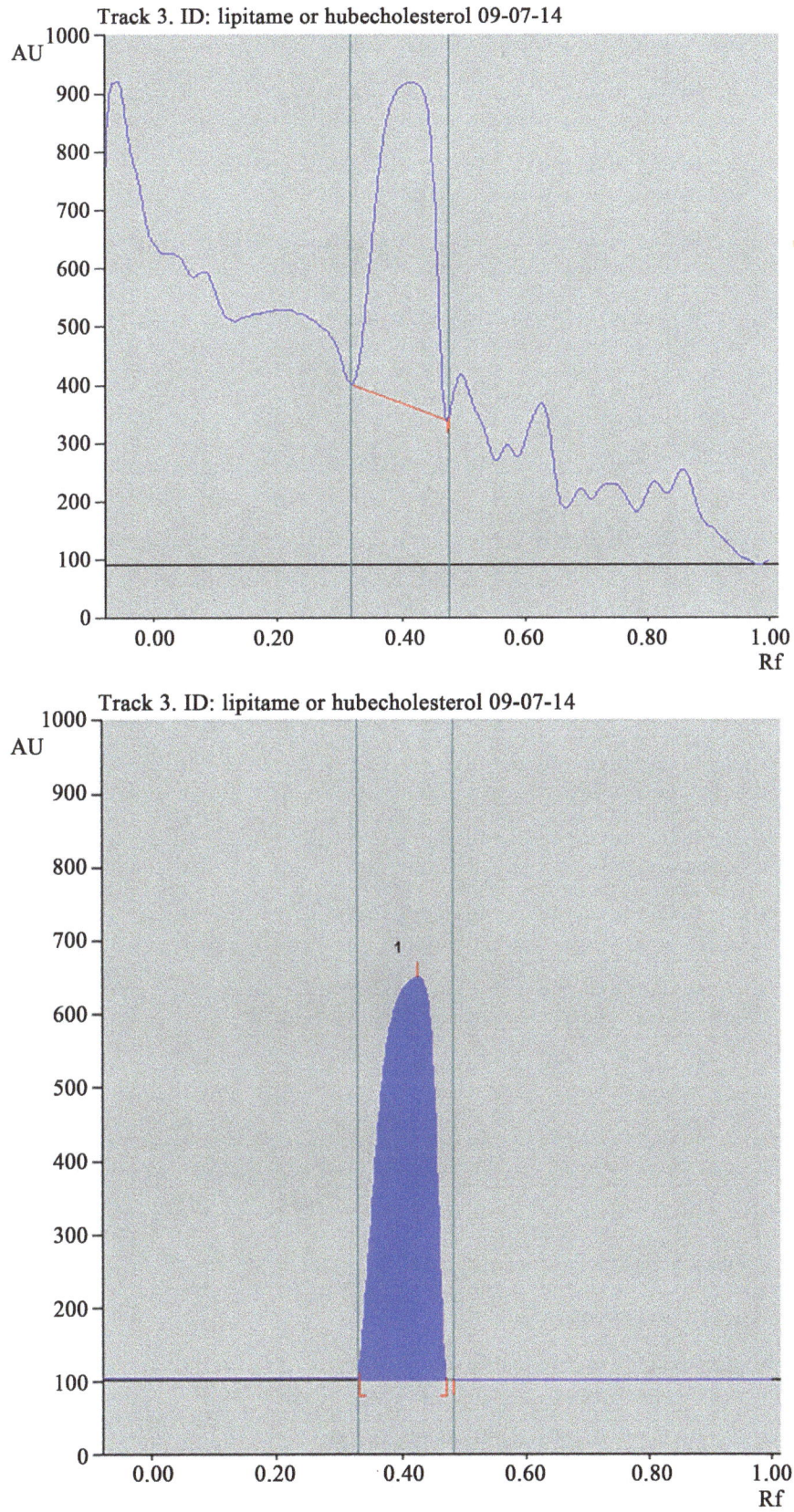

Figure 2. Peak response of gallic acid in Lipitame tablet.

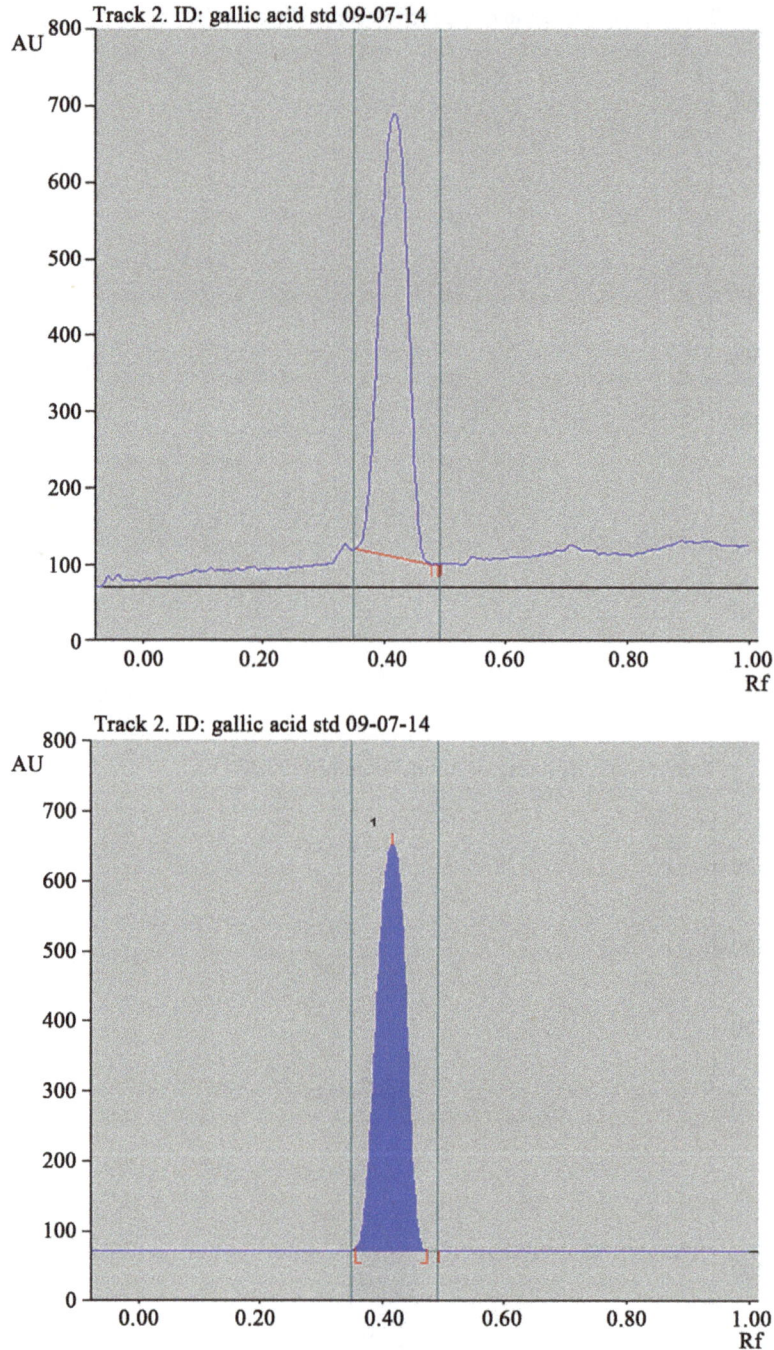

Figure 3. Peak response of gallic acid STD.

4. Results and Discussion

The quantity of gallic acid in Lipitame tablets is as follows:

$$X = \frac{34847.966 \times 4.0 \times 0.904 \times 10 \times 5 \times 99 \times 0.986}{17727.866 \times 2.5454 \times 10 \times 5 \times 100} = 2.72587 \, \text{mg/tablet}$$

The gallic acid content was also tested in a tablet containing high gallic acid (positive controls) and a tablet which did not contain gallic acid (negative controls) with the same method and comparable results were observed, confirming the quantification of gallic acid in the formulation (see **Figure 4**).

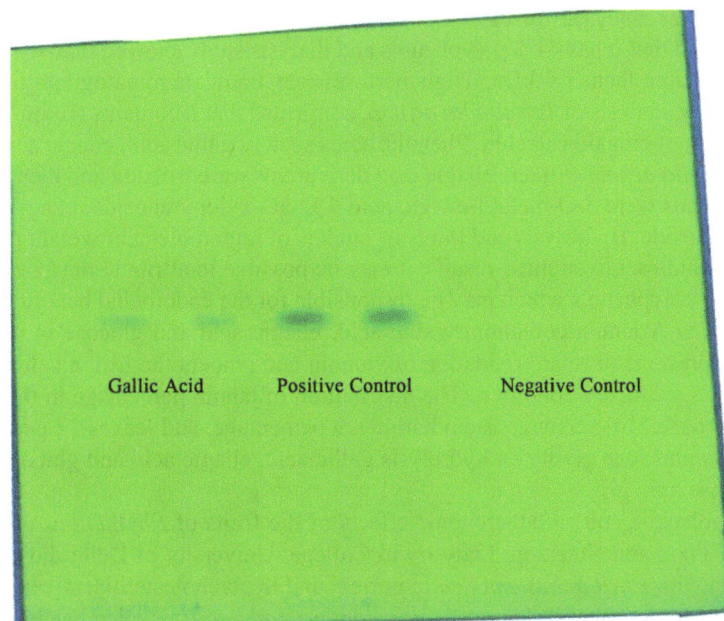

Figure 4. TLC image of Gallic acid, positive and negative control.

Standardization of specific biologically active gallic acid component was identified as material in the poly herbal formulation and quantitative analysis cover identification of chemical components where as quantitative assay measure the identification and level of bio marker in the extract establish the standard of that particular compound for validation. Lipitame is a poly herbal formulation designed by the candidate for clinical trials delineated here with in this research based study. So as to standardized the procedure of the finished tablet product and there in the four different herbal drugs such as *Terminalia arjuna*, *Terminalia belerica*, *Commiphora mukul* and *Phyllanthus emblica*. The formulation organoleptic and physic-chemical characteristics such as identification by TLC, foreign matter, total ash, acid insoluble ash, alcohol; soluble extraction and water soluble extraction are adequately presented herewith. Physico-chemical evaluation such as appearance, pH determination plays a significant role in the quality assessment. The identification with quantitative reaction and preparation of 0.1% alcohol solution exhibit the indication polarity concern of plant materials. TLC was done to augment the determination of gallic acid components and there in the identification was located. All these values show that the physic-chemical parameters adopted the values were within the limits and repeated experiments confirmed the verification. HPLC was performed to confirm the quantitative and qualitative presence of gallic acid for validation. The present standardization under taken reveal compliance with all the physic-chemical and analytical procedures, therefore it is concluded that Lipitame tablets is well standardized product at the base line parameters. As Lipitame consists of *Terminalia arjuna*, *Terminalia belerica*, *Commiphora mukul* and *Phyllanthus emblica* and where as all the three *Terminalia arjuna*, *Terminalia belerica* and *Phyllanthus emblica* contains gallic acid, therefore in the quantitative estimation gallic acid is well represented in different chromatogram. The gallic acid also inhibit the different forms of microbiological organisms so it is useful as well in diabetic dyslipidemia.

If these analytical profiles compared with the work of Modi *et al.* where Zeal cough syrup employing physico-chemical test and bioassay marker compounds agree with quality and potency [1]. In another study Desai and coworker validated the, manufacturing procedure of Vasu cough syrup with the poly herbal formulation for compliance for their reproducibility [2]. The work done by Khadair and associates validation analysis of hederacoside C, the marker of Ivy plant and percentage recovery was given as 99.6% [3]. In a patent of cough syrup the extract of *Adhatoda vasica* along with *Hedychium* spp. and *Curcuma* spp. cough syrup has been validated in greater details [4]. Therefore, Lipitame tablets standardization fall under the specific guide lines of quality herbal medicine and in line with different as mentioned earlier follow the prerequisite for global harmonization.

The bark of *Terminalia arjuna* is known for its heart-health benefits in ayurvedic literature. This has been further supported by *in vivo* studies on animal and human volunteers. But there is no detailed study on identification of the active ingredients such as polyphenols. Polyphenols possesses antioxidant properties and are well-known health actives, it is important to characterise polyphenols in *Terminalia arjuna*. Aqueous extract of *Ter-*

minalia arjuna bark was analysed for its composition and molecular weight distribution by dialysis. Compositional analysis revealed that it has 44% polyphenols and dialysis study showed that 70% of the polyphenols have molecular weight greater than 3.5 kDa. High performance liquid chromatography and liquid chromatography-mass spectrometry analysis of *Terminalia arjuna*, confirmed that it contains flavon-3-ols such as (+)-catechin, (+)-gallocatechin and (−)-epigallocatechin. Phenolic acids such as gallic acid, ellagic acid and its derivatives were also found in *Terminalia arjuna* extract. Ellagic acid derivatives were isolated and their spectral studies indicated that isolated compounds were 3-O-methyl-ellagic acid 4-O-aD-xylopyranoside, ellagic acid and 3-O-methyl ellagic acid 3-O-rhamnoside. Hydrolysis and thiolysis studies of high molecular weight polyphenols indicated that they are proanthocyanidins. Given these results, it may be possible to attribute the heart-health effects of *Terminalia arjuna* to these polyphenols which may be responsible for the endothelial benefit functions like tea [5].

Phyllanthus emblica A tannin containing gallic acid, ellagic acid and glucose in its molecule and naturally present in the fruit, prevents or retard oxidation of vitamin and renders the fruit a valuable antiscorbutic activity in the fresh as well as in the dry condition. The distribution of tannin percentage in the plant is as follows: fruit 28 percentage, twig bark 21 percentage, stem bark 8 - 9 percentage, and leaves 22 percentage respectively. The fruit contains two tannins, one giving on hydrolysis gallic acid, ellagic acid and glucose and the other giving ellagic acid and glucose only [6].

The anticholesterolaemic and antiatherogenic effects of the fruits of *Phyllanthus emblica* have been studied. The Department of Food and Nutrition, Lady Irwin College, University of Delhi did the research over the supplementation of diet with *Phyllanthus emblica* in normal and hypercholesterolaemic men aged 35 - 55 years and found to be effective hypocholesterolemic [7]. *Phyllanthus emblica* fruit juice has been proved to be hypolipidemic at the Department of Home Science (Food and Nutrition), University of Rajasthan, Jaipur, India. The fruit juice was administered at a dose of 5 ml/kg body weight per rabbit per day for 60 days reduced serum cholesterol, triglycerides, phospholipids and LDL levels by 82%, 66%, 77% and 90% respectively [8]. Similarly, the ethanol extract of *Phyllanthus emblica* at a dose of 10 or 20 mg/kg body weight/day for 20 days to rats fed 1% cholesterol diet significantly reduced total, free and LDL-Cholesterol levels in a dose-dependent manner [9]. Flavonoid extracts from the fruits of *Phyllanthus emblica* inhibited synthesis and enhanced degradation of cholesterol via increased hepatic HMG-CoA reductase [10]. In another study, the fruit juice of *Phyllanthus emblica* shown to reduce the oxidative stress induced by ischemic-reperfusion injury (IRI) in rat heart in three different doses 250, 500, 750 mg/kg for 30 days. These changes were due to increased production of myocardial endogenous antioxidants like superoxide dismutase (SOD), catalase and glutathione peroxidase (GPx) in rat [11]. Another study shown the dried fruit powder to be hypolipidemic in rabbits by reducing 42%, 29% and 31% of total cholesterol, triglycerides and LDL-Cholesterol and by increasing 33% of HDL-Cholesterol and reducing 38% of plaque areas in vascular system [12]. *Phyllanthus emblica* aqueous extract also reduces cholesterol in alloxan-induced diabetic rats along with glucose levels [13]. In another study in rabbits for 12 weeks showed increased lipid mobilization and catabolism and retarded deposition of lipids in the extrahepatic tissue [14].

Terminalia chebula fruit contains about 30% of an astringent substance called chebulinic acid, tannic acid about 20% to 40%, gallic acid, resin and some purgative principle of the nature of anthraquinone [15].

Terminalia chebula has been analyzed for its antioxidant activity at different magnitudes of potency [16]. Chebulanin of *Terminalia chebula* has its inhibitory effects on the lipid peroxidation and the production of superoxide radicals in the body [17]. It also possessed hypocholesterolemic activity against cholesterol-induced hypercholesterolemia and atherosclerosis in rabbits [18].

In conclusion, a HPTLC method has been developed and it can be used for the quantitative determination of gallic acid in lipitame tablet. Its mean advantages are its simplicity accuracy and selectivity. This method can also be used conveniently for the estimation of gallic acid in other herbal preparations and may be utilized for standardization purpose.

5. Conclusion

In this study for medicinal plants component, *Terminalia arjuna*, *Terminalia belerica*, *Commiphora mukul* and *Phyllanthus emblica* were formulated for the indication of diabetic dyslipidemia activity. TLC of extract and gallic acid reference standard were carried out. The R_f value (0.4) of gallic acid spot in both extract and reference standard was found comparable under UV light at 254 nm. Quantitative and spectrophotometric estimation of gallic acid was found between the range of 0.035% and 0.07%. HPLC in Liptame tablets was determined as 0.3 mg per 10 ml. The analytical profile of Lipitame tablets and that in gallic acid have been validated to prove that Lipitame tablets in different batches confirmed the verification.

References

[1]   Modi, J., Soni, H., Pandya, K., Patel, G. and Patel, N. (2014) A Detail Phyto-Chemical Evaluation of Herbo-Mineral Formulation Used in Respiratory Diseases. *Journal of Pharmacognosy and Phytochemistry*, **2**, 36-42.

[2]   Desai, L., Oza, J. and Khatri, K. (2012) Prospective Process Validation of Polyherbal Cough Syrup Formulation. *Journal of Advanced Pharmaceutical Technology & Research*, **2**, 225-231.

[3]   Khdair, A., Mohammad, M.K., Tawaha, K., Al-Hamarsheh, E., AlKhatib, H.S., Al-khalidi, B., Bustanji, Y., Najjar, S. and Hudaib, M. (2010) A Validated RP HPLC-PAD Method for the Determination of Hederacoside C in Ivy-Thyme Cough Syrup. *International Journal of Analytical Chemistry*, **2010**, Article ID: 478143, 5 p.

[4]   Herbal Formulation Comprising Extracts of Adhatoda, Hedychium and Curcuma as Cough Syrup, WIPO Patent Application (2005) WO/2005/077393 Kind Code: A1.

[5]   Saha, A., Pawar, V.M. and Jayaraman, S. (2012) Characterisation of Polyphenols in *Terminalia arjuna* Bark Extract. *Indian Journal of Pharmaceutical Sciences*, **74**, 339-347.

[6]   Said, H.M. (1970) Emblica Officinalis. In: *Hamdard Pharmacopoeia of Eastern Medicine*, The Times Press, Karachi, 383.

[7]   Jacob, A., Pandey, M., Kapoor, S. and Saroja, R. (1988) Effect of the Indian Gooseberry (Amla) on Serum Cholesterol Levels in Men Aged 35 - 55 Years. *European Journal of Clinical Nutrition*, **42**, 939-944.

[8]   Mathur, R., Sharma, A., Dixit, V.P. and Varma, M. (1996) Hypolipidaemic Effect of Fruit Juice of *Emblica officinalis* in Cholesterol-Fed Rabbits. *Journal of Ethnopharmacology*, **50**, 61-68. http://dx.doi.org/10.1016/0378-8741(95)01308-3

[9]   Kim, H.J., Yokozawa, T., Kim, H.Y., Tohda, C., Rao, T.P. and Juneja, L.R. (2005) Influence of Amla (*Emblica officinalis* Gaertn.) on Hypercholesterolemia and Lipid Peroxidation in Cholesterol-Fed Rats. *Journal of Nutritional Science and Vitaminology*, **51**, 413-418.

[10]   Anila, L. and Vijayalakshmi, N.R. (2002) Flavonoids from *Emblica officinalis* and *Mangifera indica*—Effectiveness for Dyslipidemia. *Journal of Ethnopharmacology*, **79**, 81-87. http://dx.doi.org/10.1016/S0378-8741(01)00361-0

[11]   Rajak, S., Banerjee, S.K., Sood, S., Dinda, A.K., Gupta, Y.K., Gupta, S.K. and Maulik, S.K. (2004) *Emblica officinalis* Causes Myocardial Adaptation and Protects against Oxidative Stress in Ischemic-Reperfusion Injury in Rats. *Phytotherapy Research*, **18**, 54-60. http://dx.doi.org/10.1002/ptr.1367

[12]   Liu, L., Li, B. and Wang, L. (2005) Effect of *Emblica officinalis* on Formation of Atherosclerotic Plaque in Hypercholesterolemia Rabbits. *Applied Journal of General Practice*, **2**, 97-98.

[13]   Qureshi, S.A., Asad, W. and Sultana, V. (2009) The Effect of Phyllanthus Emblica Linn on Type-II Diabetes, Triglycerides and Liver-Specific Enzyme. *Pakistan Journal of Nutrition*, **8**, 125-128. http://dx.doi.org/10.3923/pjn.2009.125.128

[14]   Mand, J.K., Soni, J.L., Gupta, P.P. and Singh, R. (1991) Effect of Amla (*Ebmlica officinalis*) on the Development of Artherosclerosis in Hypocholesterolemic Rabbits. *Journal of Research and Education in Indian Medicine*, **10**, 1-7.

[15]   Pharmacopoeia Committee (2003) Monographs on Herbal Drugs of Unani Medicine. Drugs Control and Traditional Medicine Division, National Institute of Health, Islamabad, Vol. 1, 530.

[16]   Kapoor, L.D. (1990) Ayurvedic Medicinal Plants. In: *CRC Handbook of Ayurvedic Medicinal Plants*, CRC Press, India, 322.

[17]   Cheng, H.Y., Lin, T.C., Yu, K.H., Yang, C.M. and Lin, C.C. (2003) Antioxidant and Free Radical Scavenging Activities of *Terminalia chebula*. *Biological & Pharmaceutical Bulletin*, **26**, 1331-1335.

[18]   Chattopadhyay, R.R. and Bhattacharyya, S.K. (2007) Plant Review *Terminalia chebula*: An Update. *Pharmacognosy Reviews*, **26**, 1331-1335.

12

Therapeutic Acupunctural Resonance: The Original Research

Adrián Ángel Inchauspe

School of Medical Sciences, National University of La Plata, Buenos Aires, Argentina
Email: adrian.inchauspe@yahoo.com.ar

Abstract

The Chinese managed to interpret not only the natural rhythms of cosmic and seasonal cycles but the chrono-biological rhythms present in human body. What since long ago was merely taken to be a pre-scientific tradition has currently become a tangible reality. Nowadays, the specific frequencies pulsating along each meridian can be measured in hertz—according to its own resonance—as Acupuncture determined thousands of years ago. Their effort to establish a taxonomic classification of all environmental and human phenomena is closely related to Mathematics propositions of Euclid Five Regular Polyhedra, in order to consolidate the axiomatic-deductive model which we can now relate to the Chinese Theory of the Five Elements and their constant changes. As presented in OMICS Group *Traditional Medicine*-2015 *Conference* in Birmingham, it could be also proved that there also exists an inescapable relationship between Pythagoras and the Mathematical foundation of the Pentatonic Chinese Musical Scale. A simple way to incorporate the ideal frequency rhythm for each channel to correct its unbalanced situation is to insert said frequencies through the needles, *by way of "antennae"*, restructuring the meridian's resonance affected and through it, of the Element it belongs to. *Therapeutic Acupunctural Resonance* therefore finds effective application when pins are used as "resonators", putting the frequency of said Element of the channel in line, so that they transmit by means of punctures pure vibratory patterns which shall recondition the Qi flow frequency which has been altered by the Chinese syndrome diagnosed to be treated.

Keywords

Five Elements, Euclid, Pythagoras, Therapeutic Acupunctural Resonance, Qi Recondition

1. Introduction

Back in early 1990s, Dr. Rupert Sheldrake's book *A New Science of Life*: *The Hypothersis of a Formative Cau-*

sation (1982) was edited in Spanish translation as *Unanuevaciencia de la vida* (Editorial Kairós-1990). Sheldrake, a member of the prestigious Royal Society-among whom theorists such as Cooke, Newton, Haley and Hawkins appear-stated his hypothesis on formative causation following the theory of morphic fields, defined as entities which organize and exert influence both on forms and behaviors of natural systems [1].

Based in turn on the Inter-Dependency theory, Sheldrake explains how-because of the co-evolution through collective information fields, *i.e.* morphic fields—every living being acquires its own organization form or pattern, nurtured by habits or thoughts that "*in-form*" the memory of species. Thus, morphic fields determine evolutional development and progress, DNA acting as "tuner" or "decoder" of that memory, providing its structures of the self-determination property [1].

It may well be the case that this theory contributes to interpreting the de-evolutional changes leading so many species to their extinction, according to the pulsating cyclical feature nature has. This enables the vital replacement of ecological niches by means of the generation of new species provided with higher adaptation capacities to their environment.

Unlike I-Ching, Sheldrake states in his works that there exists no such thing as an immutable law, but that there is a temporal reflection of habits which may be modified. In this way, morphogenetical structures conceptually evoke ancient Oriental wisdom to provide foundations to its millennial principles very much like the sacred Geometry established by Euclid as mathematical support for his own age [1] [2].

The Chinese managed to interpret not only the natural rhythms of cosmic and seasonal cycles but also the chrono-biological rhythms present in the human body [3], as we can see in **Figure 1** [2]. What not that long ago was merely taken to be an empirical rendering of a pre-scientific tradition has currently become a tangible reality. Nowadays one can measure the frequency in hertz of each energetic level—according to its own resonance-that Acupuncture had thousands of years ago determined, besides those specific pulsating along each meridian [2] [4].

Their effort to establish a taxonomic classification of all cosmic, seasonal, environmental and human phenomena [3] is closely related to Euclid's proposition for Mathematics of a *Fundamental Classification Theorem* for his Five Regular Polyhedra in order to consolidate the axiomatic-deductive model *par excellence* which we can now relate to the Chinese Theory of the Five Elements and their constant changes [5].

2. Antecedents for This Research

In August 2014, I had the privilege of presenting a hypothesis whereby Chinese Traditional Medicine (TCM) ought to be considered an exact science by tracing a parallelism between the deductions offered by Euclid for his Five Regular Polyhedra and the Theory of the Five Elements proposed by CTM [2] [5].

Euclid (330-275BC.) was a virtuous and inspired mathematician whose transcendental contributions were

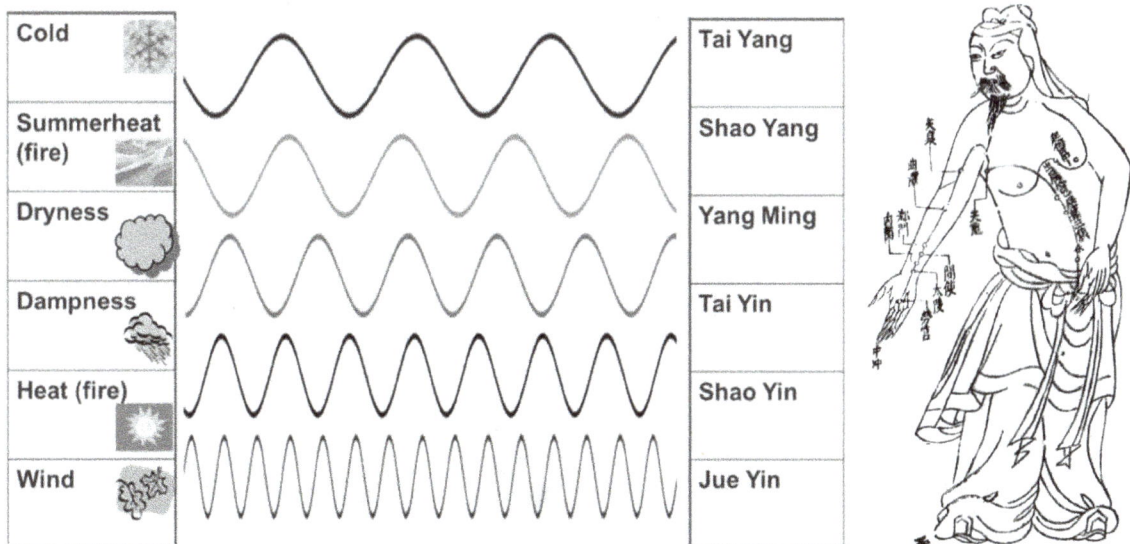

Figure 1. Vibrational frequencies along each energetic level [2].

not limited to the exact sciences (**Figure 2**) [2] but extended to human knowledge in general. The literary dissemination of his posthumous work, *Elements* has been compared—according to Prof. Pedro Miguel González de Urbaneja—to that of the Bible or Don Quixote and a perfect example of the axiomatic-deductive model of thinking [5] [6].

According to Proclus, Euclid—a disciple of Plato's Academy in Athens (**Picture 1**) [2]—was fascinated by the origin and formation of the five regular polyhedra, which he brilliantly presented in the propositions of his Book XIII, the last one of his formidable work [7].

By doing this, Euclid provided Mathematics with a perfect example of the *Classification Theorem*. Following Urbaneja's analysis, from Book VII to X Euclid analysed the geometry of the Platonic Solids; however, in Book XIII, he presented the last propositions for the Five Regular Polyhedra by taking to an optimum level Taetetus' previous line of thought as regards the Five Platonic Solids [8]. Euclid's brilliant work culminates in his last proposition (465, XIII, 18 [7]: "*...to construct the Five Regular Polyhedra inscribing them in a same sphere and then compare the angles of the resulting figures*" [2].

Thus, a sequential definition of those bodies started, beginning by the tetrahedron (XI, 12); the cube (XI, 25); the octahedron (XI, 26); the icosahedron (XI, 27) and the dodecahedron (XI, 28), finding the rates in the angles and then in succession the figures corresponding to each Solid (**Table 1**)—in Pérez de Urbaneja's words—"*with unique geometric genius*" [8].

Thus the famous diagram was introduced showing step by step each of the preceeding propositions (**Figure 3** and **Figure 4**) [7]. Once his Fundamental Theorem was established and demonstrated he was able to assert "*Geometry has ruled that, even though there might exist an infinite number of polygonal shapes, the number of (possible) regular polyhedra is five, not one more, not one few*" (**Figure 5**) [7] [8].

From that moment on, Euclid was devoted to obtaining the faces of such Five Dimensional Solids by determining their configuration in space.

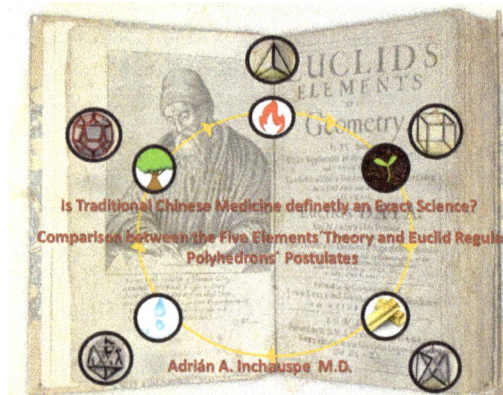

Figure 2. A caption of the August 2014 powerpoint presentation [2].

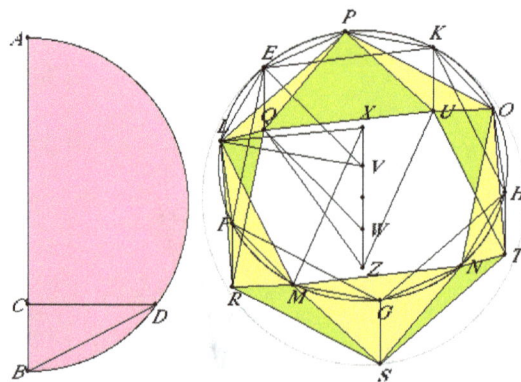

Figure 3. Euclid's elements. Book XIII—Preposition 16.

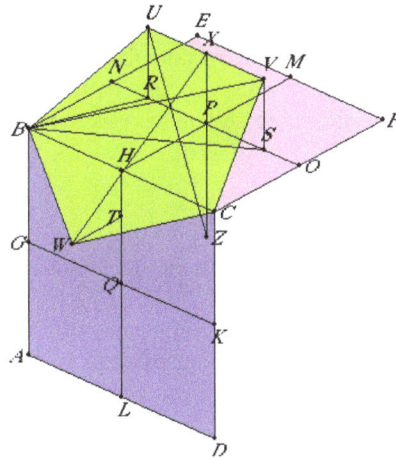

Figure 4. Euclid's elements. Book XIII—Preposition 17.

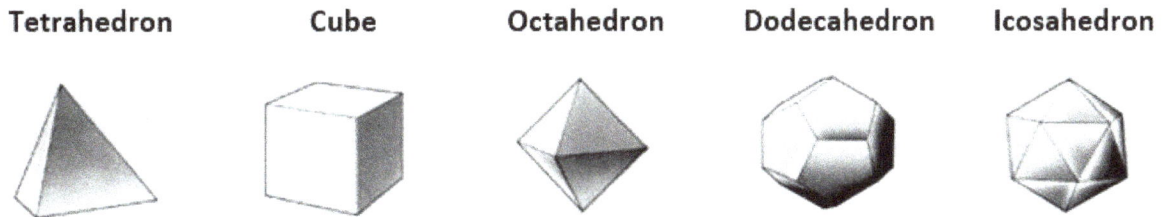

Figure 5. Source: The Five Regular Polyhedra. Euclid. *Elements*. Book I-IV: "General introduction: The constitution of the elements" 1. Gantry Axiomatic, pp. 48-65. [Translated title] Classic Gredos's Library. Madrid, Spain, 2000. Spanish.

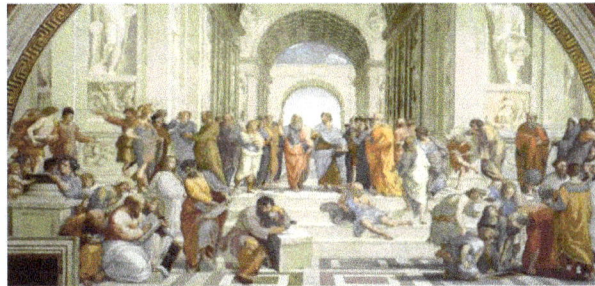

Picture 1. R. Sanzio's The School of Athens [La scuola di Atene, 1510-1511] [2].

Table 1. Euclid's elements. book XIII—Preposition 18th; pp. 355-56. Gredos Classical Library. Madrid, Spain, 2000 [7].

Polyhedron	Proposition	Edge
Tetrahedron	XIII. 13	$\dfrac{2R\sqrt{6}}{3}$
Cube	XIII. 14	$R\sqrt{2}$
Octahedron	XIII 15	$\dfrac{2R\sqrt{3}}{3}$
Icosahedron	XIII 16	$\dfrac{R\sqrt{10}\left(5-\sqrt{5}\right)}{5}$
Dodecahedron	XXX 17	$\dfrac{R\left(\sqrt{5}-\sqrt{3}\right)}{3}$

In a simple demonstration he then concluded that [9] "I am able to state that—other than the figures herein presented—no other figure with equilateral or equiangular angles can be constructed".

W. Dunham's words seem suitable corollary to this part of the work, which I here transcribe: "Euclid has proved no logical argument can produce more than these wonderful images, leaving a mathematically irrefutable document that has lasted for 2300 years so far" [10].

2.1. Euclid's Theoretical Background

Which antecedents did Euclid use as basis for his geometric propositions? Which the stepping stones that enabled such marvelous conclusions?

We have previously mentioned that Euclid was a disciple of Plato's at the Academy in Athens and in the roots of his master's research he seemed to have found inspiration for his deductions [11].

Plato's *Timaeus* (**Picture 2**) is, in fact a work comparable to the Biblical Genesis, where another version of the creative Chaos is offered, analogous to the archaic Chinese vision on the origin of Creation. Plato wrote [11]:

Once his theory on the formation of Dimensional Solids was established, Plato stated *a sequence in the order of Creation*, thus giving origin to the Fundamental Classification Theorem [8] [11]:

The solid figure of the pyramid (tetrahedron) is element and germ of Fire; the second one in the order of creation (octahedron) represents Air, and the third one (icosahedron) is Water; Finally, a cubic form was given to Earth, for this element is the most difficult one to move about, the most tenacious one and its bases are the most solid ones […] Therefore, we had to strive in order to compose those four types of bodies of extraordinary beauty and state that we have captured Nature (**Figure 6**) [11].

2.2. Pythagoras' Theoretical Background

"Everything is conformed by numbers"
Pythagoras

As introduced in last OMICS Group *Traditional Medicine-2015 Conference* in Birmingham, UK, very much like the relationship existing among the Five Elements of Chinese Medicine and Euclid's Five Regular Polyhedra

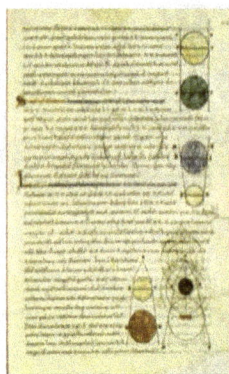

"*Before the Creation, there were no measures or proportions. When God started to put order into the Universe, He first created Fire, Water, Earth and Air...*"

"*First, I believe-and this is beyond any possible doubt- that Fire, Earth, Air and Water are bodies ...*"

"*However, every physical form is also provided with depth ...*"; "*And it is necessary that there is an area surrounding such depth*".

"*Each side (limited by itsarea) consists of triangles...*"; "*Each triangle is developed, each with its right angle and the others, acute ones*".

Picture 2. Medieval manuscript of Calcidius' Latin translation of Plato's *Timaeus.*

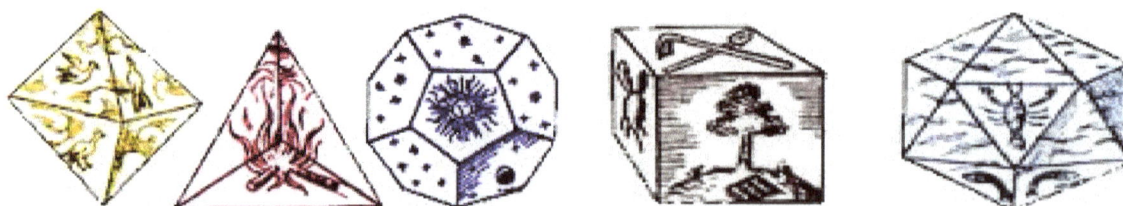

Figure 6. Euclid's elements. Source: Euclid. Elements. Book I-IV: "General introduction: The Constitution of the elements" 1. Gantry axiomatic pp. 48-65. [Translated title] Classic Gredos's Library. Madrid, Spain, 2000. Spanish.

could be proved, there also exists an inescapable relationship between Pythagoras and the Mathematical foundation of the Pentatonic Chinese Musical Scale [12].

Mathematics derives from the Greek *mathema*, which means *knowledge*. And it was Pythagoras himself who divided into four sections the exact knowledge of his time, namely: Geometry-Arithmetic-Astronomy-Music-Mathematics (**Picture 3**) [12]; this, besides the creation of the Multiplication Table, of the theorem bearing his name and the construction of the first regular pentagon, all Mathematical demonstrations through deductive reasoning.

By listening to the sound of a smith's hammer on the anvil, Pythagoras tried to conform and group the sounds he found nice to the ear as well as their combinations that is why he called them *harmonious*. According to Boethius' account, Pythagoras—who was obsessed with the problem of mathematically explaining the fixed intervals of a scale-when passing by a smith's, the musicality of the hammer striking on the anvil called his attention (**Figure 7**) [13].

After having long spent in observation, he eventually made an experiment with five hammers (**Figure 7**) [12]. The weight of four of them was in a proportion of 12, 9, 8 y 6; the fifth one, whose weight did not correspond numerically to the rest, was the one spoiling the perfection of ringing. It was withdrawn and he listened to the hammers again. The biggest of them, whose weight was twice that of the smallest one, was an octave lower. As the weight of hammers 9 and 8 corresponded to the arithmetic means and harmony respectively, from the 12 and 6 weights, Pythagoras though that those two would provide the fixed notes of the scale.

Thus, supported by his mathematical genius, Pythagoras managed to deduce the seven notes we know to date as well as its intervals (**Figure 8**). He provided arithmetical support to those concepts, establishing besides that "*the properties and relationships in musical harmony are determined by numbers.*" [13].

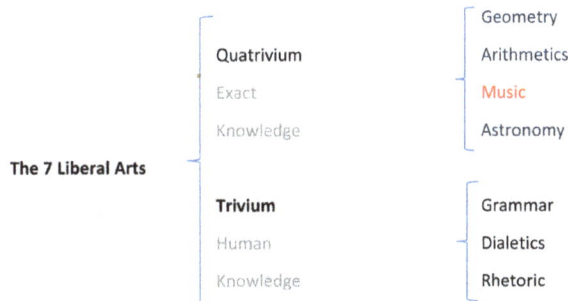

Picture 3. Seven liberal arts. Source:
http://latindecuisine.blogspot.com.ar/2010/01/las-artes-liberales-el-trivium-y-el.html   [12].

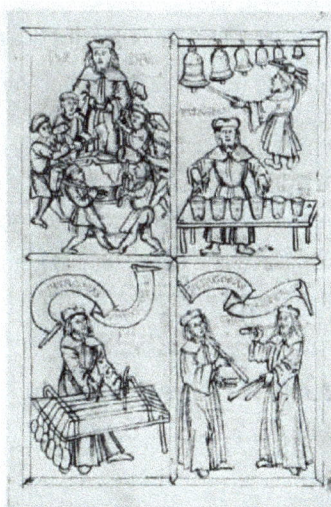

Figure 7. Pythagoras' experiment with the blacksmith five hammers. Source:
http://sauce.pntic.mec.es/~rmarti9/WebBabilonia/Biografias/Pitagoras.htm [13].

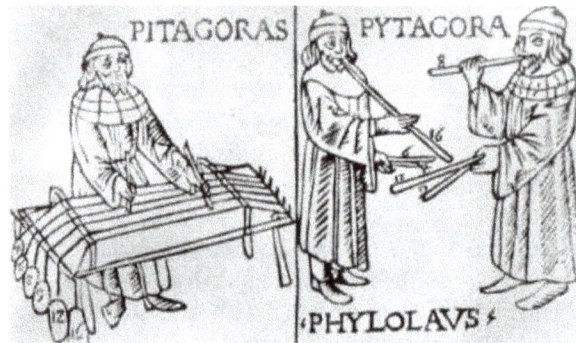

Diatonic Scale: by using strings with lengths in 1:2; 2:3 (harmonic means) and 3:4 (arithmetic means) ratios, Pythagoras verified they vibrated according to relative combinations of such *harmonious sounds*. He also found out, in the musical proportion, that geometric means between two numbers equates the geometric means between its arithmetic and harmonious means [12]:

Thus, the notes we are familiar with, namely **Do-Re-Mi-Fa-Sol-La-Si**, emerged.

Pythagoric Scale: it is based on the following arithmetic sequence. As its geometric progression was immense, they used the Circle of Fifths (**Figure 9**) [13]. When they surpassed the octave, they multiplied by two the length of the string in order to go backwards to the original octave in a 9:8 rate, e.g.,

Sol-Re-La-Mi-Si.

Ethnomusicology classifies pentatonic scales into Hemionic or Anhemitonic ones. The former possess one or more semitones; the latter, does not.

In the Diatonic Scale, the biggest interval existing between notes is the *ditone* (not to be mistaken with scales solely formed by two tones) [12].

Major Pentatonic Scale: it can be formed by a scheme of intervals starting from a concrete note as, for example:

Do-Re-Mi-Sol-La.

Another way is by eliminating degrees VI and VII (withdrawing the sequence from Fa to Si), in which case, the scale remains Do-Re-Mi-Sol-La.

Yet another way of doing this is by following the circle of fifths, counting the "just fifths" as from one prefixed one and ordering the rest as a result, e.g.:

Do-Sol-Re-La-Mi

Minor Pentatonic Scale: it is a scale related to the Major Pentatonic Scale which starts by a not which is not Do [12].

In this brief way we have determined that Chinese music derives from a *pentatonic-anhemitonic major scale*. Its sequence, established by the passing of the Generative Cycle or Cheng is:

Do-La-Mi-Re-Sol

We can notice—as Euclid did to justify the exact scientific mathematical bases for the Five Elements in Chinese Medicine—that the selection of musical notes also has a precise and exact foundation in the development of Music, as Pythagoras explained.

2.3. Retrospective Antedecents for This Research

We shall now briefly refer to a revision of pulse therapy application at specific energetic vibratory frequencies:

2.3.1. Electroacupuncture

Yoshio Manaka was one of the pioneers in employing electric current on needles, trying in this way to "align" the hyper-electro conductive point along the meridian in question. This method, known as *Ryodoraku Method* was used as diagnosis though electro-acupuncture, as well as with therapeutic purposes, based on the frequency and intensity of the stimulus (**Picture 4**) [14]:

- Low frequency and high intensity: illnesses and chronic pain
- High frequency and low intensity: acute illnesses and pain.

Manaka also established his results in a group scale, according to efficiency:

A: very efficient; B: efficient: C: inconstant; D: symptomatic (Parkinson).

There also exists a painless pediatric system, with a few punctures at only 2 mm depth, derived from the previous one, called "*Shonishin Method*" [14].

2.3.2. Acupunctural Lasertherapy

This is a new, painless and efficient acupuncture technique with a wide range of indications.

The acronym LASER (Light Amplification by Stimulated Emission of Radiation) indicates the nature of the power from a narrow beam of monochromatic, coherent light provided by a device which offers such electro-magnetic radiation (**Picture 5**) [15].

Low-power semiconducting lasers (<2 Mw) with a Gallium arsenide diode are inexpensive, efficient and small; they allow for the modulation of the emitted radiation and are used with analgesic-anti-inflammatory purposes in Acupuncture.

Other indications for lasertherapy are stress, anxiety, tobacco addiction, food disorders and other types of addiction [15].

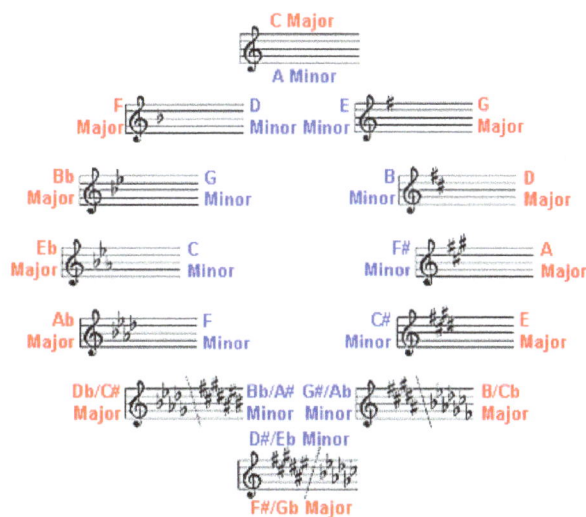

Figure 9. Cycle of fifths. Source: http://sauce.pntic.mec.es/~rmarti9/WebBabilonia/Biografias/Pitagoras.htm) [13].

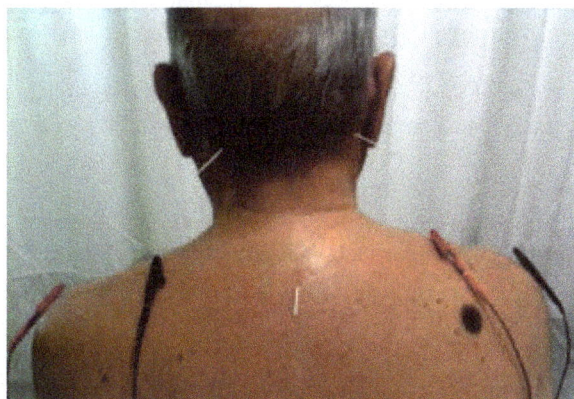

Picture 4. Electroacupuncture [14].

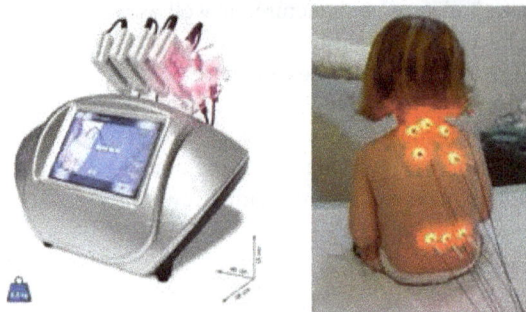

Picture 5. "Laserterapia: Tratamientos innovadores y dolencias". www.lasersalud.es [15].

Sound therapies were already present before considering the theory of *Therapeutic Acupunctural Resonance.* Anyway, let us review some of the contemporary therapies related to this concept.

1) Five ElementFusion

Taoist Spiritual Alchemy also refers to the Five Element Fusion, resorting to a sub-vocalic intonation of specific Healing Sounds for each of the affected organs-following specific positions to be adopted during the session-for each of them [16]:

2) Tama-Do

As regards this, one can read in Webster's New Encyclopaedic Dictionary (1993): Human blood cells can respond to certain sound frequencies, changing form and color. It seems that modified or sick blood cells can heal and be harmonized by sounds.Fabien Maman (French musicianand acupunctor) (**Picture 6**) [17].

Maman uses non-invasive techniques by means of tuning forks on the Command or "Shu" Acupuncture point, accepting that vibration-along the meridian-transmitsits resonance to cell DNA, which in turn resends the message to the meridian's "counterpart" (the energetic field) thus modifying or erasing negative patterns that had an impact on the structures of the physical body.

Tuning forks are tuned to the chromatic scale A = 220 Hz-bearing in mind pianos are tuned at A = 440 Hz-in order to get a deeper resonance and a more prolonged vibration.

French physicist Joel Stemheimer corroborated the tone for each meridian, for he himself was the one to discover the sound frequency of elementary particles ("*The Music of Molecules*"). The tone of the tuning fork has to be in perfect concordance with the note of the organ to be treated [17].

3) TopologySystem

At the Manaka Institute in Japan there is an efficient treatment through micro-stimulations which regulate Acupuncture meridians. Such superficial neuro-stimulation (Neas Topology System) implies a bio-electrical interface which applies an "x" signal system to the human body (**Picture 7**) [18].

Meridians are accessed via the Shu points at wrists and ankles, which generate an electrical field in the whole body. Then, electrical micropotentials are applied, which modify channel conductivity. Their efficiency was proved in cases of blood hypertension; muscle-skeletal conditions; somnolence; anxiety; anguish; pain therapy. A marked improvement of neuronal activity was noticed at the frontal and left brain (concentration-memory) [18].

As to the current therapies with sonic radiations that are accepted and applied in the Western world, we shall make a brief reference to the fundamentals of ultrasound and radiofrequency.

2.3.3. Ultrasound and Radiofrequency

We mention here these allopathic therapies which use radiation with sound or electromagnetic waves; these are closely related to the use of vibrations at specific established frequencies. Below, their main characteristics:

1) Ultrasound

The discovery of the piezoelectric effect in France at the end of 19th century by P. and J. Curie made the generation of waves viable thanks to the first ultrasound generator, built by P. Langenin and C. Chilowsky at the beginning of the 20th century. Crystals such as quartz ($Si\ O_2$) or barium titanate ($Ba\ Ti\ O_3$) are electrically polarized when compression is applied; that is, when an oscillating electric field is applied, they experience mechanical vibrations (**Picture 8**) [19]

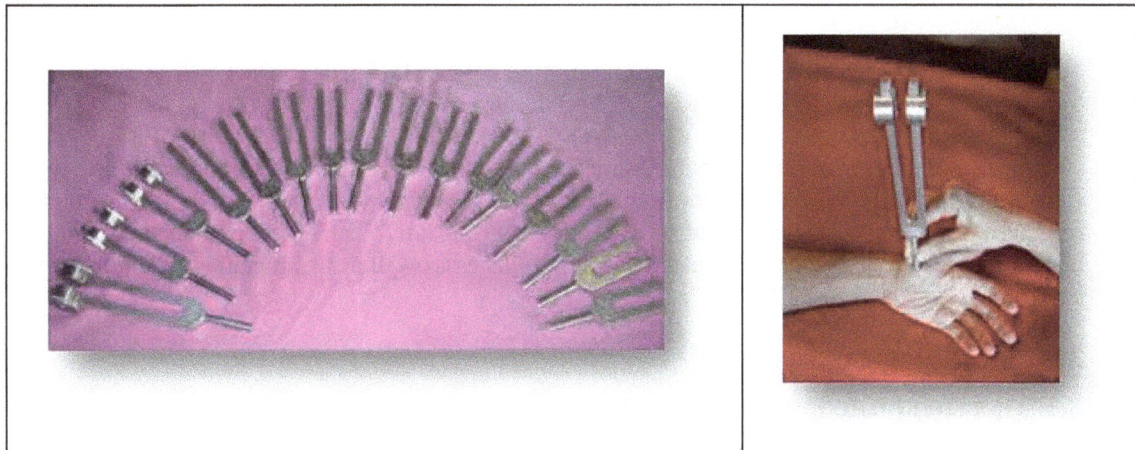

Picture 6. Mamman's tuning forks. Source: http://tama-do.com/product/tuningforks.html [17].

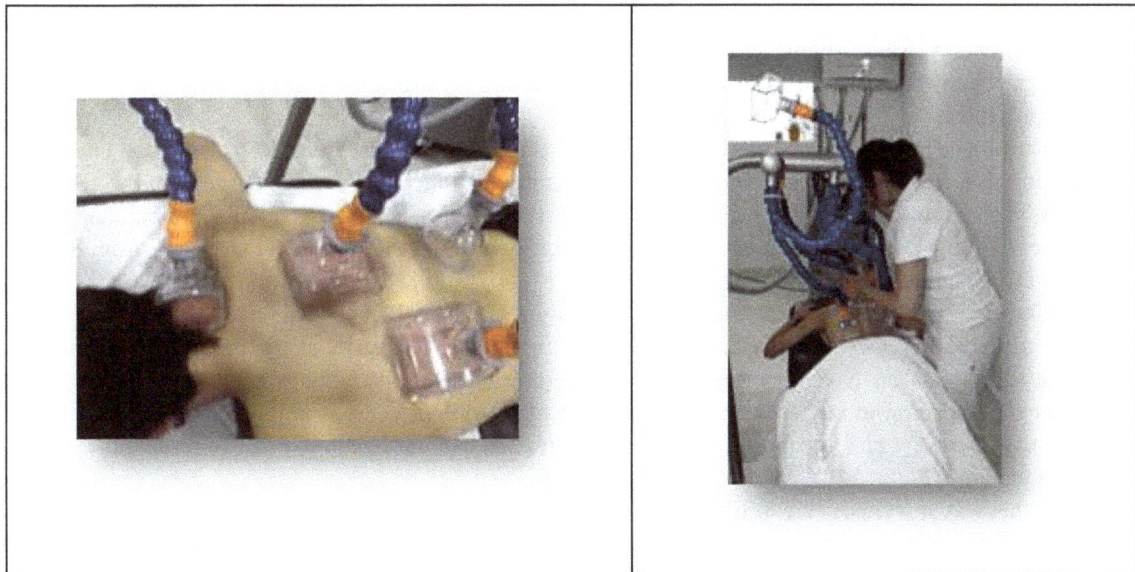

Picture 7. Topology system. Source: http://trade.nosis.com/es/www.acupunturaorekavitoria.com/1311065/s [18].

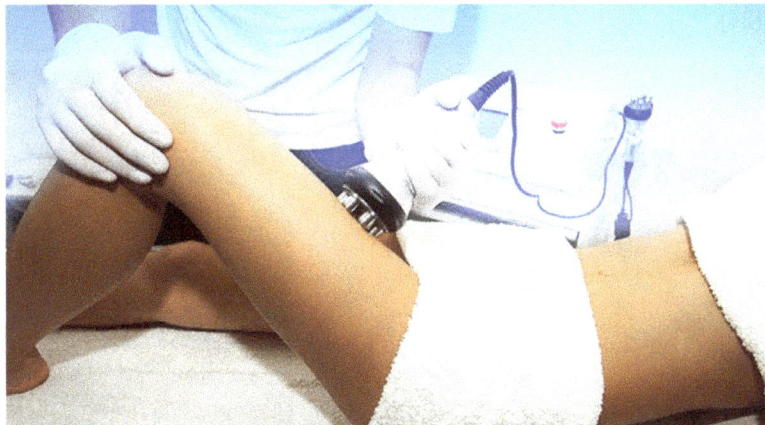

Picture 8. Therapeutic ultrasonography. Link:
http://www.astook.com/ultrasonido-para-adelgazar-o-cavitacion-ultrasonica-pros-y-contras/ [19].

If they coincide with the frequency of the vibration which is that of the tissue or organ to be treated, their width increases as a result of their resonance.

It is extensively used in Physiotherapy and Rehabilitation, for it generates beneficial metabolic changes at the level of the injury, generating heat due to the effect of ultrasound waves.

2) Radiofrequency

It consists of electromagnetic radiations simultaneously oscillating in the electric and magnetic fields; thus, an electric field is generated that changes from positive (+) to negative (−), causing a molecular rotational movement also generating heat. Heat, in turn, affects subcutaneous fatty tissue, favoring lymphatic drainage, circulation within the affected area, the formation of new collagen as well as the migration of fibroblasts (**Picture 9**) [20].

3. Methodological Approach

3.1. Therapeutic Acupunctural Resonance

After my presentation at Beijing—and once Mariano Giacobone's dissertations on the relationships between structure and function in Occidental Medicine and Traditional Chinese Medicine were known [1]—our research focused on assessing how Nature adapts the forms created to the purposes of their consecutive functions. By extrapolating concepts from TCM to biological structures, we can call the *parenchyma*, Yang, as "corporatization" of energy; while Yin makes reference to *stroma*, the structure responsible for "nurturing" matter. Likewise, we can acknowledge the different states of matter and energy, making evident the distinction between the opposite polarities.

If we transfer such concepts to human biology, as regards structure, *Yin* or *Stroma* is the one containing the support tissue; whereas, *Yang* or *Parenchyma* represents the functional organic tissue of living systems [1].

As regards this analysis of "structure function", it was André Thomas—an eminent neurologist of La Salpetriére-who first coined the concept of *muscular tone*, describing the disorders that derive from disturbing it his new research field within Neurology [21] [22].

Likewise, and regarding "structure and its function", Richard B. Fuller defined in his book *Synergetics: Explorations in the Geometry of Thinking* (1975) the notion of Tensegrity as the property "...some structures of isolated components have which are related through a tensional continuous network." [23]. However, it was Kenneth Snelson who adapted this concept to that of *Integrated Tension* in biological systems, thus redefining them as "those systems capable of absorbing compression and distension in order to resume their original structural pattern" (**Picture 10**) [24].

In this way it was possible to interpret the notion of *Integrated Tension* in the structural balance of biological models, where the connective tissue components "interconnect" the whole body through coalescence fascias and the intersticial matrix: another fundamental "collagen wiring," arranged as a body "computing web" [2]. Then, tensegritical systems make an indirect reference to membranes—at architectural biological tissue level—as "connective structures capable of providing support and resistance to torsion, compression, traction, and flexion" (**Figure 10**) [24].

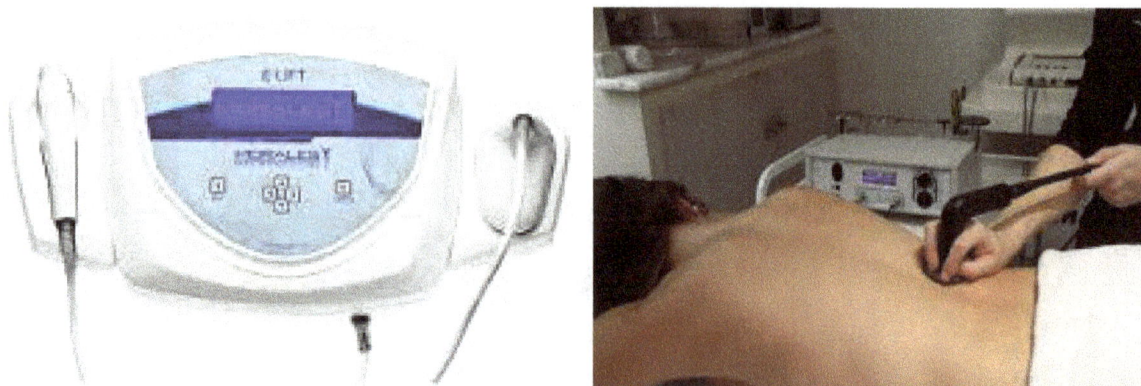

Picture 9. Radiofrequency treatment. Source: Radiofrecuencia: www.esteticasincirugia.es [20].

Thus, the notion of membrane as *fascial network* enables us to adapt the concept of *muscular tone* from Thomas to that of *cellular tone*, which in turn permits the introduction to the definition of Mechanical Transduction as a "property derived from kinetics that cells possess when bearing constant tensions on the filament of their cytoskeleton" (**Figure 11**) [1] [2].

Such knowledge-which can be made evident in physiopathology and therapeutics through the *Tendino-muscular channels*-shows the property the parenchyma has of "encoding" within its cellular DNA the heightened or diminished vibrations transmitted from the stroma nets as a "sensation of arrival and propagation of energy" (*T'chi phenomenon*) [1] [2].

This situation, known as *Kinematic Cellular Indetermination* (**Figure 12**) is also a concept which derives from kinetics and allows for interpretation of the role of (sound) stimuli which-through the connective fascia-reach and influence the expression of nuclear genoma.

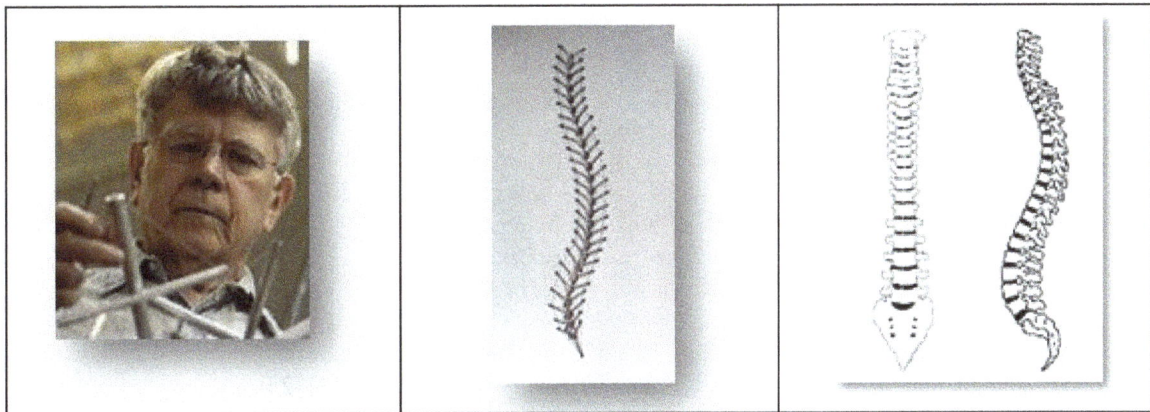

Picture 10. Comparison between tensegrity structures. Source: Gómez Jáuregui, V. "Tensegridad: Estructuras de Compresión Flotante". Cap. 1 "¿Qué es la Ten-segridad?"; pp. 1-2.
http://www.tensegridad.es/Publications/Tensegridad-Estructuras_De_Compresi%C3%B3n_Flotante_by_GOMEZ-JAUREG UI.pdf [24].

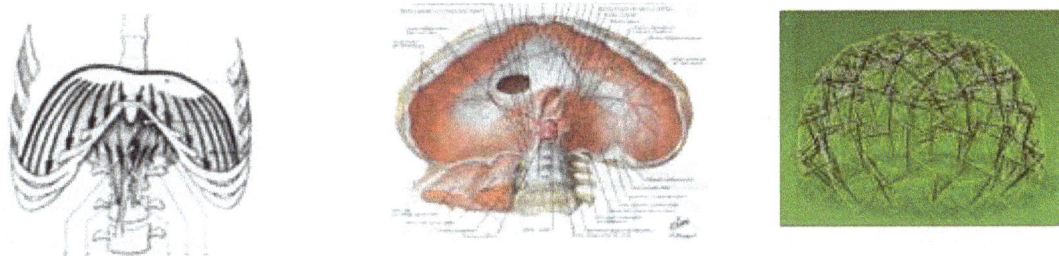

Figure 10. Biological tensegritic systems. Inchauspe, A. "Is Traditional Chinese Medicine definitely an exact science? Comparison between the oriental five elements' theory and Euclid five regular polyhedrons postulates" presented at the 2nd International conference and exhibition on traditional & alternative medicines. 2014. Beijing, China.

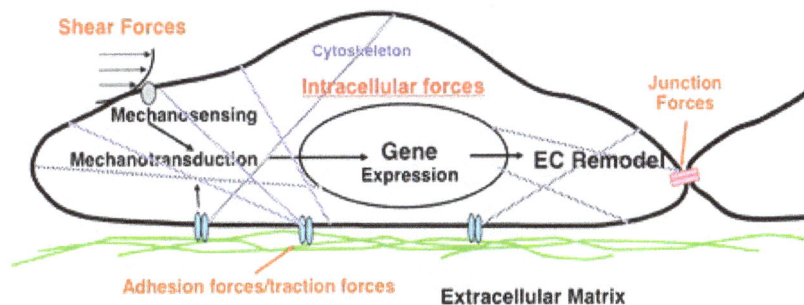

Figure 11. Use of DNA microarray technology to study gene expression. Source: http://chienlab.ucsd.edu/about.

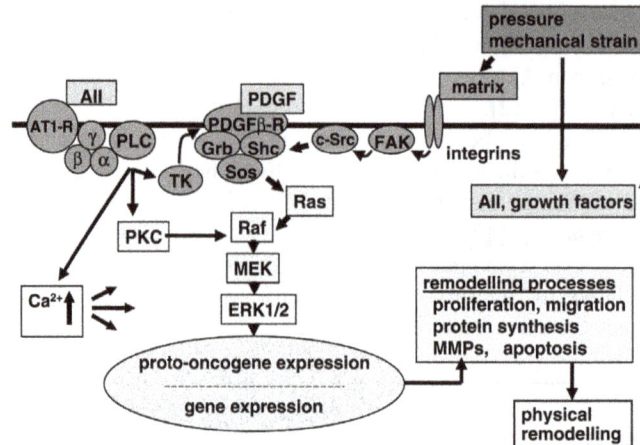

Figure 12. *Kinematic Cellular Indetermination.* Source: Mulvany MJ. Small artery remodeling in hypertension. *Curr Hypertens Rep* **4**: 49-55, 2000.

From what has been described above, this *tensional dimensional integration* enables Nature's complex bio-structural systems to "*integrate*" each of its components in order to *remain stable* and-as epitome for its adaptation capacity-recover its original structural conformation.

All of this shall guide us through—as was stated in I-Ching as the Law of Energy Transformation of Lo-monósov-Lavoisier—to an *understanding of the changes produced at physiological as well as at structural level which occur within a biological system* (the cell being the best example of this) and the way in which there can be adaptation in order to maintain an adequate internal dynamic balance [2] [25].

From the morphic resonance point of view, such morphogenetic changes constitute an example of the intrinsic dynamic balance between biological coded information within cells and the resulting Geometry in the structure and development of organisms (**Picture 11**) [1] [24].

By way of conclusion for this section, let us share a phrase from Rupert eldrake: "Morphogenetic structures add the concepts from Ancient Oriental Wisdom and Sacred Geometry as mathematical support for its own reality" [2].

3.2. Using Morphogenetic Fields in Acupuncture

Morphogenetic Fields

This theory deals with the origin of forms and the behavior of natural systems which ar self-organized by the integrated influence of their morphic fields.

Such complex biostructural systems in Nature integrate the whole with each of their components so as to keep their stability [26]. The analysis needed in order to determine the number of necessary links a determined structure has to resort to so as to remain stable is called *Kinematic Indetermination*. This knowledge aims at clearing up the doubts that structural mechanics displacement presupposes.

Likewise, *morphogenetic fields* (Boveri, 1910) [26] also refer in human beings to an area in the embryo which affects the development of certain organs. Also known as *embryological induction*, a particular cell group which shall give origin to a determined biological structure, even if transplanted to a different part of the embryo (Gilbert, 1949). This concept is often compared to that of tissue *ectopia* [26].

The general aim of a *morphogenetic field* is determined by what the particular cell group shall render even if transplanted to another part of the embryo; thus, the behavior in the development of a cell shall depend on the instructional signals from its surrounding space: they presuppose the *modular* nature of embryo cells because of their relationship genotype/phenotype [26].

According to Gilbert, it is the *morphogenetic field*-and not genes or cells, what functions as the largest ontogenetic unit, the variations of which generate the changes in biological evolution (Gilbert, 1996). Such fields describe the intrinsic relationship existing between the *biological information encoded in cells* and the *realization of the geometric form* in the development of any organism (Morozova, 2013). Following Rupert Sheldrake, both concepts converge in the modern view of morphic resonance [2].

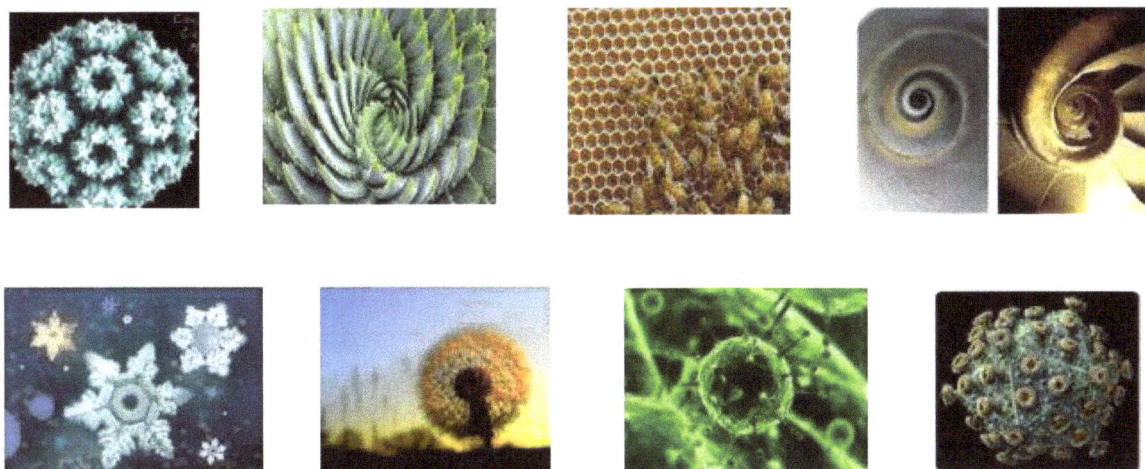

Picture 11. Geometric biological forms within morphic fields [1].

As regards morphic resonance, after having analyzed Euclid's propositions and the knowledge derived from them, such as *Multidimensional Vectorial Geometry* and those relating to biological structures, tensional dimensional integration, we find a current direct application linking morphogenetic fields theory and Chinese Acupuncture [2].

Together with the taxonomic designation proposed by Chinese medicine as regards the Five Main Elements (as Euclid had stated his Five Regular Polyhedra), the determination of corresponding musical notes—*i.e.* the vibrating frequency related to each of them-enables us to reestablish their vibration dynamics thanks to the restructure of their energetic frequency pattern along the meridian in question (**Table 2**) [2], thus:

Ever since *Zou Yen* (350-270 BC.) established the Theory of the Five Movements together with Yin/Yangas an action paradigm in Chinese Medicine, there appears minutely described, a grouping—activing very much as a general classification theorem [2]—over the various cosmic, seasonal, environmental, sensitive, emotional, organoleptic, etc. characteristics upon which the use of that information as support for action on that theory is grounded.

Consequently, as regards the sounds attributed to each of the Elements, the musical notes corresponding to each of the Five Movements are [3]:

- *Wood*: *Do*.
- *Fire*:*La*.
- *Earth*: *Mi*
- *Metal*: *Re*.
- *Water*: *Sol*.

It is worth remembering that Chinese music is pentatonic, a situation that most surely derives from its origin and integrated location within the Five Elements, which Pythagoras determines by means of his harmonic means and the *Circle of fifths* in order to exert their influence and *harmonization* on the meridians representing those Movements.

A simple way to check the incorporation of the ideal frequency rhythm for each cannel or to correct their unbalanced situation—following its Chinese syndromic diagnosis—is to insert through the needles, *by way of "antennae" capturing said frequencies*, which treat the condition, the restructuring frequency for the meridian affected and through it, of the element it belongs to.

Morphic Resonance therefore finds effective application when pins are used as "resonators" which put the frequency of the element of the channel in line, so that they transmit by means of punctures pure vibratory patterns which shall recondition the Qi flow frequency which has been altered by the Chinese syndrome diagnosed to be treated.

The way to access such harmonizing frequency might be established in different ways, for example:

- *Use the Cheng or Generative Cycle sequence, starting from Wood in cases of organs (Yin) or from Metal in case of viscerae (Yang).*

Table 2. Energetic frequency patterns in the main meridians [2].

-Lung: 824 Hz (Reininger)	-Small intestine: 791 Hz
-Large intestine: 553 Hz.	-Urinary Bladder: 667 Hz
-Stomach: 471 Hz.	-Kidney: 611 Hz
-Spleen-Pancreas: 702 Hz	-Sanjiao: 732 Hz
-Heart: 492 Hz.	-Gallbladder: 583 Hz
-Liver: 442 Hz	-Du y RenMai: 493,88 Hz.
-Pericardium/Triple Warmer Meridian: 497 Hz.	

(An example for organ tonification: *Do-La-Mi-Re-Sol*)

(An example for visceraetonification: *Re-Sol-Do-La-Mi*)

Any of these sequences can be started by stimulating each note repeatedly till its influence on the channel is assured (6 - 8 times, approximately, at 4 - 6 second intervals in between each resonance)

- *Use the manual pin turn tonification clockwise in case of tonification; and anticlockwise in cases needing-dispersal.*
- *Another way of stimulating is considering the Mother-son rule of the Five Elements, i.e. using for tonification the sound of the previous Element to that affected in the Generative Cycle, and in cases of sedation, the following one within the sequence of that cycle.*
- *Stimulation by election of the musical sound which is suitable to the constitutional biotype of the patient or according to any of the TCM's principles.*
- *Stimulation according to the pairing of meridians which establish the Six Energetic Levels conforming TCM, that is:*

Tai Yang Tai Yin

Shao Yang Jue Yin

Yang Ming Shao Yin

Lastly, one of the most efficient stimulations is the *consecutive sequence* of Therapeutic Acupunctural Resonance and, through the Chen or Generative Cycle sequence notes played in an almost uninterrupted succession (Do-La-Mi-Re-Sol) at intervals no longer than 4 - 6 seconds in between each note. This idea is supported in the five ancient Shu command points present in all the main meridians in Acupuncture, which presupposes—from TCM's perspective—the inclusion of the Five Element Theory in all meridians, thus enabling their regulation and energetic "tuning" by means of adding their sequenced resonances.

All the aforementioned is an already solved issue from the Exact Sciences. In the following scheme we can appreciate how Prof. Pedro González Urbaneja has managed to draw every inter-transformation of the Elements within the same polyhedron (**Figure 13**) [8].

In keeping with the demonstration or Euclid's regular polyhedral and the Elements of TCM, here we can see the mathematical support justifying the five elements and their sequential changes at each of the main meridians that make up our bioenergetic acupunctural map [25].

4. Results

The basics of tissue reconstruction of Therapeutic Acupunctural Resonance, supported by Mechanical Transduction, Kinematic Indetermination and Dimensional Tensional Integration which justify cell restructure and remodeling through the action of the resonance phenomenon throughout the cell's cytoskeleton (see the diagram in Euclid's work section above—**Figure 11** and **Figure 12**)

The *reverberation* produced by the musical note chosen would recompose the vibrational patter, coupling and modifying the abnormal frequency of the meridian, liberating the normal flow of energy through it. In the course of this neurosensitive transportation several patients experience an enhanced pain threshold as well as an increased pain resistance threshold, very much like when *PS* is experienced [27].

It may be worth noticing, as regards what was stated above, that certain phenomena take place, e.g. *T'chi* (*i.e.* "energy arrival") and that of a "strengthened" propagated sensation or neurosensitive transportation referred to by patients who are treated with Therapeutic Acupunctural Resonance themselves. Unlike the first one which

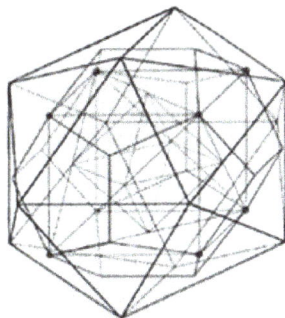

Figure 13. Inter-transformation among five regular polyhedral. Source: González Urbaneja, P. M. "Euclid's Elements—Mathematics's Bible"; "The Propositions" [Translated title] pgonzale@pie.xtec.es [8].

means: to experience a certain numbness, pain, distension, languor or heaviness [28], neurosensitive transportation shares with SP the characteristic feeling of "*something that is running*". Such "tickling" sensation could—following Edward LimChai-his—be attributed to the activation of neural fibers [29], more particularly, those of a peptidergic type [30].

Very much as the *T'chi phenomenon* is associated to pain, distension and heaviness after puncture (probably carried by type III or IV neural fibers), such *neurosensitive transportation*, which derives from the sound stimulation of the sounds corresponding to the Five Elements, appears in patients after the phenomenon mentioned above-like SP-without distinction of age, sex, race or occupation [28] in a painless way, and it is highlighted by patients when the line involving the meridians involved continues to be drawn, or is deviated from the original channel in order to reach the area affected [31].

According to TCM principles, the continuous flow of Qi through the main Acupuncture channels ensures good health in patients.

It is believed that *SP* sensation recognition could be located at Brodmann areas 3, 1 and 2. Identical deductions are made for *neurosensitive transportation*, even though it may also manifest in dissociated from cortical activity [31].

According to Bossy, "…conscious sensation is cortical; however, the organization of such sensation is to be found at the primary centers of the neural axis" [32]. According to the embryological agreement between the skin and the Central Nervous System (let us remember the neural tube is generated from ectoderm during the third week of pregnancy) when the impulse runs through medullar areas corresponding to dermic stimuli [33]. As Lópezcompares in his magnificent book: "at the medulla area (plates II and III) there exists what can be considered a 'controlpanel' which informs us on the movement of a 'train' of neural impulses generated at skin level" [34].

The feeling of relaxation and a tendency to sleep-natural consequences after an acupunctural treatment-were more deeply manifested and for a longer period. In those cases in which patients evoke flavors, aromas or any of the categories listed in taxonomies of the Five Elements [2], it is worth to carefully confront them with their medical records so that a link between the reason for consultation and the actual disease of the nosological entities each patient presents may be established.

By way of conclusion for this section, let me share what Edgardo Lópezstated about propagated sensation: "Definitively, in order for this sensation to be made manifest, it requires a chain of impulses in an inter-neural structure together with a projection phenomenon from the upper structures. This sensation makes good communication between central levels and the periphery manifest. When it emerges clinically, we may rest assured of good initial acupunctural effects." [35].

5. Discussion

A new phenomenon called *neurosensitive transportation* is equivalent to that one known as "*propagated sensation*" (*PS*) and the "*ghost limb*" sensation after amputation occurred [36]; but I would like to differentiate them from that achieved by stimulation of the pin's sound vibrations used for this technique.

Very much like PS, it does not exactly follow the somatosensory distribution of the neural territories where it is applied. It circulates slowly and bilaterally and does not restrict itself to one or more dermatomes [33] [36].

Unlike PS effect, *neurosensitive transportation* does not seem to slow down at the level of main articulations, neither because of cold nor because of pressure [30] [36].

Following the results obtained, the influence exerted by *neurosensitive transportation* may—like *PS*—reach the viscera or organ targeted for its application, thereby producing significant changes which favor the functionality of these structures when sensation reaches them [30] [37].

Now let us assess some of the formal counter indications of the therapies referred to at the beginning of this work:

Counter indications as regards acupunctural lasertherapy also list a series of situations to bear in mind:

- Retinaldamage
- Neoplastic processes (biostimulating ones and accelerators of cellular mitosis)
- Bacterial foci (acceleration and extension of the problem)
- Metal prosthesis—IUD—pacemaker (increased heat)
- Photosensitiveepilepsy
- Pro-photosensitive medicines (steroids-antimalarials-quinacrine-tetracyclines)
- Pregnancy[38].

As regards other therapies already mentioned such as ultrasound and radiofrequency, [39] it is known, for example, that the frequency used by those devices ranges between 1 to 3 megahertz (1,000,000 - 3,000,000 Hz). Such high frequency ultrasound radiation values may provoke blood cell stagnation in parallel with the ultrasound beam. Parasitical Head Radiations over 100 mW/cm^2 may even cause symptoms in those providing treatment (International Electrotechnical Committee—IEC).

Both for ultrasound as for radiofrequency there are, however, formal counter indications for therapeutic application:

- Severe heart disorders
- Coagulationdisorders
- Connective and neuro-muscular tissue diseases
- Collagenimplants
- Cancer
- Pacemakers and metal prothesis
- Pregnancy andlactation [19].

As regards *Therapeutic Acupunctural Resonance*, this simple practice:

- Does not presuppose any complication whatsoever beyond that of needle insertion (except for specific cases such as multifocal epilepsy).
- It "resets" the energetic flow in order to "unclog" obstructions and ensure the continuous flow through the channels selected for the therapeutics in question by a subjective amplification of the classical propagated sensation or *neurosensitive transportation*.
- It provides an enhanced emotional and general wellbeing, which is referred to by patients treated [40].
- Its practice has no counter indications as the conditions mentioned above and does not produce any secondary effects. The addition of this concept to classical acupuncture does in no way affect diagnosis nor the selection of points to be used, it does not delay the estimated time allotted to a patient for treatment.

Besides, it has the advantage of not muffling down sound vibrations—a situation that most often occurs when using the tuning fork directly on the points—which perpetuates stimuli on the needles (which receive sound waves like an antenna transmitting the frequency directly to the meridian in question)

In this therapeutic variation of Acupuncture, the patient has a more active role both because he is conscious and reveals new sensations to correlate with his clinical condition and because it offers a most useful *sensitive feedback* as reference of the therapeutic effect. This neurosensitive transportation effect (this denomination is used to separate it from the "pure" propagated sensation which results from classical Acupuncture) may be identified in cases of low tolerance to anxiety, where it has proved a most effective relaxation which seems to separate—however temporarily—their Space-Time problem [41].

6. Conclusions

Ultrasound and radiofrequency therapies have become ever more relevant since the 1990s for post-surgical or post-traumatic rehabilitation treatments; that fact makes the therapeutic action of specific vibratory frequencies evident to achieve those results.

There have been other suggestions of *vibratory therapies* inspired in Acupuncture (such as that of Maman, in France) [17] and the *bio-impedance of the meridians* preceding this technique, though they were developed from different scientific hypotheses.

Therapeutic Acupunctural Resonance finds its foundations in the classical principles of TCM, and in no way does it subvert any of its therapeutic principles; this is done with a view to promote the effect of punctures in order to achieve faster and more effective recoveries.

Thanks to that knowledge the Chinese might have objectified the trajectory of the classical meridians and understand the expression of more complex physiopathological reactions the body has projected onto the skin surface, notwithstanding their lack of knowledge about the fundamental role played by the Central Nervous System. Nowadays, the analgesic and regulatory effects resulting from *PS* achieved by means of the Acupunctural therapeutics are widely accepted [41].

Following the concordance of the Classification Fundamental Theorem, both what *Euclid* stated in his propositions for regular polyhedra and the principles in TCM and its Five Elements clearly show—from a theoretical point of view—that there is scientific ground to access the therapeutic manifestation of the *Morphic Resonance* phenomenon during Acupuncture sessions, as was presented last year during the World Congress of Complementary and Alternative Medicines and before the authorities of the National Medical Science Chinese Academy at Beijing.

Likewise, *Pythagoras'* proposal paved the way for the development of Music and it is thanks to his arithmetic demonstration of the harmonic means and the Circle of Fifths we were able to find scientific-mathematical support to the development of Chinese pentatonic music involving the Theory of the Five Elements that regulates their TCM. This theory was introduced in *the 3rd International Traditional Medicine* 2015 *Conferen*ce-Birmingham. United Kingdom from August 03-05, 2015 [42].

In Sheldrake's words, both Ancient Oriental Wisdom and Sacred Geometry—on flowing into Morphic Resonance—become *"causative agents in the development and maintenance of biological forms"*. To some extent, both kinds of knowledge are compatible for the concordance of the *internal dynamic balance* that encourage and keep the vital processes.

References

[1] Giacobone, M. (2009) Morphic Resonance: A New Approach from Biology. [Translated Title]. (In Spanish). http://budacuantico.blogspot.com.ar/2009/12/la-resonancia-morfica-un-nuevo-enfoque.html

[2] Inchauspe, A. (2014) Is Traditional Chinese Medicine Definitely an Exact Science? Comparison between the Oriental Five Elements' Theory and Euclid Five Regular Polyhedrons postulates. Presented at the *2nd International Conference and Exhibition on Traditional & Alternative Medicines*, 25-26 August 2014, Beijing. http://dx.doi.org/10.4172/2327-5162.s1.006

[3] Jovenich, E. (2005) Theory of Five Movements. [Translated Title]. Monograph of the Educational Department of the Argentinian Society of Acupuncture, Buenos Aires. (In Spanish).

[4] Coop. Group of Investigation of PSC Beijing (1979) A Survey of Occurrence of the Phenomenon of Propagated Sensation along Channels in the Mass and Its Basic Properties. Adv.in acup. and acup-an.

[5] Euclides (2000) *Elements*. Book I-IV: General Introduction: The Constitution of the Elements. 1. Gantry Axiomatic, 48-65. [Translated Title]. Classic Gredos's Library, Madrid. (In Spanish).

[6] Euclides (1996) *Elements*. Books I-XIII. [Translated Title]. Classic Gredos's Library, Madrid. (In Spanish).

[7] Euclides (2000) *Elements*. Book XIII: Proposition 18, 355-56. [Translated Title]. Classic Gredos's Library, Madrid. (In Spanish).

[8] González Urbaneja, P.M. "Euclid's Elements—Mathematics's Bible"; "The Propositions" [Translated Title]. (In Spanish).

[9] González Urbaneja, P.M. "Critical Study of Three Works Summit of the Mathematics Literature". Volume I: "Euclid's Elements", 168: "The Philosophical Substrate of Euclid's Elements". [Translated Title]. (In Spanish).

[10] Dunham, W. (1996) Travel through the Geniuses. 116. [Translated Title] Editorial Pyramid. Madrid. (In Spanish).

[11] Cooper, J.M. and Hutchinson, D.S., Eds. (1997) Plato: Complete Works. "Timaeus" (Or "Timaeus' Exposure"). Introduction: "Constitution of the Elements." (Translated Title). 52nd Patricio de Azcarate Edition, Volume 6, Madrid. (In

Spanish)

[12] Cecilia Tomasini. http://latindecuisine.blogspot.com.ar/2010/01/las-artes-liberales-el-trivium-y-el.html

[13] Wikipedia. http://sauce.pntic.mec.es/~rmarti9/WebBabilonia/Biografias/Pitagoras.htm

[14] Cobos Romana, R. (2013) Acupuncture, Electroacupuncture, Moxibustion and Related Techniques in the Treatment of Pain. *Revista de la Sociedad Española del Dolor*, **20**, 263-277. (In Spanish)

[15] Laser Therapy: Innovative Treatments and Ailments. (In Spanish) www.lasersalud.es

[16] Chia, M.M. (1995) Fusion of the Five Elements—Basic and Advanced Meditations to Transform Negative Emotions. Formula Four: Transforming Negative Emotions of the Bodies into Usable Energy. (Translated Title). Ed. Sirio, S.A. Málaga, 91. (In Spanish)

[17] Tama—Do. http://tama-do.com/product/tuningforks.html

[18] Topology System. http://trade.nosis.com/es/www.acupunturaorekavitoria.com/1311065/s

[19] Ultrasound Therapy. (Translated Title) (In Spanish)
      http://www.astook.com/ultrasonido-para-adelgazar-o-cavitacion-ultrasonica-pros-y-contras/

[20] Radiofrequency. (Translated Title) (In Spanish) www.esteticasincirugia.es

[21] Alix, G. "Muscle Tone and Strength". "Generalities"; Neurologic Evaluation of the Newborn". 569. (Translated Title) (In Spanish)
      http://se-neonatal.es/Portals/0/Publicaciones/EVALUACION_NEUROLOGICA_DEL_RECIEN_NACIDO[2].pdf

[22] Barraquer-Bordas, L. and Codina-Puiggros, A. Semiotics of Muscle Tone Disorders, 20. (In Spanish)
      http://www.bvsde.paho.org/texcom/revneuropsiquiatr/LBarraquer-Bordas.pdf

[23] Fuller, R.B. (1975) Synergetics: Explorations in the Geometry of Thinking.
      www.amazon.com/Synergetics-Explorations-Geometry-Buckminster-uller/dp/002541870K

[24] Gómez Jáuregui, V. Tensegrity: Structures of Floating Compression. Cap. 1 "What It Is Tensegrity?" 1-2. (In Spanish)
      http://www.tensegridad.es/Publications/Tensegridad-Estructuras_De_Compresi%C3%B3n_Flotante_by_GOMEZ-JAU REGUI.pdf

[25] Chamfrault, A. and Van Nghi, N. (1969) L Énergétique Humaine en Medecine Chinoise. Cap. I "Nociones Generales". Imprimiérede la Carente, Angoulenne, 8.

[26] Morphogenetic Field (Developmental Biology) (In Spanish)
      https://es.wikipedia.org/wiki/Campo_morfogen%C3%A9tico_(biolog%C3%ADa_del_desarrollo)

[27] Meng, Z.W. (1979) The Origin, Establishment and Prospect of the Theory of Channels. Symposium of Acupuncture and Moxibustion and Acupuncture Anaesthesia. Beijing, June 1979.

[28] López, E. (2005) Chapter 2: Neurophysiology of Acupuncture—His Mind-Body Relationship. Ed. Serendipity, Buenos Aires, 51. (In Spanish)

[29] Pan, C.C., *et al.* (1991) A Research of Correlation on Neuropeptide and Electroacupuncture Effect. *Acta Medica Sínica*, **6**, 6.

[30] Coop. Group of Investigation of PSC (1979) A Survey of Occurrence of the Phenomenon of Propagated Sensation along Channels in the Mass and Its Basic Properties. Adv. In acup, And Acup-an. Beijing, June 1979.

[31] The People's Hospital of Guangxi Zhuangzu Automous Region (1979) The Phenomenon of Propagated Sensation along Channel and the Cerebral Cortex. Department of Neurological Surgery, Adv. In acup and acup-an. Beijing, 1979.

[32] Bossy, J. (1973) Bases morphologiques et functionelles de l'analgesieacupunturale. Giornaledell Academia de Medicina de Torino, Torino.

[33] Bossy, J. (1995) Les dermalgiesreflexes. Acupuncture Course in Buenos Aires.

[34] López, E. (2005) Chapter 2: Neurophysiology of Acupuncture—His Mind-Body Relationship. Ed. Serendipity, Buenos Aires, 55. (In Spanish)

[35] López, E. (2005) Chapter 2: Neurophysiology of Acupuncture—His Mind-Body Relationship. Ed. Serendipity, Buenos Aires, 56. (In Spanish)

[36] Res. Group of Acup., Anesth. Instit. of Medic. and Pharm. of Fujian, China, 1979.

[37] López, E. (2005) Chapter 2: Neurophysiology of Acupuncture—His Mind-Body Relationship. Ed. Serendipity, Buenos Aires, 53. (In Spanish)

[38] Hernández Díaz, A. The Low-Power Laser in Current Medicine. (In Spanish)
      http://www.sld.cu/galerias/pdf/sitios/rehabilitacion-fis/(monografia._el_laser_de_baja_potencia_en_la_medicina_actua _205)_1.pdf

[39] Radiofrecuency. (In Spanish) www.tesis.uchile.cl

[40] López, E. (2005) Chapter 2: Neurophysiology of Acupuncture—His Mind-Body Relationship. Ed. Serendipity, Buenos Aires, 54. (In Spanish)

[41] Res. Group of Acup. Anaesth. Instit.of. Medic and Pharm. of Fujian. (1979) The Electroencephalographic Observations on Subjects with Marked Propagated Sensations along Channels. Adv. in Acup. and Acup-on. Beijing, June 1979.

[42] Inchauspe, A. (2015) Therapeutic Acupunctural Resonance. *Proceedings of the 3rd International Traditional Medicine 2015 Conference*, Birmingham, 3-5 August 2015.

13

Application of Customized Navigated Template for Percutaneous Radiofrequency Thermocoagulation Treatment of Primary Trigeminal Neuralgia

Peng Wang[1,2], Tiebao Gu[3], Zefeng Zhang[2], Huiqun Wu[4], Dafeng Ji[5*]

[1]Department of Pediartic Orthopaedic, Nantong Rich Hospital Affiliated to Yangzhou University, Yangzhou, China
[2]Jiangsu ZhouKe Medical Instrument Technological Co., Ltd., Nantong, China
[3]Department of Pain, Nantong Convalescence Hospital Affiliated to Nantong University, Nantong, China
[4]Medical College Affiliated to Nantong University, Nantong, China
[5]Digital Medical Center, Fudan University, Shanghai, China
Email: wangpeng1981-cool@163.com, gutb-015@sina.com, 44664383@qq.com, *13111010058@fudan.edu.cn

Abstract

Objective: To investigate the successful rate and accuracy of percutaneous radiofrequency thermocoagulation (PRT) for treatment of primary trigeminal neuralgia (PTN) with customized navigated template via three dimensional (3D) printing technique. Methods: 65 patients with PTN were recruited from January 2014 to March 2015 and randomly divided into two groups: template group (n = 28) and traditional group (n = 37). The patients in traditional group received PRT under guidance of C-arm fluoroscopy, while the ones in template group were treated with customized navigated templates. The data of time, depth and accuracy rate of puncture, the average effective dose equivalent of radiation, complications after operation were collected and analyzed. Results: No intra-operative failures occurred in the template group: the pain was alleviated immediately after operation. Accuracy rate of the template group was 100% while 96% was achieved in traditional group. However, the average time of puncture by the template was significantly reduced compared with traditional group (2.37 ± 0.64 minutes and 24.2 ± 6.55 minutes, respectively; $P < 0.001$). Meanwhile, the average effective dose equivalent of radiation was apparently reduced compared to the traditional group. The depth of puncture in operation was mostly close to the results of simulation (9.45 ± 0.58 cm and 9.33 ± 0.87 cm respectively, $P > 0.05$). No complications were observed in template group while several complications such as blooding, leakage of cerebrospinal fluid and dizziness were observed in traditional group. Conclusion: The application of customized template is advocated for improving the accuracy of PRT.

---

*Corresponding author.

Keywords

Primary Trigeminal Neuralgia, 3D Printing, Radiofrequency, Customized Template

1. Introduction

The primary trigeminal neuralgia (PTN) is a nerve disorder that causes a stabbing or electric-shock-like pain in parts of the face, which was first reported by Nicolas Andri in 1756 [1]. The pathogen of PTN is still unclear, while secondary TN is always a sequela of malformation, tumors or trauma in encephalic surgeries [2] [3].

At present, kinds of medicines and surgical operations have been utilized for the treatment of TN [3]-[9]. However, the results seem not to be completely satisfying. In many cases, drug resistant becomes more regularly and attacks become more and more resistant over time so that some patients cannot endure the side effects of high-dose medication and intolerably intense pain after clinical treatments. At last, a surgical procedure is necessary. Nonetheless, recurrence rate of pain after surgical operations is significantly high. Meanwhile, the good effects of surgical procedure depend on the experiences of surgeons and familiarities with variances of encephalic anatomy. Recently, the PRT caters for more patients' demands due to immediate pain relief, lower expense, minimal trauma and high efficacy [10]. However, several complications such as masticatory weakness, dysesthesia, and corneal numbness were also reported due to long procedure and high dose of radiation [11]. Thus, in order to promote the accuracy of PRT, various instruments such as computer temography, neuro-navigation were applied [12] [13]. But these applications are limited due to the price and unstable effects. Nevertheless, the ratio of pain relief was not as high as expected [14].

Nowadays, computer-aided surgery (CAS) has been more and more widespread and significant in the field of most surgeries [15]-[17], which could reduce risks and promote accuracy through preoperative simulation. Furthermore, more studies on 3D printing can make the ideas of CAS come true [18]-[21]. However, there is seldom applications in pain management been reported recently. The character of pain management is micro-trauma, variance of anatomic structures, which fits the advantage of CAS and 3D printing techniques.

Thus, this study aims to design a novel method to increase the ratio of the management accuracy of pain surgery. We designed a customized navigated template with Computer-Aided Design (CAD) and 3D printing according to the patient specific anatomy. The results show that the customized navigated template increased the accuracy, and reduced the procedure and the dose of radiation of PRT.

2. Patients and Methods

2.1. Patients

The study was approved by local ethics committee at the Nantong Convalescence Hospital affiliated to Nantong University. Written informed consent was made for enrolled patients. As secondary TN being excluded, 65 outpatients from Jan 2014 to March 2015 were recruited and were divided randomly into two groups: the template group and traditional group. The patients in traditional group received PRT under guidance of C-arm fluoroscopy, while the ones in template group were treated with customized navigated templates combined with C-arm fluroscopy. Basic characteristics of the two groups were shown as **Table 1**.

2.2. Surgical Procedures

All patients were received thin slice CT scanning (SIMENS AVANTO Germany). Every slice is 0.625mm thick. The scanning region is from top of the skull to maxillary. The imaging data was imported as Digital Imaging and Communications in Medicine (DICOM) files into Materialise's Interactive Medical Image Control System (MIMICS) 16.0 software (Materialise, Leuven, Belgium).

After image processing which contained thresh-holding and morphological operations, the model of encephalic and skin model were visualized (**Figure 1**), which were saved as Stereolithography (STL) files.

The diameter of foreman oval was measured (**Figure 2(a)**) and the best puncture path was simulated in 3-Matic software 8.0 (Materialise, Leuven, Belgium), meanwhile, the depth of puncture (from skin to foreman oval) was measured (**Figure 2(b)**).

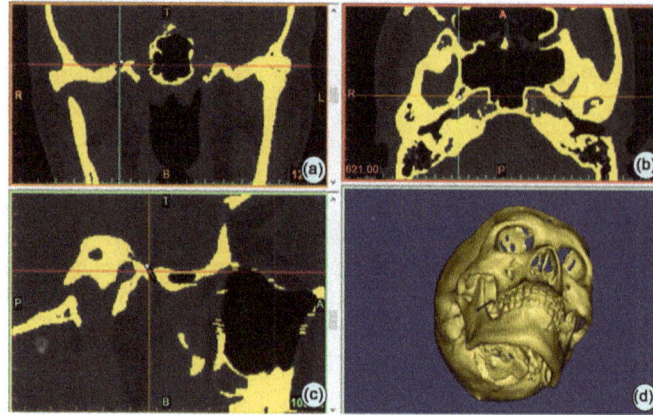

Figure 1. The DICOM data imported into MIMICS and mask of bone was threshold segmented ((a) coronal position; (b) axial position; (c) sagittal postion; (d) the reconstruction of bone).

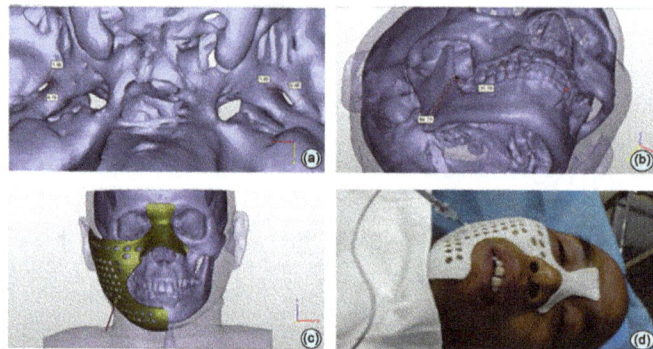

Figure 2. Model of the patient, morphology of foramen oval and digital template. (a) The morphology of foramen oval; (b) The optimum path of simulator punction; (c) the digital customized template; (d) the plate fit maxillofacial surface in operation.

Table 1. Basic characteristics comparison between two groups.

	Template group (N = 28)	Traditional group (N = 37)
Age	56.4 ± 12.7	61.2 ± 18.3
Lateralization		
right	18	21
left	8	15
bilateral	2	1
Region of pain		
V1	0	0
V2	8	11
V3	13	21
V1+V2	0	0
V2+V3	7	5
V1+V3	0	0
V1+V2+V3	0	0

With application of reverse-engineering, the osteal characteristics of face such as zygomatic arch and nasal root were picked up and the digital customized navigated template was extruded 2 mm and trimmed the edges (**Figure 2(c)**), the needle way is designed according the path from skin to foremen oval. In the end, the digital template was fabricated from 3D printing machine (ZRapid, SLA300, China).The material of template is polylactic acid which is bio-compatible without any poisonous effect.

The patient was in supine position. The maxillofacial region was sterilized by iodophor and the template was sterilized by plasma. After the puncture region was locally anaesthetized, the template was put to fit the maxillofacial surface shape (**Figure 2(d)**). According to the depth of puncture in simulation, minimal adjust was made with the guidance of the C-arm fluoscopy. When the target pot was achieved, the pain was triggered. At the same time, the following PRT operations were performed as a matter of routine as soon as possible.

2.3. Data Collection

Time of surgical process, depth and accuracy of punture was measured; meanwhile, average effective dose equivalent of radiation was recorded with Radiation detector (LK3600, ReKo China).

2.4. Statistical Analysis

SPSS13.0 was utilized in this paper. Student's-t test was used for analysis. P value less than 0.05 was considered to be statistically significant.

3. Results

1) Basic characteristics of two groups (**Table 1**).
2) The diameters of foramen ovale (**Table 2**).
3) The time of puncture and accuracy rate of operation and adverse reactions (**Table 3**).
4) The depth of puncture between simulation and real procedure (**Table 4**).

Table 2. The difference of foramen ovale between two groups.

		Template group	Traditional group
Left	length	7.13 ± 2.46^{ac}	6.28 ± 1.67
	width	3.46 ± 2.58^{bd}	2.73 ± 3.16
Right	length	6.51 ± 2.84	7.72 ± 2.19
	width	2.93 ± 2.55	3.54 ± 2.19

Note: a represents $P > 0.05$, while left length between template group and traditional group; b represents $P > 0.05$, while left width between template group and traditional group; c represents $P>0.05$, while length between left and right; d represents $P > 0.05$, while width between left and right.

Table 3. The variance of time, accuracy rate, dose of radiation and adverse reactions of puncture.

	Template group	Traditional group
Time of puncture (min)	$2.1 \pm 1.2^{**}$	20.2 ± 8.6
Total procedure time (min)	$30.5 \pm 4.6^{**}$	62.3 ± 10.4
Accuracy rate (percent)	$100^{\#}$	96
Average effective dose equivalent of radiation (mSv)	$0.152 \pm 0.003^{**}$	1.438 ± 0.032
Adverse reactions		
blooding	1	4
leakage of cerebrospinal fluid	0	2
dizzness	0	1
nausea	0	0
vomit	0	0
diplopia	0	0
Cost (RMB)	$6538.4 \pm 38.7^{\#}$	6928.3 ± 45.2

$^{**}P < 0.001$; $^{\#}P > 0.05$.

Table 4. The depth of puncture between simulation and real procedure.

	Simulation procedure	Real procedure
Depth of puncture	$9.05 \pm 0.58^{*}$	9.55 ± 0.83

$^{*}P > 0.05$.

4. Discussion

This paper provides a new method to promote the accuracy of percutaneous punction and reduces the time of repeat puncture and radiation according to the CAS and 3D printing technique apparently.

The morphological variations of foramen ovale has been described in recent studies [22] [23], but most of them noted that there was no significantly difference between two sides. However, in this study, some foreman ovales had narrow morphology, and both sides were obviously asymmetry. During the simulation, traditional puncture path could hardly get the target pot successfully. Considering this, we moved the percutaneous puncture pot laterally so that the puncture path got the target successfully without any obstacle. In this case, the surgical process time was about 1min and the routine was succeed with customized template.

Jen-Tsung Yang et al. suggested 3D reconstruction can improve the accuracy of puncture apparently [24]. However, it was necessary to adjust the tip of needle several times during operation. According to the articles [24] [25], the average time of procedure was about 20 minutes, whereas 1 to 2 minutes was spent in the template group. Moreover, the template can be stored for repetitive case. Meanwhile, several paths can be integrated in one template in case of failure from one path. In this study, a zygomatic path was finally selected and succeeded after the failure of foreman ovale path in a V2 case.

However, a patient with transient blooding appeared during the procedure, but the effect was satisfying. The authors consumed that the design of template was from the CT data, which was hardly to show soft tissue especially blood vessel. Osteal marks were only considered in this study while some important soft tissues have been ignored. This study was focused on improving the accuracy rate of PRT and reducing the dose of radiation, however, there was no significantly increase in the cost of discharge and simulation training.

5. Conclusion

The customized template can improve the accuracy of percutaneous puncture and reduce the dose of radiation for PTN.

Acknowledgements

Special thanks to the technical and administrative staff at Jiangsu ZhouKe Medical Instrument Technological Co., Ltd., thanks to Mr. Zefeng Zhang for excellent support in supplying equipment and Dr. Huiqun Wu in language management to facilitate this study.

Declaration of Interest

The authors received no financial support. However, no direct funding was received for this particular study.

References

[1]   Andre, N.A. (1756) Observations Pratiques Sur Les Maladies de L'Uretre. Chez Delaguette, Imprimeur de College et de L'Academie Roy de Chir, Paris, 318-382.

[2]   Gronseth, G., Cruccu, G., Alksne, J., Argoff, C., Brainin, M., Burchiel, K., et al. (2008) Practice Parameter: The Diagnostic Evaluation and Treatment of Trigeminal Neuralgia (An Evidence-Based Review): Report of the Quality Standards Subcommittee of the American Academy of Neurology and the European Federation of Neurological Societies. Neurology, **71**, 1183-1190. http://dx.doi.org/10.1212/01.wnl.0000326598.83183.04

[3]   Guo, Z., Ouyang, H. and Cheng, Z. (2011) Surgical Treatment of Parapontine Epidermoid Cysts Presenting with Trigeminal Neuralgia. Journal of Clinical Neuroscience, **18**, 344-346. http://dx.doi.org/10.1016/j.jocn.2010.07.110

[4]   Sindrup, S.H. and Jensen, T.S. (2002) Pharmacotherapy of Trigezminal Neuralgia. Clinical Journal of Pain, **18**, 22-27. http://dx.doi.org/10.1097/00002508-200201000-00004

[5]   Zakrzewska, J.M. and Linskey, M.E. (2014) Trigeminal Neuralgia. *BMJ Clin Evid,* pii: 1207.
http://dx.doi.org/10.1136/bmj.g474

[6]   Montano, N., Papacci, F., Cioni, B., Di Bonaventura, R. and Meglio, M. (2013) What Is the Best Treatment of Drug-Resistant Trigeminal Neuralgia in Patients Affected by Multiple Sclerosis? A Literature Analysis of Surgical Procedures. *Clinical Neurology and Neurosurgery,* **115**, 567-572. http://dx.doi.org/10.1016/j.clineuro.2012.07.011

[7]   Akram, H., Mirza, B., Kitchen, N. and Zakrzewska, J.M. (2013) Proposal for Evaluating the Quality of Reports of Surgical Interventions in the Treatment of Trigeminal Neuralgia: The Surgical Trigeminal Neuralgia Score. *Neurosurgical Focus,* **35**, E3. http://dx.doi.org/10.3171/2013.6.FOCUS13213

[8]   Gu, W. and Zhao, W. (2014) Microvascular Decompression for Recurrent Trigeminal Neuralgia. *Journal of Clinical Neuroscience,* **21**, 1549-1553. http://dx.doi.org/10.1016/j.jocn.2013.11.042

[9]   Oesman, C. and Mooij, J.J. (2011) Long-Term Follow-Up of Microvascular Decompression for Trigeminal Neuralgia. *Skull Base,* **21**, 313-322. http://dx.doi.org/10.1055/s-0031-1284213

[10]   Karol, E.A., Sanz, O.P., Gonzalez La Riva, F.N. and Rey, R.D. (1993) A Micrometric Multiple Electrode Array for the Exploration of Gasserian and Retrogasserian Trigeminal Fibers: Preliminary Report: Technical Note. *Neurosurgery,* **33**, 154-158. http://dx.doi.org/10.1227/00006123-199307000-00027

[11]   Smith, H.P., McWhorter, J.M. and Challa, V.R. (1981) Radiofrequency Neurolysis in a Clinical Model: Neuropathological Correlation. *Journal of Neurosurgery,* **55**, 246-253. http://dx.doi.org/10.3171/jns.1981.55.2.0246

[12]   Gusmão, S., Oliveira, M., Tazinaffo, U. and Honey, C.R. (2003) Percutaneous Trigeminal Nerve Radiofrequency Rhizotomy Guided by Computerized Tomography Fluoroscopy. Technical Note. *Journal of Neurosurgery,* **99**, 785-786. http://dx.doi.org/10.3171/jns.2003.99.4.0785

[13]   Xu, S.J., Zhang, W.H., Chen, T., Wu, C.Y. and Zhou, M.D. (2006) Neuronavigator-Guided Percutaneous Radiofrequency Thermocoagulation in the Treatment of Intractable Trigeminal Neuralgia. *Chinese Medical Journal (English Edition),* **119**, 1528-1535.

[14]   Erdine, S., Ozyalcin, N.S., Cimen, A., Celik, M., Talu, G.K. and Disci, R. (2007) Comparison of Pulsed Radiofrequency with Conventional Radiofrequency in the Treatment of Idiopathic Trigeminal Neuralgia. *European Journal of Pain,* **11**, 309-313. http://dx.doi.org/10.1016/j.ejpain.2006.04.001

[15]   Hirao, M., Ikemoto, S. and Tsuboi, H. (2014) Computer Assisted Planning and Custom-Made Surgical Guide for Malunited Pronation Deformity after First Metatarsophalangeal Joint Arthrodesis in Rheumatoid Arthritis: A Case Report. *Computer Aided Surgery,* **19**, 13-19. http://dx.doi.org/10.3109/10929088.2014.885992

[16]   Raaijmaakers, M., Gelaude, F., De Smedt, K., Clijmans, T., Dille, J. and Mulier, M. (2010) A Custom-Made Guide-Wire Positioning Device for Hip Surface Replacement Arthroplasty: Description and First Results. *BMC Musculoskeletal Disorders,* **11**, 161. http://dx.doi.org/10.1186/1471-2474-11-161

[17]   Modabber, A., Ayoub, N., Möhlhenrich, S.C., Goloborodko, E., Sönmez, T.T., Ghassemi, M., *et al.* (2014) The Accuracy of Computer-Assisted Primary Mandibular Reconstruction with Vascularized Bone Flaps: Iliac Crest Bone Flap versus Osteomyocutaneous Fibula Flap. *Medical Devices: Evidence and Research,* **7**, 211-217. http://dx.doi.org/10.2147/MDER.S62698

[18]   Liu, Y.F., Xu, L.W., Zhu, H.Y., Liu, S.-Y.S. (2014) Technical Procedures for Template-Guided Surgery for Mandibular Reconstruction Based on Digital Design and Manufacturing. *BioMedical Engineering OnLine,* **13**, 63. http://dx.doi.org/10.1186/1475-925X-13-63

[19]   Farzadi, A., Solati-Hashjin, M. and Asadi-Eydivand, M. (2014) Effect of Layer Thickness and Printing Orientation on Mechanical Properties and Dimensional Accuracy of 3D Printed Porous Samples for Bone Tissue Engineering. *PLoS ONE,* **9**, e108252. http://dx.doi.org/10.1371/journal.pone.0108252

[20]   Ventola, C.L. (2014) Medical Applications for 3D Printing: Current and Projected Uses. *Pharmacy and Therapeutics,* **39**, 704-711.

[21]   Parthasarathy, J. (2014) 3D Modeling, Custom Implants and Its Future Perspectives in Craniofacial Surgery. *Annals of Maxillofacial Surgery,* **4**, 9-18. http://dx.doi.org/10.4103/2231-0746.133065

[22]   Patil, J., Kumar, N., KG, M.R., Ravindra, S.S., SN, S., Nayak, B.S., *et al.* (2013) The Foramen Ovale Morphometry of Sphenoid Bone in South Indian Population. *Journal of Clinical and Diagnostic Research,* **7**, 2668-2670.

[23]   Khairnar, K.B. and Bhusari, P.A. (2013) An Anatomical Study on the Foramen Ovale and the Foramen Spinosum. *Journal of Clinical and Diagnostic Research,* **7**, 427-429. http://dx.doi.org/10.7860/jcdr/2013/4894.2790

[24]   Yang, J.T., Lin, M., Lee, M.H., Weng, H.H. and Liao, H.H. (2010) Percutaneous Trigeminal Nerve Radiofrequency Rhizotomy Guided by Computerized Tomography with Three-Dimensional Image Reconstruction. *Chang Gung Medical Journal,* **33**, 679-683.

[25]   Luo, F., Shen, Y., Wang, T., Meng, L., Yu, X.T. and Ji, N. (2014) 3D CT-Guided Pulsed Radiofrequency Treatment for Trigeminal Neuralgia. *Pain Practice,* **14**, 16-21. http://dx.doi.org/10.1111/papr.12041

14

Lily bulb Nectar Produces Expectorant and Anti-Tussive Activities, and Suppresses Cigarette Smoke-Induced Inflammatory Response in the Respiratory Tract in Mice

Hoishan Wong[1], Shiyu Zou[2], Jiangping Li[2], Chungwah Ma[2], Jihang Chen[1], Poukuan Leong[1], Hoiyan Leung[1], Wingman Chan[1], Kamming Ko[1*]

[1]Division of Life Science, Hong Kong University of Science and Technology, Hong Kong, China
[2]Infinitus (China) Company Ltd., Guangzhou, China
Email: [*]bcrko@ust.hk

Abstract

Air pollutants pose a major environmental threat to the respiratory system. Pathogen invasion and the exposure to particulate matters in atmospheric air, particularly, cigarette smoke (CS), have been found to be associated with acute and chronic respiratory diseases, including asthma. Therefore, the search for agents that can protect the respiratory system against potentially harmful substances is of interest in preventive health. *Lily bulb* Nectar (LBN), which contains *Lily bulb*, *Pyrus pyrifolia* N., *Siraitia grosvenorii* and *Apricot kernel* as its ingredients, is a health supplement intended to improve the wellness of the respiratory system in humans. *Lily bulb*, *Pyrus pyrifolia* N., *Siraitia grosvenorii* and *Apricot kernel* are commonly prescribed for the treatment of respiratory tract disorders such as bronchitis, pneumonia and cough in the practice of traditional Chinese medicine. Pharmacological studies have shown that these herbs can produce beneficial effects on the respiratory tract or even the lungs. In the present study, we investigated the effects of LBN on mouse respiratory tract function under normal and challenged conditions. LBN was first examined for its expectorant and anti-tussive activities in mice. The effect of LBN on long-term exposure to CS was also investigated. Our findings showed that long-term LBN treatment enhanced the expectorant activity and suppressed the SO_2-induced coughing in mice. LBN treatment also suppressed the CS-induced inflammation in the respiratory tract, as assessed by differential cell count and cytokine production. In conclusion, long-term LBN consumption may produce beneficial effects on the respiratory tract function in humans, particularly in the face of challenge by irritants in the inhaling air.

---

[*]Corresponding author.

Keywords

Lily bulb, Expectoration, Anti-Tussion, Anti-Inflammation

1. Introduction

Atmospheric air, which is the main source of oxygen, is essential for the survival of aerobic organisms. In addition to nitrogen, oxygen, carbon dioxide and trace amounts of other gases, the inhaled air also contains many air pollutants, of which the over-exposure poses a threat to the well-being of respiratory system [1] [2]. The lungs, which provide the gas exchange surface of our body, are exceptionally vulnerable to such insult because of the close proximity to the potentially harmful substances in the inhaled air [3] [4]. Air pollutants, including particular matters (PMs), especially PMs smaller than 2.5 micrometer (also known as fine PMs), and airborne microbial pathogens, can impair the functioning of the respiratory system by physical irritation and/or the induction of inflammatory response in the respiratory tract [5] [6]. The air microbes and pollutants were also found to be associated with a broad spectrum of acute and chronic illnesses, such as lung cancer, chronic obstructive pulmonary disease, asthma and even cardiovascular diseases [7]. To cope with these challenges, the lungs are equipped with sophisticated defense mechanisms, which operate in a coordinated fashion to expel foreign particles from the respiratory tract.

Mucociliary clearance and coughing are two of the defensive mechanisms that mechanically remove foreign particles from the respiratory tract [8] [9]. Conducting airways, including nasal passage and tracheobronchial tree, are covered with a layer of mucus secreted by goblet cells, submucosal glands and clara cells. The mucous blanket provides a surface for the deposition of inhaled particles. The particle-laden mucus, also known as sputum, is transferred by the coordinated movement of cilia to the naso-/oropharynx where it is swallowed [8] [9]. Cough reflex is triggered by mechanical or chemical stimuli on the epithelium of larynx or tracheobronchial tree. It prevents the accumulation of mucus secretion and thus helps eliminate the inhaled particles from the lower respiratory tract [8] [9]. However, while mucociliary clearance and coughing are effective in removing most of the inhaled particles in healthy individuals, their clearance efficiency is far from sufficient when the respiratory system is affected by the exposure to cigarette smoke (CS), which exists as the most frequently occurring air pollutant [10].

CS, with over 4000 chemical components, is the major etiological factor of chronic lung inflammation [11]-[14]. The CS-induced lung inflammation is mediated by a complex mechanism that involves various types of cells and inflammatory mediators, in which redox-sensitive signaling pathway plays a primary role [15]. The exposure of respiratory system to CS leads to an increased production of reactive oxygen species (ROS) by NADPH oxidase [16]-[18]. The ROS, in turn, triggers the release of pro-inflammatory cytokines, such as tumor necrosis factor-α (TNF-α) [19] [20], via the mitogen-activated protein kinase (MAPK) and nuclear factor kappa-light-chain-enhancer of activated B cells (NF-κB) signaling pathways. TNF-α, together with other chemokines, facilitates the recruitment of effector cells, including macrophages, neutrophils and lymphocytes, to eliminate foreign particles mainly by phagocytosis [21]. The effector cells, after being exposed to CS, lead to further and excessive production of inflammatory substances/enzymes that cause an increase in mucosal secretion and destructions of collagen and elastin, with the resultant decline in respiratory function of the lungs [22].

Lily bulb (the flower bulb of *Lilium brownie* F. E. Brown var. *viridulum* Baker, *Lilium lancifolium* Thunb. and *Lilium pumilium* DC.), *Pyrus pyrifolia* N. (a member of the Rosaceae family and Pomaceae tribe), *Siraitia grosvenorii* (a herbaceous perennial vine of the Cucurbitaceae family), and *Apricot kernel* (the dried and mature seed of *Prunus armeniaca* L. and *Prunus ameniaca* L. var. Ansu Maxim.) are listed in the Chinese Pharmacopoeia (2010) as medicinal plants. According to the theory of traditional Chinese medicine, these herbs produce "Yin-nourishing" and "Lung-moistening" effects, and are therefore commonly prescribed for the treatment of bronchitis, pneumonia and cough in the practice of traditional Chinese medicine [23]-[29]. Their beneficial effects on respiratory system were also demonstrated in recent pharmacological studies. Oral administration of the aqueous extracts of *Lily bulb* and *Siraitia grosvenorii* suppressed the SO_2-induced coughing in mice, as evidenced by the reduced number and delayed onset of SO_2-induced coughing, and improved tracheobronchial expectorant action [28] [30]. The cough relieving and phlegm expelling activities could also be observed in *Apri-*

cot kernel-pretreated mice through which hydrocyanic acid, a metabolite of amygdalin in *Apricot kernel*, reflexively stimulated the respiratory center in the brain of the pretreated animals [29]. Moreover, *Lily bulb* was found to exhibit anti-inflammatory activity on lipopolysaccharide-stimulated Raw 264.7 mouse macrophages, presumably by down-regulating the NF-κB and extracellular signal-regulated kinases (ERK)/c-Jun N-terminal kinases (JNK) signaling pathways [23].

Lily bulb Nectar (LBN), which is comprised of *Lily bulb*, *Pyrus*, *Siraitia grosvenorii* and *Apricot kernel*, is a health supplement intended to improve the wellness of the respiratory system in humans. In the present study, we investigated the effect of LBN on tracheobronchial expectorant action by phenol red secretion test in mice. The anti-tussive and anti-inflammatory activities were also examined in the mouse model of SO_2-induced coughing and CS-induced inflammation in the respiratory tract.

2. Materials and Methods

2.1. Chemicals

Ammonium chloride (NH_4Cl) was purchased from Nacalai Tesque Inc. (Kyoto, Japan). Cigarettes (Camel; filters, Japan Tobacco Inc.) were purchased from local distributors. Concentrated sulfuric acid (H_2SO_4) was purchased from BDH Reagents & Chemicals (Poole Dorset, UK). Phenol red and sodium bisulfite ($NaHSO_3$) were purchased from Sigma (St. Louis, MO). Dextromethorphan hydrobromide (DH) was purchased from Santa Cruz Biotechnology (Santa Cruz, CA). ELISA kits for immunoglobulin G (IgG), interleukin-8 and secretory immunoglobulin A (sIgA) were purchased from Cusabio Biotech Co., Ltd. (Suffolk, UK), whereas ELISA kits for interleukin-6 (IL-6) and TNF-α were purchased from Life Technologies (Grand Island, NY).

2.2. LBN Preparation

LBN is a syrup preparation comprising water extracts of *Lily bulb*, *Pyrus pyrifolia* N., *Siraitia grosuenorii*, and *Apricot kernel*. The commercial product was manufactured and supplied by Infinitus (China) Company Ltd., Guangzhou, China.

2.3. Animal Care

Male adult Balb/c mice were used for the assessment of expectorant and anti-tussive activities, whereas male adult ICR mice were used for examining the CS-induced pulmonary immune response. Animals (~8 weeks of age; 25 - 30 g) were randomly assigned to 4 groups, respectively, with 5 - 10 animals in each. LBN, at daily doses of 2.46, 8.20, 24.6 g/kg (with human equivalent dose being 8.20 g/kg), was administered intragastrically 5 days per week for 4 weeks (*i.e.*, a total of 20 doses). Control animals received the vehicle (water) only. All experimental procedures were approved by the Research Practice Committee (Hong Kong University of Science and Technology) (Animal Protocol Approval No. 2013064; Approved Date: 12 November 2013; Experiment Duration: 3 years).

2.4. Measurement of Expectorant Activity

The tracheobronchial expectorant activity was measured by phenol red secretion test. NH_4Cl, which was used as a positive control, was administered intragastrically at 1 g/kg for 3 consecutive days. Twenty-four h after the last dosing with vehicle/LBN/NH_4Cl, phenol red [suspended in 0.9% saline (w/v)] was administered intraperitoneally, at a dose of 500 mg/kg. The mice were sacrificed 30 min after phenol red injection and the tracheas were carefully excised. All connective tissues and traces of blood were removed from the excised trachea. Half-centimeter of the trachea was cut out, and was then incubated in 0.5 mL 0.9% saline (w/v) with 100 µL 1 M NaOH for 30 min with thorough mixing by vortexing. After the incubation, the absorbance at 550 nm of the solution was measured. The amount of phenol red eliminated through tracheobronchial secretion was calculated using a calibration curve of phenol red [31]-[35].

2.5. Anti-Tussive Activity

Coughing was induced by SO_2 and the frequency of coughing was recorded [36] [37]. The experimental set-up is shown in **Figure 1**. Briefly, the mouse was put into chamber B and 0.2 mL concentrated H_2SO_4 was added

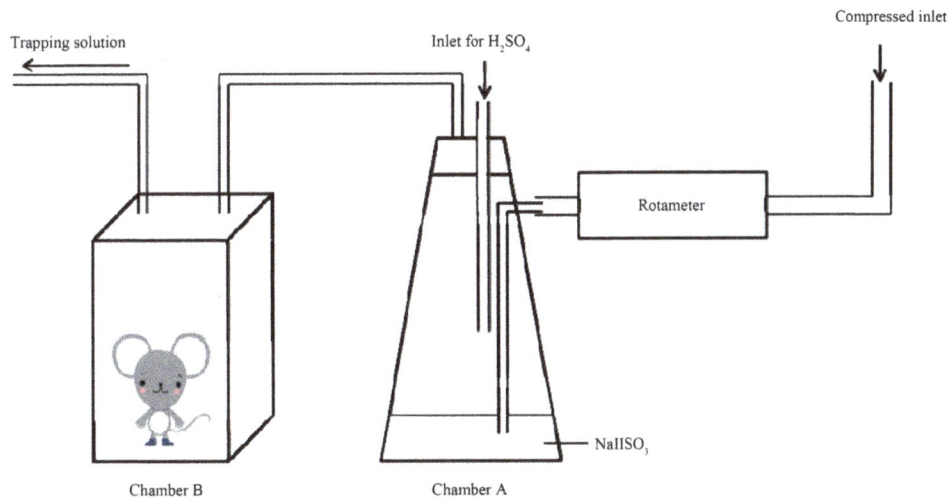

Figure 1. Experimental set-up of anti-tussive assay.

into chamber A which contained 500 mg/mL NaHSO$_3$ in distilled water. The generated SO$_2$ was flushed into chamber A by compressed air at a flow rate of 5 L/min. The mouse in chamber B was then exposed to SO$_2$ for 30 s and withdrawn from the chamber thereafter. One minute after the withdrawal, the number of coughing of the mouse was counted until up to 5 min post-exposure. The concentration of SO$_2$ was determined by spectro-photometric method and the average concentration of SO$_2$ used in this experiment was found to be 207 ± 23.3 mg/m^3. DH was administered 30 min prior to the SO$_2$ exposure to serve as a positive control for the suppression of SO$_2$-induced tussive activity.

2.6. CS Challenge

Camel cigarettes (containing 10 mg tar and 0.8 mg nicotine per cigarette) were used to produce CS. A cage with 5 mice was placed into a container (57 × 41.8 × 34.8 cm) connecting to a circulation pump (see **Figure 2**). The container was closed tightly immediately after the cigarette was ignited. Mice were exposed to CS flowing through the container for 6 min (one cigarette burning time was equal to one session). For the experiment with differential cell counts, mice were exposed to CS during the last 11 days of LBN administration, wherein mice were exposed to CS ten sessions per day, five days per week. For the experiment with measurements of cyto-kines and immunoglobulins, mice were exposed to CS during the last 4 days of LBN administration, wherein mice were exposed to CS ten sessions per day.

2.7. Collection of Bronchoalveolar Lavage Fluid (BALF)

Twenty-four h following the last exposure to CS, the BALF was collected from ketamine-anesthetized mice by cannulating the upper part of the trachea using 27-G syringe. The lavaging procedure was done once with 1 mL phosphate-buffered saline-type A (PBS-A) for measurements of cytokines and immunoglobulins and twice with a total of 1.6 mL PBS-A for differential cell counts.

2.8. Differential Cell Counts

The collected BALF in PBS-A samples were centrifuged at 1000× g for 10 min at room temperature. The total number of leukocytes was counted using a hemocytometer. Differential cell counts were determined by staining the cells on a glass slide with Giemsa-Wright stain. More than one hundred cells per slide were counted and the percentages of macrophages, neutrophils and lymphocytes with respect to the total number of cells were esti-mated [38]-[40].

2.9. Measurements of Cytokines and Immunoglobulins in BALF

For measurements of cytokines and immunoglobulins, BALF samples were collected and centrifuged at 2150× g

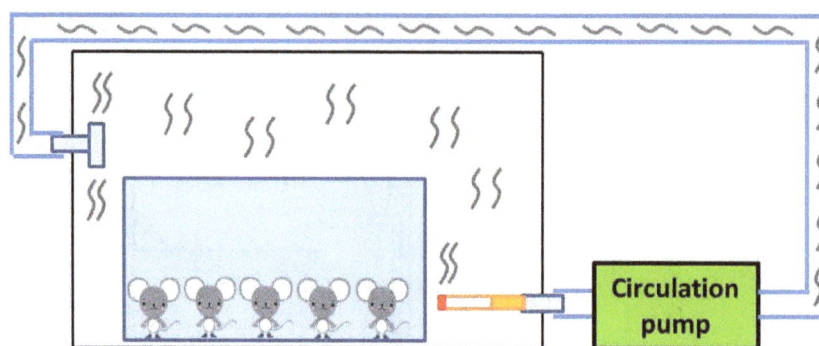

Figure 2. Experimental set-up for CS challenge.

for 10 min at 4°C. The supernatants were used for analyses. Levels of IL-6, TNF-α, IL-8, IgG and sIgA in BALF were measured using ELISA kits [38]-[45].

3. Results

Long-term treatment with LBN at daily doses of 2.46 to 24.6 g/kg did not produce any detectable changes in body weight in mice, with or without exposure to CS, when compared with the respective untreated control (data not shown).

Whereas NH_4Cl caused an increase in expectorant activity by 105% in mice, long-term LBN treatment, at a daily dose of 24.6 g/kg, significantly increased the expectorant activity by 30%, when compared with the untreated control (**Figure 3**).

The exposure to SO_2 caused coughing response in mice, with 196 coughs from 1 - 5 min post-exposure (**Figure 4**). Treatment with DH, at a dose of 10 mg/kg, significantly suppressed the SO_2-induced coughing by 33%. Long-term treatment with LBN caused a dose-dependent suppression in SO_2-induced coughing, with the number of coughs being significantly reduced by 42% at a daily dose of 24.6 g/kg (**Figure 4**).

While long-term LBN treatment did not produce any detectable changes in total cell count, macrophage number and lymphocyte number in the BALF of mice, CS exposure for 11 days caused significant decreases in total cell count (26%) and macrophage number (10%) as well as an increase in lymphocyte number (by 10-fold), when compared with the non-CS exposed control (**Figure 5**). Long-term LBN treatment restored the CS- induced decreases in total cell count (by 100%) at a daily dose of 8.20 g/kg and in the number of macrophage (by 23%) at a daily dose of 24.6 g/kg. The CS-induced increase in lymphocyte number was suppressed by LBN treatment (by 45%) at a daily dose of 24.6 g/kg. However, neither LBN treatment nor CS exposure produced any detectable changes in neutrophil number in the BALF of mice.

Long-term LBN treatment did not cause any detectable changes in IL-6, IL-8, sIgA, IgG and TNFα levels in the BALF of mice (**Figure 6**), whereas 4-day CS exposure increased the levels of IL-6 (25%), IL-8 (1.79 fold), sIgA (1.33 fold), IgG (26%) and TNF-α (22.7%). Long-term LBN treatment at a daily dose of 2.46 g/kg completely inhibited the CS-induced increase in IL-6 level. The CS-induced increase in sIgA level was largely suppressed by LBN treatment by 85%. LBN treatment also inhibited the CS-induced increase in IgG (94%) and TNF-α (125%) levels at daily doses of 8.20 and 24.6 g/kg, respectively. However, LBN treatment did not produce any detectable change in the CS-induced increase in IL-8 level (**Figure 6**).

The tracheobronchial expectorant activity was assessed as described in materials and methods. Data were expressed in percent control with respect to vehicle-treated control [amount of expectorant of control (μg/mL) = 2.07 ± 0.15]. Values given are mean ± SEM, with n = 5 to 10.

The extent of SO_2-induced tussive activity was measured as described in materials and methods. Data were expressed in percent control with respect to vehicle-treated control [number of coughing of control = 196.45 ± 14.61]. Values given are mean ± SEM, with n = 5 to 10.

BALF was collected and cells were quantified as described in materials and methods. Data were expressed in percent control with respect to vehicle-treated control [percent cell count of control = 84107.14 ± 3572.64 (total cell count); 236.67 ± 20.36 (macrophages) 2.62 ± 0.38; (lymphocytes) and 4.23 ± 1.19 (neutrophils)]. Values given are mean ± SEM, with n = 5 to 10.

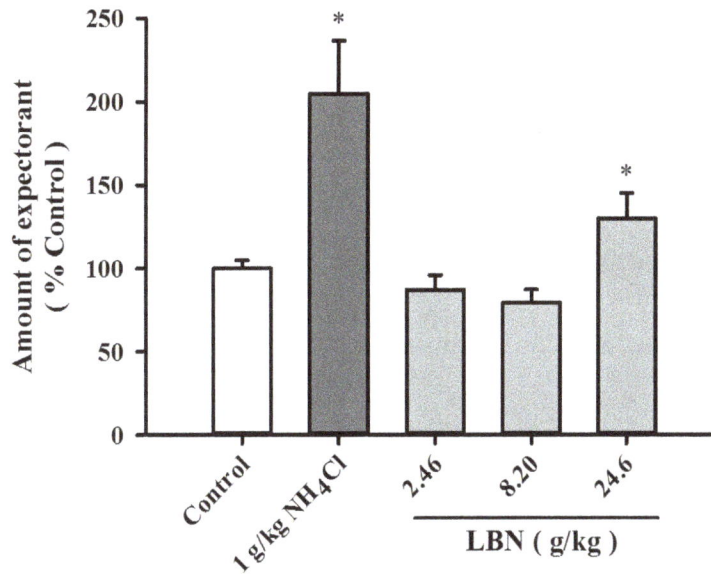

Figure 3. The Effects of long-term LBN treatment on the expectorant activity in Balb/c mice. *Significantly different from vehicle control (p < 0.05).

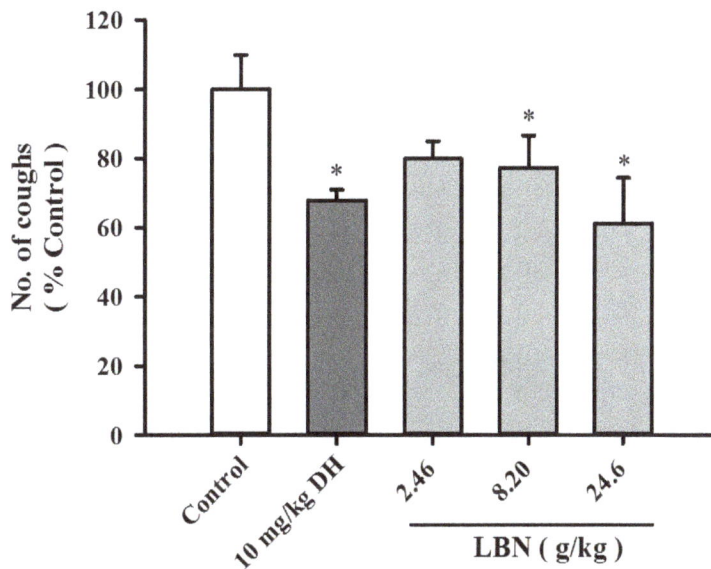

Figure 4. The effects of long-term LBN treatment on SO_2-induced tussive activity in Balb/c mice. *Significantly different from vehicle control (p < 0.05).

The amount of pro-inflammatory cytokines and immunoglobulins were measured as described in materials and methods. Data were expressed in percent control with respect to non-CS vehicle control [control values = 10.02 ± 0.91 pg/mg protein (IL-6); 16295.73 ± 2623.85 pg/mg protein (IL-8); 18.52 ± 1.09 pg/mg protein (TNF-α); 10233.67 ± 493.26 (IgG) and 204.14 ± 15.24 ng/mg protein (sIgA)]. Values given are mean $\pm$ SEM, with n = 5 to 10.

4. Discussions

Results obtained from the present study showed that long-term treatment with LBN enhanced the expectorant activity in mice, as assessed by tracheobronchial clearance of the intraperitoneally-injected phenol red. The expectorant action is characterized by increased secretion and hydration of sputum for more efficient sputum re-

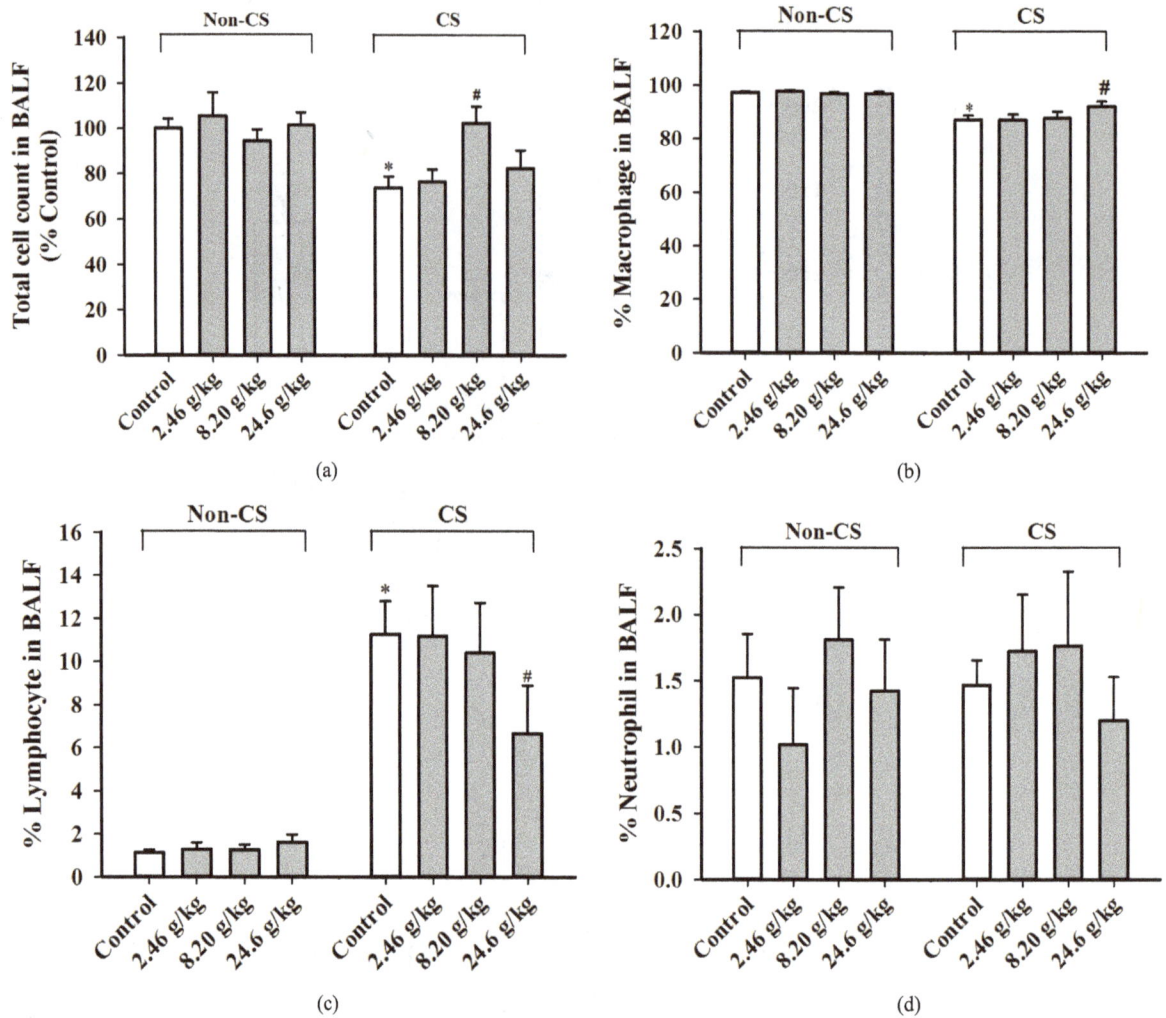

Figure 5. Effects of long-term LBN treatment with or without 11-day CS exposure on total and differential cell counts in BALF of ICR mice. *Significantly different from vehicle-treated control; #significantly different from CS-exposed vehicle control ($p < 0.05$).

moval via mucociliary transport in the respiratory tract [46] [47]. Long-term LBN treatment was also found to produce anti-tussive activity against SO_2-induced coughing in mice. While coughing secures the removal of mucus, noxious substances and infectious particles from the respiratory tract, persistent coughing, which affects over 40% of non-smokers in the United States and Europe, presents psychological and social burdens, as well as contributes to the spread of airborne microbes [48]-[51]. The cough-relieving activity of LBN, therefore, has clinical implications in suppressing the hypersensitivity of coughing provoked by mildly irritating or innocuous stimuli [52].

The beneficial effect of LBN on the respiratory tract was also evidenced by its action on CS-induced lung inflammation in mice. CS exposure caused significant increases in pro-inflammatory cytokines (IL-8, IL-6 and TNF-α) and the subsequent recruitment of lymphocytes in mouse respiratory tract, indicative of a localized inflammation in the lungs. Long-term LBN treatment reduced the CS-induced elevations in pro-inflammatory cytokines and the associated lymphocyte infiltration, suggesting a reduction in the degree of CS-induced lung inflammation in mouse respiratory tract. Inflammation is a defensive mechanism that protects tissues against pathogenic invasion [53]. Nevertheless, depending on the extent and characteristic of inflammation, it may also result in the functional impairment in relevant tissues/organs, presumably through macrophage-/leukocytes-released ROS and the associated protease activities [54] [55]. In this regard, while the CS exposure caused significant decreases in total and macrophage cell counts in BALF, possibly due to oxidative stress-induced cell death

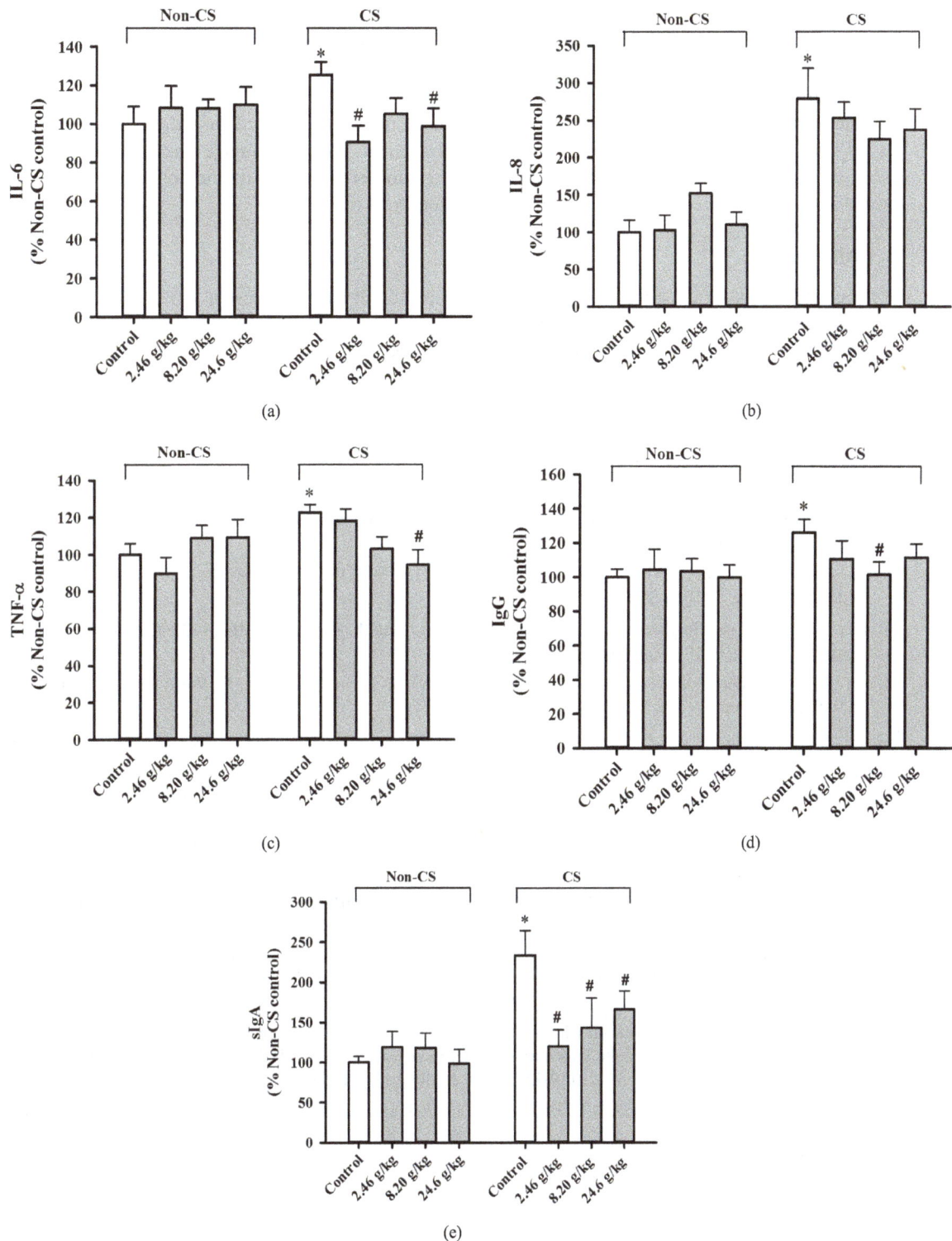

Figure 6. The effects of long-term LBN treatment with 4-day CS exposure on cytokines and immunoglobulins in BALF of ICR mice. *Significantly different from non-CS vehicle control; #significantly different from CS-exposed vehicle control (p < 0.05).

in mouse respiratory tract during inflammation [54], the anti-inflammatory action of LBN was paralleled by its ability to suppress such decreases, suggests the potential beneficial effect of LBN on innate immunity in CS-exposed animals. In addition, a marked increase in lymphocyte number in BALF of CS-exposed mice was likely related to the increases in levels of IgG and sIgA, which are the two most abundant types of antibodies in the mucosal lining of respiratory tract. These antibodies, when acting in concert with effector cells, can eliminate foreign particles from mouse respiratory tract, possibly through the induction of both antibody-dependent cell-mediated cytotoxicity and intracellular antibody-mediated proteolysis of foreign particles [56]. The reduced extent of the CS-induced IgG and sIgA secretion in LBN-treated CS-exposed mice was likely an effect secondary to the anti-inflammatory activity of LBN. The findings, therefore, implicate the potential use of LBN for the prevention of CS-induced inflammation in the respiratory tract in humans.

5. Conclusion

In conclusion, long-term LBN treatment produced expectorant and anti-tussive activities in mouse respiratory tract. It also suppressed the CS-induced lung inflammatory response in mice. The mechanisms by which LBN produces these effects remain to be investigated. Taken together, LBN may serve a health supplement for safeguarding the function of the respiratory system, particularly in the respiratory tract.

References

[1]   Mayer, H. (1999) Air Pollution in Cities. *Atmospheric Environment*, **33**, 4029-4037.
      http://dx.doi.org/10.1016/S1352-2310(99)00144-2

[2]   Kampa, M. and Castanas, E. (2008) Human Health Effects of Air Pollution. *Environmental Pollution*, **151**, 362-367.
      http://dx.doi.org/10.1016/j.envpol.2007.06.012

[3]   Seaton, A., Godden, D., MacNee, W. and Donaldson, D. (1995) Particulates Air Pollution and Acute Health Effects.
      http://dx.doi.org/10.1016/S0140-6736(95)90173-6

[4]   Brunekreef, B. and Holgate, S.T. (2002) Air Pollution and Health. *The Lancet*, **360**, 1233-1242.
      http://dx.doi.org/10.1016/S0140-6736(02)11274-8

[5]   Review of Evidence on Health Aspects of Air Pollution—Revihaap Project (2003) World Health Organization Regional Office for Europe, Denmark.

[6]   Rackley, C.R. and Stripp, B.R. (2012) Building and Maintaining the Epithelium of the Lung. *Journal of Clinical Investigation*, **122**, 2724-2730. http://dx.doi.org/10.1172/JCI60519

[7]   Wargo, J., Wargo, L. and Alderman, N. (2006) The Harmful Effects of Vehicle Exhaust: A Case for Policy Change. Environment and Human Health, Inc., North Haven.

[8]   Green, G.M., Jakab, G.J., Low, R.B. and Davis, G.S. (1977) Defense Mechanisms of the Respiratory Membrane. *The American Review of Respiratory Disease*, **115**, 479-514.

[9]   Tamura, S. and Kurata, T. (2004) Defense Mechanisms against Influenza Virus Infection in the Respiratory Tract Mucosa. *Japanese Journal of Infectious Disease*, **57**, 236-247.

[10] Ma, W.J., Sun, Y.H., Jiang, J.X., Dong, X.W., Zhou, J.Y. and Xie, Q.M. (2014) Epoxyeicosatrienoic Acids Attenuate Cigarette Smoke Extract-Induced Interleukin-8 Production in Bronchial Epithelial Cells. Prostaglandins Leukotrienes and Essential Fatty Acids.

[11] Pessina, G.P., Paulesu, L., Corradeschi, F., Luzzi, E., Stefano, A.D., Tanzini, M., Matteucci, G. and Bocci, V. (1993) Effects of Acute Cigarette Smoke Exposure on Macrophage Kinetics and Release of Tumour Necrosis Factor Alpha in Rats. *Mediators of Inflammation*, **2**, 119-122. http://dx.doi.org/10.1155/S0962935193000171

[12] Finch, G.L., Nikula, K.J., Chen, B.T., Barr, E.B., Chang, I. and Hobbs, C.H. (2002) Effect of Chronic Cigarette Smoke Exposure on Lung Clearance of Tracer Particles Inhaled by Rats. *Fundamental and Applied Toxicology*, **24**, 76-85. http://dx.doi.org/10.1006/faat.1995.1009

[13] Sekine, T., Sakaguchi, C. and Fukano, Y. (2014) Investigation by Microarray Analysis of Effects of Cigarette Design Characteristics on Gene Expression in Human Lung Mucoepidermoid Cancer Cells NCI-H292 Exposed to Cigarette Smoke. *Experimental and Toxicological Pathology*, **67**, 143-151.

[14] Liu, M.H., Lin, A.H., Lu, S.H., Peng, R.Y., Lee, T.S. and Kou, Y.R. (2014) Eicosapentaenoic Acid Attenuates Cigarette Smoke-Induced Lung Inflammation by Inhibiting ROS-Sensitive Inflammatory Signaling. *Frontiers in Physiology*, **5**, 440. http://dx.doi.org/10.3389/fphys.2014.00440

[15] Phipps, J.C., Aronoff, D.M., Curtis, J.L., Goel, D., O'Brien, E. and Mancuso, P. (2010) Cigarette Smoke Exposure Impairs Pulmonary Bacterial Clearance and Alveolar Macrophage Complement-Mediated Phagocytosis of *Streptococcus pneumoni*a. *Infection and Immunity*, **78**, 1214-1220. http://dx.doi.org/10.1128/IAI.00963-09

[16] Kirkham, P.A., Spooner, G., Ffoulkes-Jones, C. and Calvez, R. (2003) Cigarette Smoke Triggers Macrophage Adhesion and Activation: Role of Lipid Peroxidation Products and Scavenger Receptor. *Free Radical Biology and Medicine*, **35**, 697-710. http://dx.doi.org/10.1016/S0891-5849(03)00390-3

[17] van der Vaart, H., Postma, D.S., Timens, W. and ten Hacken, N.H. (2004) Acute Effects of Cigarette Smoke on Inflammation and Oxidative Stress: A Review. *Thorax*, **59**, 713-721. http://dx.doi.org/10.1136/thx.2003.012468

[18] Liu, M.-H., Lin, A.-H., Lee, H.-F., Ko, H.-K., Lee, T.-S. and Kou, Y.R. (2014) Paeonol Attenuates Cigarette Smoke-Induced Lung Inflammation by Inhibiting ROS-Sensitive Inflammatory Signaling. *Mediators of Inflammation*, **2014**, Article ID: 651890. http://dx.doi.org/10.1155/2014/651890

[19] Churg, A., Dai, J., Tai, H., Xie, C. and Wright, J.L. (2002) Tumor Necrosis Factor-Alpha Is Central to Acute Cigarette Smoke-Induced Inflammation and Connective Tissue Breakdown. *American Journal of Respiratory and Critical Care Medicine*, **166**, 849-854. http://dx.doi.org/10.1164/rccm.200202-097OC

[20] Churg, A., Zay, K., Shay, S., Xie, C., Shapiro, S.D., Hendricks, R. and Wright, J.L. (2002) Acute Cigarette Smoke-Induced Connective Tissue Breakdown Requires Both Neutrophils and Macrophage Metalloelastase in Mice. *American Journal of Respiratory Cell and Molecular Biology*, **27**, 368-374. http://dx.doi.org/10.1165/rcmb.4791

[21] Karimi, K., Sarir, H., Mortaz, E., Smit, J.J., Hosseini, H., De Kimpe, S.J., Nijkamp, F.P. and Folkerts, G. (2006) Toll-Like Receptor-4 Mediates Cigarette Smoke-Induced Cytokine Production by Human Macrophages. *Respiratory Research*, **19**, 66. http://dx.doi.org/10.1186/1465-9921-7-66

[22] Li, J., Zhou, W., Huang, K., Jin, Y. and Gao, J. (2014) Interleukin-22 Exacerbates Airway Inflammation Induced by Short-Term Exposure to Cigarette Smoke in Mice. *Acta Pharmacologica Sinica*, **35**, 1393-1401. http://dx.doi.org/10.1038/aps.2014.91

[23] Guo, Z. and Jiang, S. (2004) Pharmacological Activities and Therapeutic Applications of *Lily bulbs*. *Acta Chinese Medicine and Pharmacology*, **32**, 27-29.

[24] Kwon, O.K., Lee, M.Y., Yuk, J.E., Oh, S.R., Chin, Y.W., Lee, H.K. and Ahn, K.S. (2010) Anti-Inflammatory Effects of Methanol Extracts of the Root of *Lilium lancifolium* on LPS-Stimulated Raw264.7 Cells. *Journal of Ethnopharmacology*, **130**, 28-34. http://dx.doi.org/10.1016/j.jep.2010.04.002

[25] Lee, E., Yun, N., Jang, Y.P. and Kim, J. (2013) *Lilium lancifolium* Thunb. Extract Attenuates Pulmonary Inflammation and Air Space Enlargement in a Cigarette Smoke-Exposed Mouse Model. *Journal of Ethnopharmacology*, **149**, 148-156. http://dx.doi.org/10.1016/j.jep.2013.06.014

[26] Hwang, Y., Yang, M. and Pyo, M. (2008) Effects of Heated Pear Juice on the Proliferation and Cytokines Production of Mouse Splenocytes *in Vitro*. *Journal of Cancer Prevention*, **13**, 68-73.

[27] Lee, Y.G., Cho, J.Y., Kim, C., Lee, S., Kim, W., Jeon, T., Park, K. and Moon, J. (2013) Coumaroyl Quinic Acid Derivatives and Flavonoids from Immature Pear (*Pyrus pyrifolia* Nakai) Fruit. *Food Science and Biotechnology*, **22**, 803-810. http://dx.doi.org/10.1007/s10068-013-0148-z

[28] Zhang, H. and Li, X.H. (2011) Research Advance of Pharmacological Effects and Toxicity of *Siraitia grovenorii* (Swingle) C. Jeffrey. *Chinese Agricultural Science Bulletin*, **27**, 430-433.

[29] Wang, D. (2002) [Pharmacological and Clinical Applications of *Apricot kernel*]. *Primary Journal of Chinese Materia Medica*, **16**, 61-62.

[30] Wang, X. (2009) Therapeutic Applications of *Lily bulbs*. *Aerospace Medicine*, **19**, 151.

[31] Coppi, G. and Gatti, M.T. (1989) A Method for Studying Expectorant Action in the Mouse by Measurement of Tracheobronchial Phenol Red Secretion. *Farmaco*, **44**, 541-545.

[32] Knowles, M.R. and Boucher, R.C. (2002) Mucus Clearance as a Primary Innate Defense Mechanism for Mammalian Airways. *The Journal of Clinical Investigation*, **109**, 571-577. http://dx.doi.org/10.1172/JCI0215217

[33] Canning, B.J. (2010) Afferent Nerves Regulating the Cough Reflex: Mechanisms and Mediators of Cough in Disease. *Otolaryngologic Clinics of North America*, **43**, 15-25. http://dx.doi.org/10.1016/j.otc.2009.11.012

[34] Zheng, F., Liu, W., Zheng, Y. and Li, W. (2011) Comparison of Expectorant Effect of Total Phatycosides and Secondary Saponin from the Roots of *Platycodon grandiflorum*. *Journal of Jilin Agricultural University*, **7**.

[35] Zhao, S.G. and Wang, L. (2009) Investigation of the Effects of Acidic Extracts from *Ganoderma lucidum* Fermentation Broth on Chronic Bronchitis. *Mycosystema*, **28**, 832-837.

[36] Zou, L., Liang, C., Qiu, F. and Tao, X. (2002) Antitussive and Antiasthmatic Action of Wu-Hu-Tang. *Chinese Journal of Experimental Traditional Medical Fromulae*, **8**, 38-39.

[37] Zhang, D. (2011) Methods and Evaluation of Animal Models of Induced Cough. *Acta Neuropharmacologica*, **1**, 35-42.

[38] Angrill, J., Agusti, C., De Celis, R., Filella, X., Rañó, A., Elena, M., De La Bellacasa, J.P., Xaubet, A. and Torres, A. (2001) Bronchial Inflammation and Colonization in Patients with Clinically Stable Bronchiectasis. *American Journal*

of Respiratory and Critical Care Medicine, **164**, 1628-1632. http://dx.doi.org/10.1164/ajrccm.164.9.2105083

[39] Uren, T.K., Johansen, F.E., Wijburg, O.L., Koentgen, F., Brandtzaeg, P. and Strugnell, R.A. (2003) Role of the Polymeric Ig Receptor in Mucosal B Cell Homeostasis. *The Journal of Immunology*, **170**, 2531-2539. http://dx.doi.org/10.4049/jimmunol.170.5.2531

[40] Moghaddam, A.S., Shabani, M., Fateminasab, F. and Khakzad, M.R. (2005) Level of Nitric Oxide in Bronchoalveolar Lavage Fluid of Asthmatic mice Model. *Iranian Journal of Immunology*, **2**, 103-110.

[41] Goncalves, C.T.R., Goncalves, C.G.R., de Almeida, R.M., Lopes, F.M., dos Santos Durao, A.C., dos Santos, F.A., da Silva, L.F., Marcourakis, T., Castro-Faria-Neto, H.C., Vieira Rde, P. and Dolhnihkff, M. (2012) Protective Effects of Aerobic Exercise on Acute Lung Injury Induced by LPS in Mice. *Critical Care*, **16**, R199-R209. http://dx.doi.org/10.1186/cc11807

[42] Li, W., Deng, G.C., Li, M., Liu, X.M. and Wang, Y.J. (2012) Roles of Mucosal Immunity against *Mycobacterium tuberculosis* Infection. *Tuberculosis Research and Treatment*, **2012**, Article ID: 791728. http://dx.doi.org/10.1155/2012/791728

[43] Mushaben, E.M., Brandt, E.B., Khurana Hershey, G.K. and Le Cras, T.D. (2013) Differential Effects of Rapamycin and Dexamethasone in Mouse Models of Established Allergic Asthma. *PLoS ONE*, **8**, e54426. http://dx.doi.org/10.1371/journal.pone.0054426

[44] Chandler, J.D., Min, E., Huang, J., Nichols, D.P. and Day, B.J. (2013) Nebulized Thiocyanate Improves Lung Infection Outcomes in Mice. *British Journal of Pharmacology*, **169**, 1166-1177. http://dx.doi.org/10.1111/bph.12206

[45] Okada, S., Hasegawa, S., Hasegawa, H., Ainai, A., Atsuta, R., Ikemoto, K., Sasaki, K., Toda, S., Shirabe, K., Takahara, M., Harada, S., Morishima, T. and Ichiyama, T. (2013) Analysis of Bronchoalveolar Lavage Fluid in a Mouse Model of Bronchial Asthma and H1N1 2009 Infection. *Cytokine*, **63**, 194-200. http://dx.doi.org/10.1016/j.cyto.2013.04.035

[46] Rubin, B.K. (2007) Mucolytics, Expectorants, and Mucokinetic Medications. *Respiratory Care*, **52**, 859-865.

[47] Rubin, B.K. (2014) Secretion Properties, Clearance, and Therapy in Airway Disease. *Translational Respiratory Medicine*, **2**, 6. http://dx.doi.org/10.1186/2213-0802-2-6

[48] De Blasio, F., Virchow, J.C., Polverino, M., Zanasi, A., Behrakis, P.K., Kilinç, G., Balsamo, R., De Danieli, G. and Lanata, L. (2007) Cough Management: A Practical Approach. *Cough*, **7**, 7.

[49] Chung, K.F. (2011) Chronic "Cough Hypersensitivity Syndrome": A More Precise Label for Chronic Cough. *Pulmonary Pharmacology and Therapeutics*, **24**, 267-271. http://dx.doi.org/10.1016/j.pupt.2011.01.012

[50] Yousaf, N., Montinero, W., Birring, S.S. and Pavord, I.D. (2013) The Long Term Outcome of Patients with Unexplained Chronic Cough. *Respiratory Medicine*, **107**, 408-412. http://dx.doi.org/10.1016/j.rmed.2012.11.018

[51] Ryan, N.M. and Gibson, P.G. (2014) Recent Additions in the Treatment of Cough. *Journal of Thoracic Disease*, **6**, S739-S747.

[52] Dicpinigaitis, P.V., Canning, B.J., Garner, R. and Paterson, B. (2015) Effect of Memantine on Cough Reflex Sensitivity: Translational Studies in Guinea Pigs and Humans. *Journal of Pharmacology and Experimental Therapeutics*, **352**, 448-454.

[53] Janeway, C.A., Travers, P., Walport, M. and Shlomchik, M.J. (2001) Immunobiology: The Immune System in Health and Disease. Grand Science, New York.

[54] Aoshiba, K., Tamaoki, J. and Nagai, A. (2001) Acute Cigarette Smoke Exposure Induces Apoptosis of Alveolar Macrophages. *American Journal of Physiology: Lung Cellular and Molecular Physiology*, **281**, L1392-L1401.

[55] van der Vaart, H., Postma, D.S., Timens, W. and Ten Hacken, N.H.T. (2004) Acute Effects of Cigarette Smoke on Inflammation and Oxidative Stress: A Review. *Thorax*, **59**, 713-721. http://dx.doi.org/10.1136/thx.2003.012468

[56] Goldman, A.S. and Prabhakar, B.S. (1996) Medical Microbiology. University of Texas Medical Branch, Galveston.

15

Differential Insertion Depths of Filiform Needle, Concept and Application

Lei Li*, Clara W. C. Chan, Kwai Ching Lo

School of Chinese Medicine, The University of Hong Kong, Hong Kong, China
Email: *llie@hku.hk

Abstract

In this paper, the background, evolution, basic meaning, clinical application and the detail operating procedures of the differential insertion depth in filiform needle acupuncture were discussed based on the classical expositions of the *Yellow Emperor's Canon of Medicine*. It is believed that the differential insertion depth reflects the basic idea of expelling the evil Qi from the body in the application of traditional acupuncture. Since the site of evil invasion has different shades, the position of evil Qi and correct differentiation has become the operation key points of needle insertion. Apart from this, the *Yellow Emperor's Canon of Medicine* has further associated the clinical application of filiform needle insertion depth with the seasonal change of Yin and Yang, the body built of the patients, the nature of the diseases, the heat or cold pathogenic factors of the illness, the excess and deficiency of the patient, and the reinforcing and reducing function of acupuncture. These elaborations have greatly enriched the basic content of acupuncture and laid a systematic theoretical foundation of filiform needle operation. The differential insertion depth in acupuncture has its specific meaning, the emphasis of insertion depth of filiform needle with its differentiated clinical implication exemplifies the perceptual thinking features of traditional acupuncture and typical reveals the uniqueness of Chinese civilization.

Keywords

Yellow Emperor's Canon of Medicine, Traditional Acupuncture, Differential Insertion Depths of Filiform Needle

1. Introduction

Differential Insertion depths are a basic integral part of traditional acupuncture. It describes the appropriate in-

---

*Corresponding author.

sertion depths of filiform needle and the related clinical implications.

Acupuncture is the main instrument used by *Yellow Emperor's Canon of Medicine* to describe and explain the theories and therapeutic principles of Traditional Chinese Medicine. *Yellow Emperor's Canon of Medicine* has established the basic theories, and thoroughly discussed the principles and treatment methods of acupuncture and moxibustion. It is therefore recognized as the most influential classic doctrine in the development history of acupuncture. Based on the relevant content of *Yellow Emperor's Canon of Medicine*, this paper has explored and discussed the background, evolution, basic meaning, and clinical implications of applying differential insertion depths in filiform needle treatment, with the aim of providing a framework of reference for today's scientific and clinical researches.

2. The Origin of "Differential Insertion Depths" of Filiform Needle

The application of differential insertion depths in filiform needle treatment has reflected the fundamental belief of Ancient Chinese that acupuncture was used to expel evil Qi from the body.

Ancient Chinese believed that disease was primarily the consequence of spirits haunting, or ancestral punishment or taboo violation. Hence, the disease was located exactly where the haunted site was and expelling spirits from the haunted location in the body was the principal guideline to heal.

During the early stage of developing the theory of acupuncture, the basic concept was that evil spirits invaded the body and hid in the acupoints, or "painful points", which formed a relatively superficial structure. They were visible to the naked eye, close to the blood vessels and easy to locate at the body surface. Stone wedges, horns, needles, moxibustion and massage were the major tools and techniques, which the ancient Chinese applied to dispel the evil spirits at the acupoints [1].

In the era when *Yellow Emperor's Canon of Medicine* took shape, which is commonly believed to be between the Warring States period (475-221BC) and the early Han dynasty (206BC-220AD), with the invention of Nine Needles and filiform needles becoming particularly popular in clinical application, the common understanding of the nature and structure of acupoints changed, and the concepts of acupoints and meridians began to merge. Acupoints were perceived as the locations where the Qi of the human body gathered and dispersed, and also the stage where the righteous Qi and evil Qi competed against each other. The concept of the causes of diseases also evolved: instead of evil spirits haunting the human body, diseases were attributed to various pathogenic reasons. However, using acupuncture to dispel evil Qi has remained the key concept throughout *Yellow Emperor's Canon of Medicine*.

When evil Qi invades the human body, the affected locations are naturally at different depths. Hence, the key purpose of acupuncture treatment is to reach the exact location, specifically the exact depth of the location where the evil Qi resides so as to effectively dispel the evil Qi from the body.

3. The Basic Meaning of Differential Insertion Depths

The concept of differential insertion depths of filiform needle, as expounded in *Yellow Emperor's Canon of Medicine*, placed special emphasis on determining the insertion depths to take account of 1) the nature of the evil Qi resided in the acupoints and 2) the depth where the evil Qi was resided.

As mentioned in *Spiritual Pivot: Nine Needles and Twelve Yuan*:

"When Qi has invaded the Channels, Xieqi (Evil-Qi) is in the upper, Zhuoqi (Turbid-Qi) is in the middle and Qingqi (Lucid-Qi) is in the lower. So needling the Acupoints located in the depressions eliminate Xieqi (Evil-Qi), needling the Zhongmai eliminates Zhuoqi (Turbid-Qi) and deep needling when the disease is superficial leads to internal invasion of Xieqi (Evil-Qi) and worsening of the disease." [2]

It clearly explained that the pathogenic Qi resided in the acupoint could be differentiated into Xieqi, Zhuoqi and Qingqi, and these pathogenic Qi resided at different depths. Hence, the inserted needle needs to reach the appropriate depth in order to dispel the pathogenic Qi. If the needle is inserted deeper than is appropriate, it could lead the pathogenic Qi to go deeper and aggravate the disease.

A similar concept was also discussed in *Plain Conversation: Discussion on Regulation of Channels*:

"If the disease is in the Channel, it can be treated by regulating blood; if the disease is in the blood, it can be treated by regulating the Collaterals; if the disease is in the Qi Phase, it can be treated by regulating the Wei (Defensive-phase); if the disease is in the muscles, it can be treated by regulating the muscles; if the diseases is in the sinews, it can be treated by regulating the sinews; if the disease is in the bone, it can be treated by regu-

lating the bone." [3]

This is to say that pathological changes caused by different diseases will take place in specific parts of the body. The filiform needle must reach the specific locations where the pathological changes take place in order to heal. *i.e.* If the changes take place in the blood, the blood needs to be recuperated; if the changes affect the Qi, the Qi needs to be regulated; if it happens to the sinew or bone, the respective affected parts should be strengthened accordingly.

It was mentioned in *Spiritual pivot: Application of Needles*:

"*The key of needling lies in the reasonable application of the needles. The nine kinds of needles have different usages. They are either long, or short, or large, or small. They are used for different purposes. Wrong use of them cannot cure diseases. Deep insertion of needles in treating superficial diseases will damage muscles and cause skin abscess. Shallow insertion of the needle in treating deeply located diseases will, instead of expelling pathogenic factors, cause superlative ulcer. The use of large needle in treating mild diseases will excessively reduce Qi and worsen the disease. The use of small needle in treating severe disease cannot expel pathogenic factors and cure the disease.*"

It was also mentioned in *Plain Conversation: Discussion on the essential of Acupuncture*:

"*Huandi said: 'I'd like to know the essentials of needling.' Qibo answered: 'Diseases are either external or internal and needling can be either shallow or deep. To treat diseases, needles should be inserted into the required depth, neither too deep nor too shallow. If it is inserted too deep, it will cause internal damage; if it is inserted too shallow, it will cause external stagnation, giving rise to the invasion of Xieqi (Evil-Qi). Hence improper depth of needling brings about great disaster that affects the Five Zang-Organs, and leads to serious diseases. That is why it is said that diseases are located sometimes in the body hair and Rouli (Muscular-Interstices), sometimes in the skin, sometimes in the muscles, sometimes in the Channels, sometimes in the sinews, sometimes in the bones and sometimes in the bone marrow.*

So in needling the surface of body and Rouli, care should be taken not to impair the skin. Impairment of the skin disturbs the lung, leading to Wennue (Warm-Malaria) in autumn with symptoms of chills and aversion to cold. In needling the skin, care should be taken not to impair muscles. Impairment of muscles will disturb the spleen, leading to abdominal distension and fullness and anorexia in the last eighteen days in each season, amounting to seventy-two days altogether. In needling muscles, care should be taken not to impair the Channels. Impairment of the Channels disturbs the heart, leading to heart pain in summer. In needling the Channels, care should be taken not to impair the sinews. Impairment of the sinews disturbs the liver, leading to febrile diseases and flaccidity of sinews in spring. In needling the sinews, care should be taken not to impair the bones. Impairment of the bones disturbs the kidney, leading to abnormal distention and lumbago in winter. In needling the bones, care should be taken not to impair the marrow. Impairment of the marrow reduces the marrow, leading to weakness of the legs and lassitude of the body. So the patient does not like to move."

Both paragraphs have clearly explained why there should be different depths of needle insertion. The differentiation should be made according to the depth and precise location of the targeted organ or tissue. If the pathological changes happened in the inner area, then the needle should penetrate deeply; if the pathological changes took place near the body surface, the needle should be inserted shallowly. Should the acupuncturist be unable to insert the needle to the appropriate depth, like inserting the needle to a shallow area when the pathological change happened in the inner body, or inserting the needle deeper than the area of pathological change, adverse consequences will occur.

In *Spiritual Pivot: Application of Needles*, an acupuncture methodology named "*triple needling to induce Guqi*" was discussed. It divided needle insertion depths into three levels, namely the intradermal, subcutaneous and the muscle levels, and mentioned that the depth of needle puncture should be decided according to the depth of the exact locations of the evil Qi and righteous Qi. This is probably the most classic discussion on differential insertion depths in The *Yellow Emperor's Canon of Medicine*.

As mentioned in *Spiritual pivot: Application of Needles*:

"*The needling method known as triple needling for inducing Guqi (Food-Qi) means to puncture the skin first to dissipate Yangxie (Yang-Evil); then puncture a little deeper into the muscles without reaching the muscular interstice in order to remove Yinxie (Yin-Evil); and finally deepen the needle into the muscular interstice to conduct Guqi (Food-Qi). That is why the book titled Needling Methods says, 'Shallow needling is used at first to expel Xieqi (Evil-Qi) and promote blood circulation; deep needling is then used to discharge Xie (Evil) from the Yin phase; and extreme deep needling finally is used to conduct Guqi (Food-Qi).' The reason is just what is mentioned above."*

This is to say that the needle should first be inserted into the shallow part of the selected acupoint to dispel the evil Qi of yang phase which resided there; then the needle should be inserted deeper to dispel the evil Qi of yin phase. After all the evil Qi is expelled, the needle could then be inserted even deeper to conduct the righteous Qi. By doing so, the disease could be healed and the Qi and blood of the local area could be regulated and normality could be regained.

The purpose of applying differential insertion depths in acupuncture is to dispel the evil Qi in the local area, this is the fundamental meaning of utilizing differential insertion depths in acupuncture as mentioned in *Yellow Emperor's Canon of Medicine.*

4. The Interpretation and Expansion of the Concept of Differential Insertion Depths of Filiform Needles in Yellow Emperor's Canon of Medicine

Although the fundamental consideration of utilizing differential insertion depths in acupuncture is to dispel the localized evil Qi, *Yellow Emperor's Canon of Medicine* has further expanded its implication in clinical application. Apart from the exact location where the evil Qi resides, *Yellow Emperor's Canon of Medicine* suggested that in deciding the insertion depths of the needle, reference should also be made to the yin and yang balance of the four seasons, the body built of the patients, the nature of the diseases, the heat or cold pathogenic factors of the illness, the excess and deficiency of the patient, and the reinforcing and reducing function of acupuncture. The concept of differential insertion depths of the filiform needle is thus related to all aspects of the clinical practice of acupuncture.

It was mentioned in *Spiritual Pivot: Beginning and End*:

"The invasions of pathogenic factors into the body vary in depth in different seasons. In spring, pathogenic factors tend to attack hairs; in summer, pathogenic factors tend to attack the skin; in autumn, pathogenic factors tend to attack muscular interstices; and in winter, pathogenic factors tend to attack tendons and bones. Thus the treatment of these diseases with needling should be done according to changes of seasons. So to use needling therapy to treat obese patients, the methods used in autumn and winter should be used; to use needling therapy to treat thin patients, the methods used in spring and summer should be used."

This clearly explained that evil Qi resides in different parts of the human body as the seasons change. Therefore, when to conduct acupuncture treatment, the insertion depth of the filiform needle should be decided according to the seasons. Shallow needling should be applied in spring, summer and deep needling should be applied in fall, winter. When treating obese patients, deep needling like those to be used in fall and winter seasons should be applied, and when treating thin patients, shallow needling like those to be used in spring and summer should be applied.

A similar concept was mentioned in *Spiritual pivot: Yin and Yang, Lucidity and Turbidity*:

"So in needling the Yin Channels, the needles should be inserted deeply and retained for a longer period of time; in needling the Yang Channels, the needles should be inserted shallowly and with-drawn quickly."

This further explained that in treating diseases occurred in the Yin Phase, the needle should be inserted deeply and retained longer, whereas in treating diseases occurred in the Yang Phase, the needle should be inserted shallowly and withdrawn quickly.

As mentioned in *Spiritual pivot: Beginning and Ending*:

"Pain is usually caused by accumulation of pathogenic cold and therefore belongs to Yin Syndrome and pain which is deeply rooted and cannot be felt by pressure with a fingers also pertains to Yin Syndrome. These kinds of Yin Syndrome can be treated by deep needling. Itching is a problem pertaining to Yang and should be treated by shallow needling."

This suggested that all pain syndromes including those where the hurting locations could not be identified are diseases of Yin and need to be dealt with by inserting the needle deeply. All diseases manifest as itching belong to Yang, and need to be dealt with by inserting the needle shallowly.

As discussed in *Spiritual pivot: Abnormality, Normality, Obesity and Emaciation*:

"People who are in the supreme of life and whose blood and Qi are sufficient, skin is solid, when attacked by Xie (Evil), can be treated by deep insertion and longer retention of the needles. This is the way to deal with heavy people. Their shoulders and armpit are usually broad, their muscles are thin and skin is thick and black, their lips are plump and thick, their blood is blackish and turbid, the Qi in their body is unsmooth and slow in

flowing. This kind of people tends to keep forging ahead and is also generous to others. To use acupuncture therapy to treat this kind of people, the needles should be inserted deeply and retained for a longer period of time. At the same time the frequency of needling can be increased.

Huangdi said, 'How to deal with thin people then?' Qibo said, 'Thin people are characterized by thin skin, light color emaciated muscles, thin lips, low voice, clear blood and swift Qi. So the Qi tends to be exhausted and the blood tends to be damaged. To use acupuncture to treat this kind of people, the needle should be inserted shallowly and swiftly.'

Huangdi said, 'How to deal with average people?' Qibo said, 'They can be treated by regulating respectively according to the degree of whiteness and blackness of the skin. Those who are honest and sincere with regular features and whose blood and Qi are in harmony can be treated by needling without violating the common practice.'

Huangdi said, 'How to deal with strong people?' Qibo said, 'Strong people are usually characterized by solid bones, chubby and strong muscles and relaxed and nimble joints. If they move slowly, it is usually due to un-smooth flow of Qi and turbidity of blood. To treat this kind of people with needling, the needle should be inserted deeply and retained for a longer period of time. And the frequency of needling also should be increased. If they move swiftly, it indicates that the Qi is slippery and the blood is clear. To treat this kind of people with needling, the needle should be inserted shallowly and withdrawn swiftly.'

Huangdi asked, 'how to deal with babies?' Qibo said, 'Babies are characterized by thin muscles and skin, shortness of Qi and weakness of blood. So to treat babies with needling therapy, the filiform needles should be used. The needles should be inserted shallowly and withdrawn quickly. Such a treatment is performed once the other day.'"

This illustrated that needle should be inserted deeply for fat person and shallowly for the thin person and babies. The depth of needle insertion should be decided according to the patient's overall conditions when acupuncture is applied to a normal person.

As discussed in *Spiritual pivot: Root and Knot*:

"The general rule is that to treat those whose Qi is swift, the needle should be withdrawn quickly; to treat those whose Qi is unsmooth, the needle should be withdrawn slowly; to treat those whose Qi flows rapidly, the needle should be small and inserted shallowly; to treat those whose Qi is unsmooth, the needle should be big and inserted deeply. The deeply inserted needle should be retained in the acupoint while the shallowly inserted needle should be withdrawn quickly."

This explained that shallow needling technique should be applied if the Qi and blood of the patient flows swiftly and smoothly, while deep needling technique should be applied if the Qi and blood of the patient flows unsmoothly or became stagnated.

As mentioned in *Spiritual pivot: Symptoms of Zangfu-Organs due to Attack of Pathogenic Factors*:

"All kinds of rapid pulse indicate cold; all kinds of slow pulse indicate heat; ... So the needling technique for rapid pulse and the related disease should be deep and the needle should be retained in the selected acupoint for a longer period of time. The needling technique for slow pulse and the related disease should be shallow and the needle should be withdrawn immediately after insertion in order to remove heat."

This explained that the patient's disease is normally hot in nature when his pulse is slow, then, shallow needling technique should be applied, on the other hand, the patient's disease is normally cold in nature when his pulse is rapid, then, deep needling technique should be applied.

As mentioned in *Spiritual pivot: Beginning and Ending*:

"Forceful pulse indicates excess of pathogenic factors which should be treated by deep needling in order to expel evil *Qi. Weak pulse indicates deficiency of Healthy-Qi which should be treated by shallow needling in order to prevent Jingqi (Essence-Qi) from leaking, invigorate the pulse and drain Xieqi (Evil-Qi)."*

This elucidates that the insertion depth of the needle should be deep when the patient's pulse is strong and forceful while the insertion depth of the needle should be shallow when the patient's pulse is weak.

As mentioned in *Spiritual pivot: Channels and Collecterals*:

"The heat ones can be treated by swift needling techniques; the cold ones can be treated by retaining the needles in the acupoints."

It illustrated that diseases with heat syndromes should be treated by shallow needling technique and the needle should be withdrawn quickly, whereas diseases with cold syndromes should be treated by deep needling technique with the needle retained in the acupoint for a considerably longer period of time.

As mentioned in *Spiritual pivot: Beginning and Ending*:

"*Reinforcing and reducing techniques should be performed according to the conditions of pulse. If the pulse is forceful, the needles should be inserted deeply. After the withdrawal of the needle, the needled acupoint is not pressed immediately in order to drain Xieqi (Evil-Qi). If the pulse is weak, the needles should be inserted shallowly in order to invigorate the pulse. After the withdrawal of the needle, the acupoints should be pressed immediately to prevent invasion of Xieqi (Evil-Qi).*"

This clearly explained that the insertion depth of the needle should be shallow and the acupoint should be pressed immediately after the withdrawal of needle when the goal of the acupuncture was to reinforce the Righteous Qi. Whereas, the insertion depth of the needle should be deep and the acupoint should not be pressed immediately if the goal of the acupuncture was to dispel or reduce the Evil Qi.

The differential insertion depths of filiform needles in Yellow Emperor's Canon of Medicine are hereby classified in **Table 1**.

The appropriate insertion depths of filiform needle therefore become an important part of clinical acupuncture practice. In general, if the pathological changes in the interior, the needle should be penetrated deeply; if the lesion occurs near the surface, the needle should be inserted shallowly. For example, in treating lumbago due to kidney deficiency, it should be deep needling; in treating fever caused by exogenous pathogens, it should be shallow needling; wry eye and mouth should be shallow needling, abdominal distension and diarrhea should be deeply needling.

The extensive use of differential insertion depths has vastly enriched the essential content of the application technique of filiform needle in acupuncture, which in turn, laid a solid foundation for the theoretical and systematic approach of the filiform needle application technique.

5. The Combined Needling Techniques and Differential Insertion Depth(s) of Filiform Needles in Yellow Emperor's Canon of Medicine

Various types of combined needling techniques were discussed in *Yellow Emperor's Canon of Medicine*, like the five needling methods which correspond to the five Zang-Organs; nine ways of needling to deal with the nine kinds of pathological changes and the twelve methods of needling to correspond to the twelve meridians discussed in *Spiritual Pivot: Application of Needles*.

Most of these combined needling techniques have incorporated the concept of differential needle insertion depths such as the five needling methods corresponding to the five Zang-Organs:

"*There are five needling methods to correspond to the five Zang-Organs. The first one is called 'Banci' (half needling) which means to insert needle superficially and withdraw the needle quickly without damaging the muscles. This way of needling, just like pulling body hair, is used to expel evil Qi from the skin. The second one is called 'Baowenci' (leopard spot needling) which means to insert the needles into the left, the right, the anterior and posterior regions around the affected part. In such a treatment the needles must be inserted into the*

Table 1. The differential insertion depths of filiform needles in Yellow Emperor's Canon of Medicine.

Classification	Shallow needling	Deep needling
Position of evil Qi	Superficial body	Deep body
Seasons	Spring and summer	Autumn and winter
Body built of patients	Thin	Fat
Qi and blood running	Fast and smoothly	Slowly and unsmoothly
Pulse manifestation	Slow and weak	Rapid and strong
Nature of diseases	Yang syndrome	Yin syndrome
Pain and itch	Itch	Pain
Heat or cold of illness	Heat syndrome	Cold syndrome
Excess and deficiency of patients	Deficiency syndrome	Excess syndrome
Reinforcing and reducing manipulations	Reinforcing method	Reducing method

Channels for the purpose of bloodletting. Such a treatment corresponds to the heart. The third one is call 'Guanci' (joint needling) which means to directly needle the joints in the four limbs and the distal part of the tendon to treat Jinbi (Bi-syndrome of tendons). Cares should be taken to avoid bleeding. Such a treatment corresponds to the liver. It is also called 'Yuanci' and 'Qici'. The fourth one is called 'Heguci' (Tri-directional needling) which appearing like the talon of a chicken, means to insert the needle deep into the muscular interstices to treat Jibi (Bi-Syndrome of muscle). Such a treatment corresponds to the spleen. The fifth one is called 'Shuci' (transmitted needling) which means to insert and withdraw the needle perpendicularly. The needle is inserted deep onto the bone to treat Gubi (Bi-Syndrome of bone). Such a treatment corresponds to the kidney."

When utilizing needling techniques which correspond to the five body parts, the acupuncturist will divide the acupoints into five levels according to the respective positions of skin, muscle, vein, tendon and bone, and insert the needle to the appropriate depth to treat the pathological changes in the lung, heart, liver, spleen and kidney systems respectively.

Again take for example the "Jingci", "Luoci", "Fenci" and "Maoci" of the nine ways of needle application to treat various pathological changes.

"Jingci which means to puncture that part of the large Channel that connects with the Collateral."

"Luoci which means to puncture the small Collaterals to let out the blood."

"Fenci which means to puncture the part between muscles."

"Maoci which means to puncture the skin beneath which there is floating Bi-Syndrome."

The needle needs to reach the Channels in "Jingci" and thus it is a deep needling technique. The needle needs to reach the Collaterals in "Luoci", thus it is a shallow needling technique. The needle is targeted to reach the muscle layer in "Fenci", thus it is a deep needling technique and the needle is targeted to reach the skin in "Maoci" and thus, it is a shallow needling technique.

Similarly, "Huici", "Qici", "Yangci", "Zhizhenci", "Shuci", "Duanci", "Fuci" and "Zanci" of the twelve Channels corresponding needling technique also incorporate the concept of differential insertion depths:

"Huici (extended needling), which means to insert the needles around the spasm of muscles. The needles are lifted and thrusted forwards or backwards to relax muscles and treat Jinbi (Bi-Syndrome of tendons)."

"Qici (triple needling), which means to insert one needle perpendicularly into the affected part and two more beside to treat cold disease with small scale and deep penetration of Qi (pathogenic factor)."

"Yangci (scattered needling), which means to insert one needle first into the centre of the affected part and then four more around. The needles are inserted shallowly to treat cold disease that involves a large region."

"Zhizhenci (direct needling), which means to pinch the muscle and insert the needle into it. This way of needling is used to treat cold disease with shallow location."

"Shuci (transmitting needling), which means to insert and withdraw the needle perpendicularly. Usually fewer Acupoints are selected and punctured deeply. This way of needling is used to treat the disease marked by superabundance of Qi and severity of heat."

"Duanci (gradual needling), which used to treat Gubi (Bi-Syndrome of the bone), means to insert the needle deep into the bone, slightly shake the needle and deepen the insertion till the needle reaches the bone. Then the needle is manipulated upward and downward to rub the bone."

"Fuci (floating needling), which means to insert the needle superficially beside the affected part in order to treat cold spasm of muscle."

"Zanci (supplemental needling), which means to insert and withdraw the needle perpendicularly. Usually several needles are inserted superficially to let out blood. Such a way of needling is used to treat carbuncle and swellings."

"Huici" is to insert the needle to the tendon; "Qici" targets to treat cold disease with small scale and deep penetration of Qi; "Shuci" is to insert the needle deeply in a few acupoints; "Duanci" is to insert the needle deeply to the bone to treat Bi-Syndrome of bone. These are all considered to be Deep Needling techniques. On the other hand, "Fuci" is to insert the needle to the superficial layer of the muscle; "Zanci" inserts the needles superficially to release blood; "Yangci" is to insert the needle shallowly to release the evil Qi; and "Zhizhenci" is to pinch the skin and insert the needle horizontally. These are all considered to be Shallow Needling techniques.

When the concept of differential insertion depths is applied to the combined needling techniques, special emphasis is put on the nature of diseases; the exact location of the pathological changes; the severity of the diseases and the changes of application techniques. It revealed, from a different angle, the high flexibility and wide clinical application of the filiform needle treatment and the fundamental purpose of acupuncture as dispelling the evil Qi from the body. Thus, it is an integral part of the fundamental knowledge of filiform needle operation.

6. Conclusion

Filiform needle treatment in traditional acupuncture emphasizes the clinical implications of differential insertion depths. It is a classic example of intuitive direct visualization, which is a unique characteristic of Chinese civilization. Based on the conditions of the diseases, different insertion depths are applied, and it has greatly broadened the spectrum of application techniques of acupuncture using filiform needles. The comprehensive discussion of differential insertion depths in *Yellow Emperor's Canon of Medicine* has greatly expanded the clinical application of filiform needle treatment. The concept of differential insertion depths has not only enriched the content of filiform needle treatment, but also well integrated with the reinforcing and reducing needling technique to lay the systematic theoretical foundation of filiform needle treatment. Various well-known needle manipulation techniques have developed in the later years, like "Shaoshanhuo (Heat-producing Needing)", "Toutianliang (Cool-producing Needing)", "Qinglongbaiwei (Green Dragon Shaking Tail)", "Baihuyaotou (White Tiger Shaking Head)", "Cangguitanxue (Dark-green Tortoise Seeking for Cave)" and "Chifengyingyuan (Red Phenix Meeting Resource)", etc. are all the interpretation and development of the concept of differential insertion depths in the *Yellow Emperor's Canon of Medicine*.

References

[1]   Li, L., Yau, T. and Yau, C.H. (2012) What is the Origin of Acupoint. *Journal of Acupuncture and Tuina Science*, **10**, 125-127. http://dx.doi.org/10.1007/s11726-012-0587-8

[2]   Anonymous (1956) The Spiritual Pivot (Copied Print). People's Health Publishing House, Beijing.

[3]   Anonymous (1956) Yellow Emperor's Internal Classics: Plain Conversation (Copied Print). People's Health Publishing House, Beijing.

16

Vulvodynia Treated with Acupuncture or Electromyographic Biofeedback

Oroma B. Nwanodi*, Melanie M. Tidman

Department of Interdisciplinary Health Studies, A. T. Still University Arizona School of Health Sciences, Mesa, USA
Email: *o.nwanodi@juno.com

Abstract

First, second, and third line medical treatments of vulvodynia are of limited efficacy. Surgical resection, the fourth line treatment of vulvodynia, may have unforgiving sequela. Therefore, acupuncture and electromyographic (EMG) biofeedback could bridge between medical and surgical treatments of vulvodynia. Of note, EMG biofeedback is more frequently recommended in treatment algorithms for vulvodynia than is acupuncture. Trials of acupuncture for unprovoked vulvodynia demonstrate variable efficacy, whereas trials of EMG biofeedback for provoked vulvodynia demonstrate consistent efficacy. Trials of acupuncture for treatment of provoked and unprovoked vulvodynia using identical acupoints, a vulvar algesiometer for objective pain measurement, and standardized, validated, tools for outcome assessment are needed. Such trials may enable comparison of acupuncture to EMG biofeedback for the treatment of provoked and unprovoked vulvodynia. Similarly, trials of EMG biofeedback for treatment of unprovoked vulvodynia would increase the knowledge base of EMG biofeedback for treatment of vulvodynia.

Keywords

Acupuncture, Biofeedback, Electromyography, Vestibulodynia, Vulvodynia

1. Introduction

This article is a clinical review article on vulvodynia for health care providers including physical therapists, with an interest in alternative, complementary, holistic, or integrated medicine. As the target audience's knowledge base may not focus on gynecology, following the introductory section the relevant anatomy will be reviewed.

The purpose of this review article is to determine whether acupuncture and electromyography (EMG) bio-

---

*Corresponding author.

feedback have comparable efficacy in the treatment of vulvodynia or vestibulodynia. A secondary goal is to identify why the American guideline for treatment of vulvodynia does not support usage of acupuncture whereas the British guideline supports usage of acupuncture. Additionally, future study options for the treatment of vulvodynia with acupuncture that may use a vulvar algesiometer will be identified. To this end, the pathophysiology, classification, evaluation, and treatments of vulvodynia will be reviewed. Such review should clarify the pathophysiologic basis of vulvodynia, which contributes to the biologic plausibility of both acupuncture and EMG biofeedback for treatment of vulvodynia. Second, the efficacy of acupuncture for treatment of vulvodynia will be presented. Third, the efficacy of EMG biofeedback for treatment of vulvodynia will be reviewed. Fourth, an attempt will be made to determine the comparative treatment efficacy of these two treatment modalities. Such elucidation of comparative efficacy or lack thereof, between acupuncture and EMG biofeedback may reconcile the different recommendations for the treatment of vulvodynia in the American and British guidelines.

1.1. Definition of Terminology

Vulvodynia, a chronic, disabling, burning, discomfort of the vulva was first described in 1976, and given distinction as a discrete clinical entity by the International Society for the Study of Vulval Disease (ISSVD) in 1985 [1]. Initially, vulval vestibulitis was regarded as a distinct disorder from vulvodynia. However, in 2005 the ISSVD reclassified vulval vestibulitis as vestibulodynia, a localized vulvodynia [2].

1.2. Prevalence and Comorbidities

Provoked vestibulodynia has a prevalence of 12% of women [3]. Vestibulodynia is found in 15% of gynecology patients [4]. Immunologic, infectious, inflammatory, neoplastic, and neurologic pathologies should be excluded prior to making a diagnosis of vulvodynia [1] [2] [5]. Anxiety, depression, interstitial cystitis, irritable bowel syndrome, and sexual dysfunction are co-morbidities of vulva pain syndromes [1] [3] [6]. Provoked vestibulodynia is significantly associated with chronic fatigue syndrome (odds ratio [OR] = 2.78), depression (OR = 2.99), fibromyalgia (OR = 2.15), irritable bowel syndrome (OR = 1.86), urinary tract infections (OR = 6.15), and yeast infections (OR = 4.24) [3]. Vulvodynia is known to impair partner intimacy [1] [7], presumably via contribution to the development of dyspareunia [8], hypoactive sexual desire, orgasmic dysfunction, and vaginismus [6].

2. Methods

The PubMed database was searched on August 31, 2013, with the terms "acupuncture treatment vulvodynia", "electromyographic biofeedback vulvodynia", "acupuncture treatment vulvar vestibulitis", and "electromyographic biofeedback vulvar vestibulitis", yielding 10 English language articles. Eight articles were found from the reference lists of the first 10 articles. Three references were sought as original sources of standardized testing instruments. Two references were taken from prior work for neurological background, and one reference for anatomy (**Figure 1**). Of these, three studies on acupuncture and four studies on EMG biofeedback will be reviewed (**Table 1**).

3. Anatomy, Pathophysiology, Classification, Evaluation, and Treatment of Vulvodynia

3.1. Anatomy

The vulva is bounded cephalad by the mons pubis, bilaterally by the lateral margins of the labia majora, and caudad by the anus [9]. Within the vulva, the vestibule is demarcated bilaterally by the labia minora forming Hart's line, cephalad by the clitoris, caudad by the posterior fourchette and fossa navicularis, and in depth by the vaginal introitus [10] [11]. Being contained within the vulva, the vestibule may not be exposed to all the stimuli which the larger vulva is exposed to.

3.2. Pathophysiology

The vulva is primarily innervated by the pudendal nerve plexus from S3 and S4 [12]. Cephalad and lateral portions of the vulva derive innervation from the ilioinguinal, genitofemoral, and posterior femoral cutaneous nerves from L1, L1 and L2, and S1 to S3 respectively [13]. Vulvar pain may be transmitted via rapid, myelin

Table 1. Description of studies included in the review.

Study/ Year	Study Design	Subject Sources/ Diagnosis	Treatment of Interest	Treatment Frequency	Number of Subjects	Outcome Measures	Follow-Up	Results
Reference [1]/1999	Quasi-experimental. No blinding, control group(s), or randomization	Vulval clinic/ vulvodynia	Acupuncture Spleen meridian points 6 & 9, liver meridian point 3, large intestine meridian point 4	Once weekly for 10 weeks	12 women aged 18 - 68 years; all completed treatment	VAS pain score (range not given) and adapted QOL questionnaire scores	5 weeks after last treatment session	Three groups of subject response: good, short-term, and non-responders
Reference [17]/2001	Quasi-experimental. No blinding, control group(s), or randomization	Adolescent health center/ vestibulitis	Acupuncture 4 local and 2 distal points were always used, an additional 2 - 5 points couldalso be used	Once or twice weekly for 10 treatments in total	14 women aged 19 - 26 years; 13 completed treatment	VAS pain score of 0-10, negative/positive QOL questionnaire	11 subjects at 3 months after last treatment session	Statistically significant changes to negative and positive QOL factors p = 0.01 and p = 0.001
Reference [3]/2009	Quasi-experimental No blinding, control group(s), or randomization	Gynecology clinic /provoked vestibulodynia	Acupuncture 10-20 points from the forehead to the knees	Twice weekly for 10 treatments in 5 weeks	8 women aged 21 - 49 years. Mean age 30 years.	FSFI, PCS, PVAQ, and investigator developed pain report	None	Statistically significant improvement in pain with manual genital stimulation on the FSFI, p = 0.05
Reference [12]/1995	Quasi-experimental No blinding, control group(s), or randomization	Vulval clinic/vulvar vestibulitis	EMG biofeedback In-home pelvic floor muscle exercises with vaginal sensor, portable EMG biofeedback instrument, computerized EMG data acquisition	Twice daily for an average of 16 weeks	33women aged 21 - 45 years. Mean age 31.5 years.	Subjective pain scale of 0-10, frequency of coitus, EMG amplitude for contraction, relaxation, and rest periods	6 months	Decreased resting pelvic muscle tension and instability by 68% and 62%. Decreased subjective pain by 83%. Coitus resumed by 78% of abstainers
Reference [8]/2001	Block randomization. Non-blinded. Control groups of group cognitive behavior therapy, vestibulectomy	Media advertisement and referrals/ dyspareunia due to vulvar vestibulitis	EMG biofeedback In-home pelvic floor muscle exercises with vaginal sensor, portable EMG home trainer, computerized EMG data acquisition	Twice daily for 12 weeks	29 per group. Mean age 26.8 years. Total of 9 subjects overall discontinued	PRI and sensory scales of the McGill Pain Questionnaire, frequency of coitus, Derogatis Sexual Functioning Inventory, Brief Symptom Inventory	6 months	Intention-to-treat analysis statistically significant pain reduction in each group, greatest in vestibulectomy group.
Reference [22]/2001	Quasi-experimental No blinding, control group(s), or randomization	Clinic/vulvar vestibulitis	EMG biofeedback In-home pelvic floor muscle exercises with vaginal sensor, portable EMG home trainer, computerized EMG data acquisition	Twice daily for 11 months	29 women aged 25 - 48 years	Subjective pain scale of 0 - 10 for assessment of dyspareunia. EMG amplitude for contraction and relaxation	None	Significant decrease in pain for 84.7% of subjects. Coitus resumed by 69% of subjects
Reference [23]/2006	Joint computer generated randomization, control group given 2% topical lidocaine gel and 5% lidocaine ointment	Two vulvar clinics/vulvar vestibulitis	EMG biofeedback In-home pelvic floor muscle exercises with vaginal sensor, portable EMG home trainer, computerized EMG data acquisition	Twice daily for 4 months	23 women per group	Negative/positive QOL questionnaire, PRIME MD, Short Form 36, VAS 0 - 100 pain scale, Vulvar pressure pain threshold measured by vulvar algesiometer calibrated for 3 - 1000 grams force	6 and 12 months	Equivalent improvement in vestibular pressure pain thresholds, QOL, and coitus were achieved by each treatment group.

EMG, Electromyography; FSFI, Female Sexual Function Index; PCS, Pain Catastrophizing Scale; PRI, Pain Rating Index; PVAQ, Pain Vigilance and Awareness Questionnaire; PRIME MD, Primary Care Evaluation of Mental Disorders; QOL, Quality of Life; VAS, Visual analogue scale.

ated, A-δelta fibers with encephalin mediated spinal cord synapses between inhibitory communication cells and Waldeyer cells connected with the spinothalamic tract and serotonin mediated descending pain inhibitory channels [1]. An initial painful stimulus to the vulva can cause central pain sensitization.

In central pain sensitization the dorsal horn neurons are hypersensitized to any subsequent vulval stimulus [14]. Meaning that, after the initial provocation to the vulva, nociceptor thresholds are lowered and hyperalgesia occurs [7]. Now, progressively reduced stimuli can generate an increasingly greater pain response [7]. Distal-

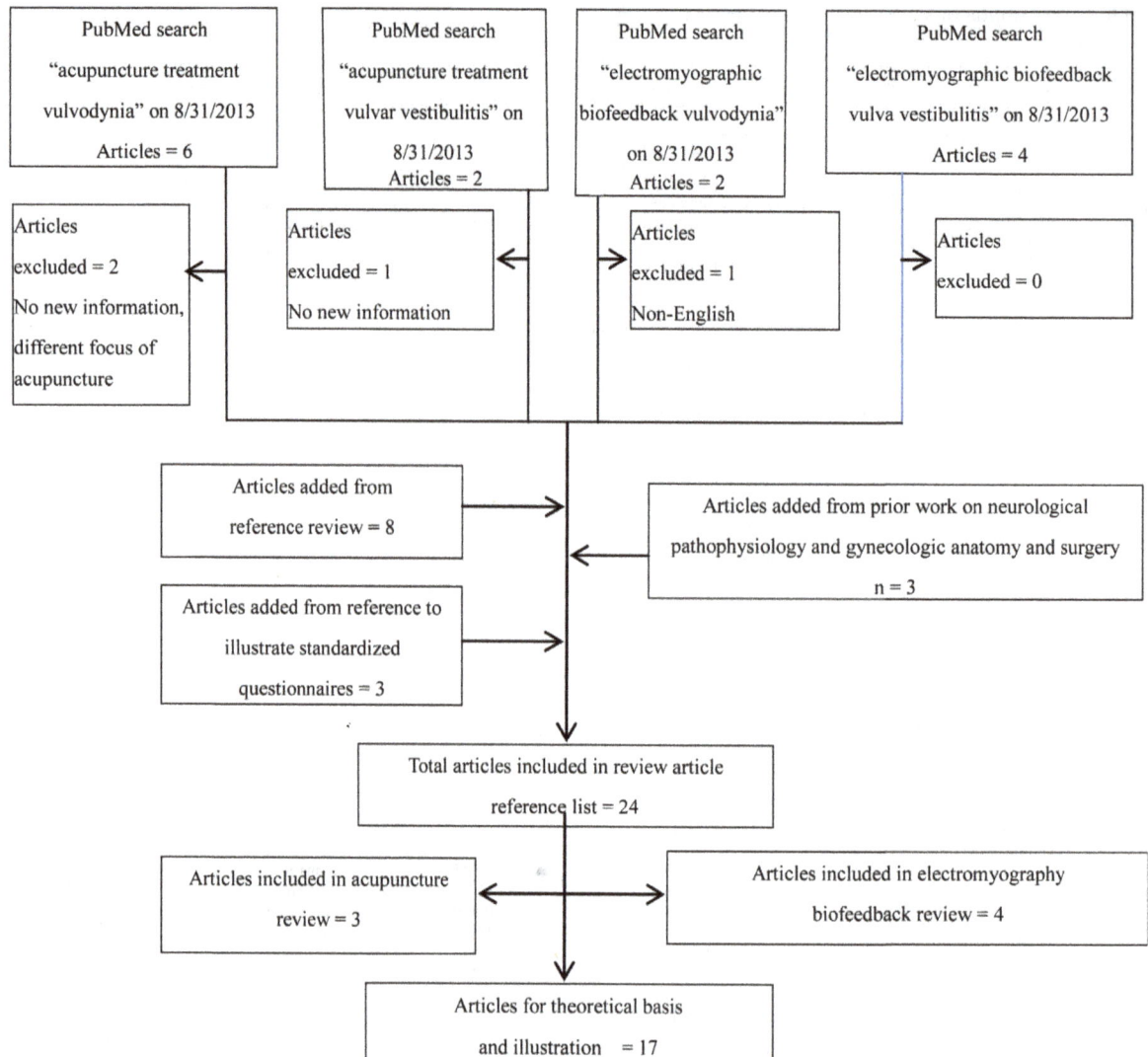

Figure 1. Article selection flow chart.

stimuli may elicit a response previously derived from local stimuli. The nociceptor field of reception increases with central sensitization and hyperalgesia [7]. Allodynia follows when nociceptors respond to what would ordinarily be non-noxious stimuli [7]. Persistent pelvic floor muscle stimulation may progress into contracture of the pubovaginalis and puborectalis portions of the pubococcygeus muscle [7] which receive innervation from S3 and S4 via the pudendal nerve [12]. Unprovoked myofascial pain ensues [7]. Baseline vulval electromyography (EMG) of healthy female controls averages 1 - 2 μV RMS [12]. Women with provoked vulvodynia have baseline EMG of 2.5 μV RMS, whereas women with unprovoked vulvodynia demonstrate further increased voltage of 3 - 5 μV RMS [12]. The progressive increase in vulva EMG voltage from healthy controls with normal pain sensation may reflect disease progression from central sensitization with hyperalgesia in provoked vulvodynia, to allodynia in unprovoked vulvodynia.

Alternatively, the concept of cross-talk pain from visceral inflammation postulates that normally inactive mucosal afferents of the bladder, urethra, and vagina are activated when sympathetic nervous system synapses are shared with afferents from viscera including the distal large intestines and rectum [14]. The pudendal dorsal root ganglia of S2 through S4 are shared with parasympathetic pelvic splanchnic nerves innervating the vagina and cervix, the inferior hypogastric plexus (from which the pelvic nerves derives) innervating the uterus and cervix, sympathetic sacral splanchnic nerves, and the vagal nerve which innervates the vagina, cervix, and uterus.

The ilioinguinal, genitofemoral, and posterior femoral cutaneous nerves share the inferior mesenteric ganglia with the lumbar splanchnic nerve from T12. In turn, the least splanchnic nerve from T12 shares the celiac and superior mesenteric ganglia with the greater and lesser splanchnic nerves. Therefore, innervation deriving from T12 can expose vulva innervation to stimuli from the ascending and transverse colon, kidney, liver, small and large intestines, spleen, stomach, and pancreas [15].

Up to 15% of afferents combine somatic and para-sympathetic motor activity permitting neurogenic sensitization, upregulation, and neurogenic inflammation in organs distant from the original inciting event, resulting in cross-talk pain [14] [16]. The anatomic location and etiologic pathophysiology of vulvodynia described above are important determinants of classification of vulvodynia and extent to which surgical treatment may eventually be recommended.

3.3. Classification of Vulvodynia

The ISSVD distinguishes between generalized vulvodynia of the entire vulva and localized vulvodynia pertaining to specific parts of the vulva [2]. Vestibulodynia is a localized vulvodynia of the vestibule anatomically described above [10] [11]. Generalized and localized vulvodynia may be provoked by nonsexual stimuli, sexual stimuli, or a combination thereof. Alternatively, generalized and localized vulvodynia may be unprovoked, or may result from a combination of provocation and non-provocation based on the described theories of central sensitization, allodynia, and cross-talk.

According to Friedrich's criteria, vestibulodynia involves six months of vestibular erythema, elicitation of pain upon application of pressure to the vestibulum, and extreme pain upon vulva penetration [17]. The classifications of provoked or unprovoked vulvodynia and vestibulodynia may affect treatment of refractory cases.

3.4. Evaluation of Vulvodynia

On physical exam, pain is elicited by the poorly reproducible operator dependent application of a cotton swab to the vulva [10] [11]. Therefore, a vulvar algesiometer (**Figure 2**) that measures pressure pain was developed [18]. Using four vulvar locations (**Figure 3**) for the vulvar algesiometer a correlation was found between 25 patients' subjective reports of pain and objective vulvar algesiometer scores. Post-treatment patients were able to tolerate increased force setting of the vulvar algesiometer force probe [18].

3.5. Treatment of Vulvodynia

Initially, vulvodynia and vestibulodynia are treated identically. Acute vulvodynia of less than three months du-

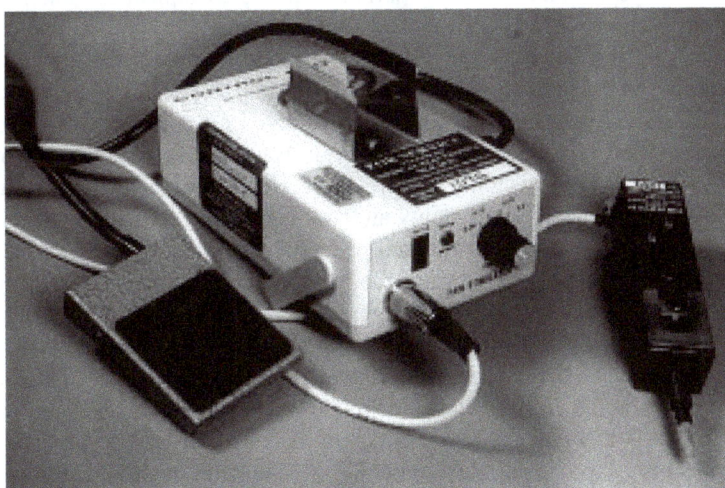

Figure 2. V ulvar algesiometer. Reproduced with permission from Eva, L.J., Reid, W.M.N., MacLean, A.B., & Morrison, G.D. (1999) Assessment of response to treatment in vulvar vestibulitis syndrome by means of the vulvar algesiometer. American Journal of Obstetrics and Gynecology, 181 (1), 99 - 102 (**Figure 1**).

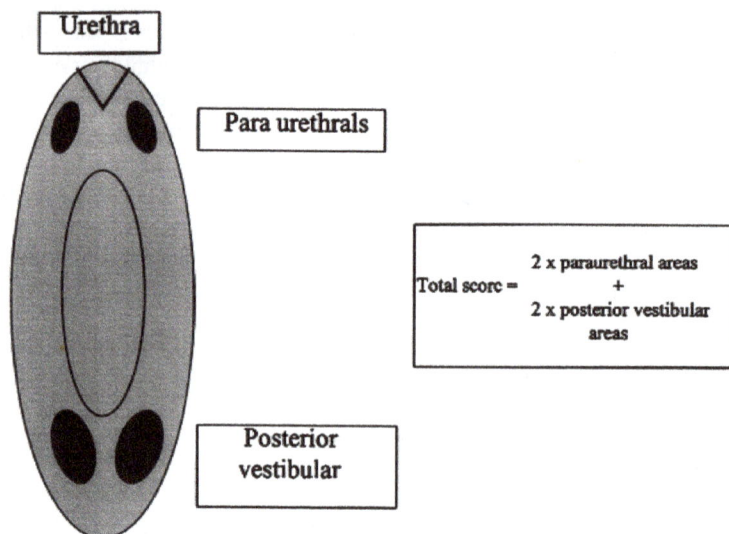

Figure 3. Positions of Application of Vulvar Algesiometer Probe. Reproduced with permission from Eva, L.J., Reid, W.M.N., MacLean, A.B., & Morrison, G.D. (1999) Assessment of response to treatment in vulvar vestibulitis syndrome by means of the vulvar algesiometer. American Journal of Obstetrics and Gynecology, 181(1), 99-102 (**Figure 2**).

ration may be treated by lifestyle changes such as the removal of irritant stimuli, suppression of inflammation and neuropathic pain [1] [5]. Bacterial and viral sexually-transmitted diseases, candidiasis, and urinary incontinence should be treated if identified. Usage of douches, harsh soaps, perfumed feminine hygiene products, propylene glycol or polyethylene glycol containing lubricants and spermicide, and tampons may provide irritant stimulus and should be discontinued [1] [5]. Underlying chronic conditions including interstitial cystitis and lichen sclerosis should be identified and treated if present. Topical steroids may be over-used by patients and are not recommended [5] [9] [12]. However, emollients and non-irritative lubricants may be used [1] [5]. These are all first line treatments.

Oral antidepressants and anticonvulsants form second line treatment [5]. Injectable anesthetic and steroid combinations are used as third line treatment when topical treatments provide inadequate relief [5]. Refractory vestibulodynia with dyspareunia achieving partial response to topical anesthetics may be more successfully treated with vestibulectomy than is unprovoked vestibulodynia [2]. Vulvectomy is the surgical alternative for refractory vulvodynia. Vestibulectomy involves the excision of painful tissue within the vestibule. Vestibulectomy is less extensive than a perineoplasty which additionally excises perineal tissue close to the anus [5]. Anatomically more extensive, vulvectomy is preferably reserved for patients with vulvar cancer. A complete or almost complete resolution of refractory vestibulodynia was achieved by 68% of participants in a randomized controlled trial (RCT) of vestibulectomy [3]. However, by six months post-procedure success rates start to decline to as low as 40 percent [10].Vulvectomy and vestibulectomy are major surgeries with the possibility of intractable post-operative adhesion formation and pudendal neuralgia [13]. Given the irreversible invasiveness of fourth line treatments of vulvodynia and vestibulodynia: vulvectomy, vestibulectomy, and perineoplasty; there is need for less invasive, reversible, alternative treatments of vulvodynia and vestibulodynia. Acupuncture and EMG biofeedback may be alternative treatments of vulvodynia and vestibulodynia.

For refractory vulvodynia, the American vulvodynia guideline recommends biofeedback and physical therapy, including electromyographic (EMG) biofeedback [5]. Acupuncture is absent from the American vulvodynia guideline [5]. Yet, the British Society for the Study of Vulval Diseases Guideline Group includes acupuncture as a possible treatment for unprovoked vulvodynia [2]. Acupuncture is efficacious as treatment of pain in dysmenorrhea, fibromyalgia, headache, lumbago, myofascial pain, and osteoarthritis [3]. Of note, while the efficacy of acupuncture for the above ailments is comparable to that of mainstream medical treatments, much fewer adverse events are encountered with usage of acupuncture than with mainstream medical treatments [3] [17]. Therefore, it is biologically plausible that acupuncture may be a safe, efficacious treatment of vulvodynia, including vestibulodynia, a local vulvodynia.

Given that currently available medical treatments do not adequately treat vulvodynia, there is room for additional effective treatment modalities of vulvodynia absent the systemic adverse events frequently associated with oral medications. Moreover, the vulvar algesiometer provides for objective, noninvasive assessment of vulvar pain that may be more highly regarded than subjective visual analogue scales (VAS) for determining efficacy of different treatment modalities for vulvodynia [18]. Clinical trials may specifically select cases of either provoked or unprovoked vulvodynia or vestibulodynia for study. Now that the vulvar algesiometer is available, an objective pain measurement may be used in clinical studies.

4. Efficacy of Acupuncture for Treatment of Vulvodynia

Penetration of acupuncture needles at acupoints by rotation or thrusting triggers numbness or fullness in the patient, referred to as "de chi" which in turn activates the release of opioid peptides[3] [17]. Acupuncture increases the concentration of β endorphins [1]. Acupuncture mediated opioid peptide β endorphin release is confirmed by opioid antagonist naloxone reversal of analgesia following acupuncture [1]. Therefore, acupuncture could alter the response of spinal cord synapses to afferent sensation of rapid, myelinated, A-δelta fibers in vulvodynia and vular vestibulitis [1].

Increased localization of analgesics or healing promoting substances at the target site facilitated by acupuncture in turn, increase rates of transmission of electromagnetic signaling from the brain [3]. Additionally, acupuncture may promote immune and central nervous system functioning [3]. Like longitude and latitude which traverse the entire globe, acupuncture meridians traverse the entire body. Meridians are energy pathways through the body, used by both acupuncture and bioenergy medicine. The acupuncture meridians of the liver, kidney, and spleen pass through the genitalia, permitting distant acupoints on the liver, kidney, and spleen meridians to elicit a therapeutic response at the vulva [3]. These acupuncture meridians echo the described interrelations between the ilioinguinal, genitofemoral, posterior femoral, and pudendal nerves that innervate the vulva, and the splanchnic nerves that innervate the liver, kidney, and spleen via sharing of the inferior mesenteric ganglia with the lumbar splanchnic nerve from T12. Thus, based on cross-talk, it is biologically plausible that acupuncture for treatment of vulvodynia and vestibulodynia need not be performed directly on the vulva or vulval vestibule.

Reference [1] performed a case series of 12 patients with unprovoked vulvodynia. Four acupoints were used weekly for 10 weeks. Two of 12 patients achieved good response, three of 12 patients achieved short-term response; seven of 12 patients were non-responders [1]. Standardized questionnaires for outcome determination were not used [1]. A pilot study of 14 women with vestibulodynia treated with acupuncture used ten treatments performed by a physiotherapist with more than 10 years of experience [17]. Each treatment done at one to two week intervals used at least six acupoints (**Table 1**), with 1 - 3 mechanical rotations for a total of 30-45 minutes [17]. Again, standardized questionnaires for outcome determination were not used [17]. Before treatment, after treatment, and three months post treatment VAS vulvar pain scores for patient-provoked vulvar pain were recorded for negative outcomes: the three major disabling effects of vestibulodynia as determined by each participant, and for positive outcomes such as "desire" and "joy of living" [17]. Statistically significant improvement of median VAS for both negative and positive outcomes occurred immediately after treatment with p = 0.004 and p = 0.04 respectively [17]. Three months post treatment a continued statistically significant but slightly changed improvement persisted with p = 0.01 for negative outcomes and p = 0.001 for positive outcomes [17].

Subsequently, reference [3] performed a pilot trial of acupuncture for treatment of provoked vestibulodynia with eight patients. Two traditional Chinese medicine practitioners (TCMs) performed 10 one-hour long acupuncture sessions utilizing 10 - 20 needles inserted from the forehead to the knees within five weeks. Reference [3] used standardized questionnaires for outcome determination. The Female Sexual Function Index (FSFI) [19], the Pain Catastrophizing Scale (PCS) [20], and the Pain and Vigilance Awareness Questionnaire (PVAQ) [21] were administered prior to initial treatment, then after the fifth and tenth treatments [3]. Following each treatment session, the investigators administered an investigator-selected questionnaire with 10 point Likert scale ranking. Analysis of reference 3 yielded a single statistically significant finding attributable to small sample size: pain reduction with manual genital stimulation (p = 0.05) [3].

5. Efficacy of Electromyographic Biofeedback of Pelvic Floor Musculature for Treatment of Vulvodynia

Physiotherapy with biofeedback has efficacy of up to 83% pain reduction in the treatment of provoked vulvodynia due to hypertonicity of the pelvic floor [3] [12]. Reference [12] performed an initial assessment in office, then studied 33 women using a surface EMG single user vaginal sensor with a separate portable EMG biofeedback machine at home on a twice daily basis with six intermittent in-office surveillance visits over 16 weeks. If necessary EMG biofeedback from accessory muscles of the abdomen, buttocks, and legs, as well as videotaped demonstration of pelvic floor muscle contractions were used to elicit correct pelvic floor muscle contraction. Patients learned to hold pelvic floor muscle contractions for one, ten, and 60 seconds. Each twice daily at-home cycle comprised of 10 second contractions alternated with 10 second rests for 60 repetitions, totaling 20 minutes. At each clinic session, patients reported pain on a Likert scale with 0 representing no pain and 10 representing the worst pain. By the 16-week clinic session, pain had decreased by 83%. Patients continued twice-daily pelvic floor contraction cycles without biofeedback for at least three months. A final evaluation was performed three months thereafter. Statistically significant decrease in pain, increase in number of patients able to have sexual intercourse, increase in pelvic floor muscle strength, and decreases in EMG amplitude during relaxation periods were achieved, with $p < 0.0001$ for each variable [12].

Reference [12] was retested with a study of 29 women, five of whom had undergone vestibular surgery [22]. The investigatory team performing the retest included the lead author of the original study as a co-investigator [22]. At 11 months from treatment initiation, reduction of pain to mild or negligible ratings was achieved in 84.7% of study subjects [22]. Moreover, 75% of study subjects were sexually active 11 months from study initiation [22].

The first RCT of treatment of provoked vestibulodynia was a comparative efficacy trial of 12 weeks of group cognitive-behavioral therapy (CBT), 12 weeks of EMG bio-feedback, and vestibulectomy involving 78 initial subjects assigned to trial arms by block randomization [8]. A subject recruitment, selection, and trial completion diagram is not provided [8]. In addition to assessing nonsexual vulvar pain via a Likert scale, perceived treatment efficacy and dyspareunia per se were also assessed [8]. Additionally, the Pain Rating Index (PRI), the Sensory scale of the McGill Pain Questionnaire (MPQ, the Global Sexual Functioning score of the Sexual History Form, the Sexual Information scale of the Derogatis Functioning Inventory, and the Global Severity Index of the Brief Symptom Inventory (BSI-GSI) [8]. Intent-to-treat analysis showed that at six months post vestibulectomy, subjects had statistically significant lower pain score than EMG biofeedback subjects ($p < 0.05$). Each treatment arm had identical improvement in pain from pretreatment to six months post treatment, MPQ-PRI pain, Sensory scale of the MPQ, sexual function, sexual history, and sexual frequency, ($p < 0.01$ for each treatment arm and variable). However, the vestibulectomy arm contained seven drop-outs, whereas the CBT group did not have any drop-outs [8].

Reference [23] performed a computer randomized comparative efficacy clinical trial of EMG biofeedback versus topical lidocaine gel with 23 subjects in each arm, of which 18 subjects completed EMG biofeedback and 19 subjects completed topical lidocaine treatment. EMG biofeedback used an identical vaginal sensor as in reference [8]. EMG biofeedback, comprised of three 10-minute sessions daily comprising of ten 5-second contractions and 5-second relaxations, followed by a 60-second rest, then fifteen 10-second contractions and 10-second relaxations, ending with a 60-second contraction [23]. Vulvar algesiometers measured vestibular pressure pain thresholds, while a 0 to 100 VAS was used to record subjective pain, sexual functioning, and dyspareunia [23]. The Short form 36 (SF 36), Primary Care Evaluation of Mental Disorders (PRIME MD, and a quality-of-life (QOL) instrument were also used. Vulvar algesiometer data at four months yielded greater improvement in pressure pain thresholds for the topical lidocaine group (site A, $p = 0.008$; site B, $p = 0.007$) than the EMG biofeedback group (Site A, $p = 0.002$; Site B $p = 0.02$), but at twelve months both groups and sites have statistically identical outcomes with $p = $ non-significant for any difference. Reduction in frequency of non-coital vestibular pain was greatest for EMG biofeedback given $p = 0.003$, and was the only VAS variable with a statistically significant difference when both treatment arms were compared, $p = 0.009$ [23].

6. Comparative Efficacy of Acupuncture and Electromyographic Biofeedback of Pelvic Floor Musculature

The studies on acupuncture for treatment of unprovoked vulvodynia lacked placebo controls [1] [3] [17]. Therefore, assessment of a placebo effect when treating vulvodynia with acupuncture cannot be performed. As is commonly a difficulty in comparing trials on acupuncture, each study used different acupuncture protocols in terms of duration of individual treatments, frequency and total number of treatments, and number of acupoints [1] [3] [17]. Furthermore, different outcome assessment methods were used in each study [1] [3] [17]. A direct comparison of these three studies cannot be made.

Similarly, the studies on EMG biofeedback for provoked vulvodynia have protocol differences. References [12] and [22] used different EMG biofeedback equipment, assessment protocol software, and durations of initial treatment. Reference [8] used different EMG biofeedback equipment and treatment repetition pattern than references [12] and [22], but the same assessment software asreference [22]. Reference [23] used a different treatment repetition pattern than references [8], [12], and [22]. As references [12] and [22] did not present study data in the same format a direct comparison of results between these two studies, of which the former was ostensibly to ascertain reproducibility of the latter is not facilitated. Furthermore, references [8] and [23] used numerous assessment questionnaires. Despite this, all four trials individually support the efficacy of EMG with biofeedback in treatment of vestibulodynia whereas none of the trials on acupuncture resoundingly demonstrate efficacy of acupuncture for treatment of vulvodynia [8] [12] [22] [23]. Yet, given that women with unprovoked vulvodynia have higher resting EMG of 3 - 5 μV RMS than an average 2.5 μV RMS in women with provoked vulvodynia [12], it is unclear why none of the trials of EMG with biofeedback in vulvodynia studied women with unprovoked vulvodynia.

7. Conclusions

Consistent with the 1997 NIH finding that evidence in support of medical applications of acupuncture was weak, at present, there is insufficient data to argue for the efficacy of acupuncture for treatment of unprovoked vulvodynia, and no data on the efficacy of acupuncture for treatment of provoked vulvodynia [24]. Therefore, it is understandable that American guidelines for the treatment of vulvodynia exclude acupuncture [5]. However, the absence of adverse events from acupuncture, and suggestion of response were sufficient for the British guidelines to include acupuncture as a treatment for unprovoked vulvodynia [2]. As acupuncture and EMG biofeedback have been used to treat different forms of vulvodynia a direct comparison of the two treatment modalities cannot be made.

Vulvectomy and vestibulectomy, the treatments of last resort for provoked vulvodynia or provoked vestibulodynia have only a culminative 68% almost cured or cured rate. Therefore, additional treatments for provoked vulvodynia including provoked vestibulodynia are needed. Given the favorable adverse event profile of acupuncture, it is reasonable to thoroughly evaluate acupuncture as a mode of treatment for provoked vulvodynia. Therefore, randomized controlled trials (RCTs) of acupuncture for treatment of provoked vulvodynia are needed. Such RCTs of acupuncture for treatment of provoked vulvodynia should use clearly delineated acupoints [1] [17], a vulvar algesiometer for reproducibility of pressure pain [23], and standardized, validated, tools for outcome assessment [3]. Designed in this fashion, RCTs of acupuncture for treatment of vulvodynia could facilitate comparison of acupuncture and EMG with biofeedback for the treatment of provoked vulvodynia. Similarly, well-designed and performed trials of acupuncture for treatment of unprovoked vulvodynia would increase the body of evidence for the use of acupuncture in the treatment of vulvodynia.

Trials of EMG biofeedback demonstrate efficacy. EMG biofeedback may be less efficacious than vestibulectomy. EMG biofeedback is also less invasive than vestibulectomy, therefore, it may be prudent to recommend a trial of EMG biofeedback prior to proceeding with vulvectomy or vestibulectomy for refractory provoked vulvodynia or refractory provoked vestibulodynia.

Acknowledgements

This paper is based on coursework previously submitted to the Arizona School of Health Sciences in partial fulfillment of the requirements for the Doctor of Health Sciences Degree, A. T. Still University.

References

[1]   Powell, J. and Wojnarowska, F. (1999) Acupuncture for Vulvodynia. *Journal of the Royal Society of Medicine*, **9**, 579-581.

[2]   Mandal, D., Nunns, D., Byrne, M., Mclelland, J., Rani, R., Cullimore, J., *et al.* (2010) Guidelines for the Management of Vulvodynia. *British Journal of Dermatology*, **162**, 1180-1185. http://dx.doi.org/10.1111/j.1365-2133.2010.09684.x

[3]   Curran, S., Brotto, L.A., Fisher, H., Knudson, G. and Cohen, T. (2009) The ACTIV Study: Acupuncture Treatment in Provoked Vestibulodynia. *The Journal of Sexual Medicine*, **7**, 981-995. http://dx.doi.org/10.1111/j.1743-6109.2009.01582.x

[4]   Goetsch, M.F. (1991) Vulvar Vestibulitis: Prevalence and Historic Features in a General Gynecologic Practice Population. *American Journal of Obstetrics and Gynecology*, **164**, 1609-1614; discussion, 1614-1616. http://dx.doi.org/10.1016/0002-9378(91)91444-2

[5]   Haefner, H., Collins, M.E., Davis, G.D., Edwards, L., Foster, D.C., Hartmann, E.H., *et al.* (2005) The Vulvodynia Guideline. *Journal of Lower Genital Tract Disease*, **9**, 40-51.http://dx.doi.org/10.1097/00128360-200501000-00009

[6]   Nunns, D. and Mandal, D. (1997). Psychological and Psychosexual Aspects of Vulvar Vestibulitis. *Genitourinary Medicine*, **73**, 541-544.

[7]   Jantos, M. (2008) Vulvodynia: A Psychophysiological Profile Based on Electromyographic Assessment. *Applied Psychophysiology and Biofeedback*, **33**, 29-38. http://dx.doi.org/10.1007/s10484-008-9049-y

[8]   Bergeron, S., Binik, Y.M., Khalifé, S., Pagidas, K., Glazer, H.I., Meana, M. and Amsel, R. (2001) A Randomized Comparison of Group Cognitive-Behavioral Therapy, Surface Electromyographic Biofeedback, and Vestibulectomy in the Treatment of Dyspareunia Resulting from Vulvar Vestibulitis. *Pain*, **91**, 297-306. http://dx.doi.org/10.1016/S0304-3959(00)00449-8

[9]   McKay, M. (1992) Vulvodynia Diagnostic Patterns. *Dermatology Clinics*, **10**, 423-433.

[10]   Baggish, M.S. and Miklos, J.R. (1995) Vulvar Pain Syndrome: A Review. *Obstetrical & Gynecological Survey*, **50**, 618-627. http://dx.doi.org/10.1097/00006254-199508000-00023

[11]   Haefner, H. (2000) Critique of New Gynecological Surgical Procedures: Surgery for Vulvar Vestibulitis. *Clinical Obstetrics & Gynecology*, **43**, 689-700. http://dx.doi.org/10.1097/00003081-200009000-00028

[12]   Glazer, H.I., Rodke, G., Swencionis, C., Hertz, R. and Young, A.W. (1995) Treatment of Vulvar Vestibulitis Syndrome with Electromyographic Biofeedback of Pelvic Floor Musculature. *The Journal of Reproductive Medicine*, **40**, 283-290.

[13]   Baggish, M.S. and Karram, M.M. (2011) Atlas of Pelvic Anatomy and Gynecologic surgery. 3rd Edition, Elsevier Saunders, Saint Louis.

[14]   Bergeron, S., Binik, Y.M., Khalifé, S. and Pagidas, K. (1997) Vulvar Vestibulitis Syndrome: A Critical Review. *The Clinical Journal of Pain*, **13**, 27-42.http://dx.doi.org/10.1097/00002508-199703000-00006

[15]   What-When-How. (n.d.) The Autonomic Nervous System (Integrative Systems) Part 1. The Crankshaft Publishing. http://what-when-how.com/neuroscience/the-autonomic-nervous-system-integrative-systems-part-1/

[16]   Ustinova, E.E., Fraser, M.O. and Pezzone, M.A. (2010) Cross-Talk and Sensitization of Bladder Afferent Nerves. *Neurourology and Urodynamics*, **29**, 77-81.http://dx.doi.org/10.1002/nau.20817

[17]   Danielsson, I., Sjöberg, I. and Östman, C. (2001) Acupuncture for the Treatment of Vulvar Vestibulitis: A Pilot Study. *Acta Obstetricia et Gynecologica Scandinavica*, **80**, 437-441. http://dx.doi.org/10.1034/j.1600-0412.2001.080005437.x

[18]   Eva, L.J., Reid, W.M.N., MacLean, A.B. and Morrison, G.D. (1999) Assessment of Response to Treatment in Vulvar Vestibulitis Syndrome by Means of the Vulvar Algesiometer. *American Journal of Obstetrics and Gynecology*, **181**, 99-102. http://dx.doi.org/10.1016/S0002-9378(99)70442-4

[19]   Rosen, R., Brown, C., Heiman, J., Leiblum, S., Meston, C., Shabsigh, R., *et al.* (2000) The Female Sexual Function Index (FSFI): Multidimensional Self-report Instrument for the Assessment of Female Sexual Function. *Journal of Sex & Marital Therapy*, **26**, 191-208.http://dx.doi.org/10.1080/009262300278597

[20]   Sullivan, M.J.L., Bishop, S. and Pivik, J. (1995) The Pain Catastrophizing Scale: Development and Validation. *Psychological Assessment*, **7**, 524-532.http://dx.doi.org/10.1037/1040-3590.7.4.524

[21]   McCracken, L. M. (1997) "Attention" to Pain in Persons with Chronic Pain: A Behavioral Approach. *Behavior Therapy*, **28**, 271-284. http://dx.doi.org/10.1016/S0005-7894(97)80047-0

[22]   McKay, E., Kaufman, R. H., Doctor, U., Berkova, Z., Glazer, H. and Redko, V. (2001) Treating Vulvar Vestibulitis with Electromyographic Biofeedback of Pelvic Floor Musculature. *The Journal of Reproductive Medicine*, **46**, 337-342.

[23]   Danielsson, I., Torstensson, T., Brodda-Jansen, G. and Bohm-Starke, N. (2006) EMG Biofeedback versus Topical Lidocaine Gel: A Randomized Study for the Treatment of Women with Vulvar Vestibulitis. *Acta Obstetricia et Gynecologica*, **85**, 1360-1367. http://dx.doi.org/10.1080/00016340600883401

[24]   Schnyer, R., Lao, L., Hammerschiag, R., Wayne, P., Langevin, H.M., Napadow, V., *et al.* (2008) Society for Acupuncture Research: 2007 Conference Report; The Status and Future of Acupuncture Research: 10 Years Post-NIH Consensus Conference. *The Journal of Alternative and Complementary Medicine*. **14**, 859-860. http://dx.doi.org/10.1089/acm.2008.SAR-2

17

Different Acupuncture for Neurodynia and Skin Lesions with Acute Herpes Zoster

Guohua Lin[1], Yunkuan Yang[2], Hongxing Zhang[3], Lixia Li[4*], Chuyun Chen[4], Yue Liu[5], Xushan Cha[1], Qian Li[1]

[1]The First Affiliated Hospital of Guangzhou University of Traditional Chinese Medicine, Guangzhou, China
[2]Chengdu University of Traditional Chinese Medicine, Chengdu, China
[3]Wuhan NO.1 Hospital, Wuhan, China
[4]Guangzhou Hospital of Traditional Chinese Medicine, Guangzhou, China
[5]The Second Hospital of Traditional Chinese Medicine of Guangdong Province, Guangzhou, China
Email: *llixia@126.com

Abstract

Objective: To analyze the effectiveness of different acupuncture-moxibustion therapies for neurodynia and skin lesions of acute herpes zoster. Patients and Methods: From April 2007 to October 2009, 500 patients with clinical acute herpes zoster were included in the study. They were randomly divided into five groups as follow: electroacupuncture (E); electroacupuncture + cotton-pave moxibustion (EC); electroacupuncture + fire acupuncture (EF); electroacupuncture + tapping combined with cupping (ET); control group of western medicine (WM). Results: The time of staunch bleb, scab and scab-off had no obvious statistical difference in the five groups; however, five methods could obviously reduce symptoms of herpes zoster and improved general symptoms. Within five days of treatment, compared to control group, the other four methods could more quickly ameliorate the general symptom of herpes zoster, and EF was superior to EC. In addition to electroacupuncture group, the treatment groups could relieve neuralgia and shortened duration of pain, which was superior to control group treatment. In addition, within first 3 days of treatment, the efficacy of treatment with E, EF or ET was superior to that of EC, and EF was better to E. After five days or end-of-treatment, the efficiency of odynolysis by treatment with EF, ETor EC was no more than E. The incidence of neurodynia was reduced after treatment with EC, EF or ET at 30th, 60th and 90th day, and pain of postherpetic neuralgia was relived. Conclusion: It is a certain advantages for organism reparation, abatement of neurodynia, and reduction of postherpetic neuralgia by acupuncture treatment.

Keywords

Herpes Zoster, Acute, Neurodynia, Acupuncture Treatment

---

*Corresponding author.

1. Introduction

Acute herpes zoster is caused by reactivation of latent varicella zoster virus (VZV or human herpesvirus 3). The virus can persist for years in the dorsal root ganglia of cranial or spinal nerves after resolution of original infection. As cellular immunity wanes with age or immunocompromise, the virus can be transported along peripheral nerves, producing an acute neuritis [1] [2]. Herpes zoster is characterized by a painful, unilateral vesicular eruption usually in a restricted dermatomal distribution [3].

Pain associated with herpes zoster infection can be classified as acute herpetic neuralgia, subacute herpetic neuralgia, and postherpetic neuralgia [4]. Pain is the most common symptom of acute herpes zoster and may precede skin changes by days or weeks [5] [6]. Moreover, pain is typically described as a sharp or stabbing sensation, burning sensation, or even "allodynia" (pain evoked by normally non-painful stimuli such as light touch) [6].

Pain associated with herpes zoster infection can cause significant suffering, particularly in elderly persons. Symptoms may be severe enough to interfere with sleep, appetite, or sexual function. In addition, symptoms may persist from months to years and cause profound psychosocial dysfunction, disability, and despair. The difficulty in treating herpes zoster means increased costs for individuals and health services [7] [8].

The treatment of herpes zoster is aimed primarily at earlier healing of lesions and prevention of complications. Randomized controlled trials and systematic reviews have found that oral antiviral agents (acyclovir, famciclovir and valaciclovir) are effective to relive pain at 1 - 3 months and to reduce the prevalence of postherpetic neuralgia at 6 months, although the effect is moderate. These drugs must be administered within 3 days from the onset of symptoms and have a good safety profile. Netivudine has a similar effect [9]-[12]. Other drugs such as levodopa, amantadine, amitriptyline, and idoxuridine are of unknown effectiveness in preventing herpes zoster complications. Moreover, corticosteroids drug are considered to be ineffective or even harmful [12]. Drugs considered to have a moderate effect in treating established postherpetic neuralgia are gabapentin and tricyclic antidepressants [11] [13] [14].

Despite these treatment options, many patients experience refractory pain and frequent adverse effects, especially elderly patients with cardiovascular disease. Therefore, pain associated with herpes zoster infection remains a challenge for effective management. Acupuncture and other methods from Traditional Chinese Medicine such as bloodletting and moxibustion have not been evaluated for this disorder. However, some Chinese case series report good treatment results but lack rigorous design [15]-[17]. We began a pain program at our primary care institution and collected cases with herpes zoster-associated pain to determine if these techniques could be helpful. This subject has been reviewed by the ethics committee of Chengdu University of Traditional Chinese Medicine.

2. Methods

2.1. Clinical Data

Diagnostic criteria: Traditional Chinese medicine diagnostic criteria has referred to diagnostic criteria of snake strand sore in "Diagnosis curative standard of tradition Chinese medicine disease"; Western medicine diagnosis standard has referred to diagnostic criteria of herpes zoster in *Cecil Textbook of Medicine*.

Inclusion criteria: Age range was from 18 to 70 years; the patients had herpes 1 to 7 days, and were not treated with antiviral or relieve pain drugs; all patients signed the information consent form, and agreed to accept the all therapeutic methods and obey arrangement.

Exclusion criteria: Special types of herpes zoster, including herpes zoster ophthalmicus (HZO), herpes zoster oticus (HZO), herpes zoster viscera, herpes zoster meninx, generalized herpes zoster, or no rash type herpes zoster; pregnant or lactating women; patients of anaphylaxis or drug allergy; scar diathesis; primary disease or systemic failure including cardiovascular, blood vessel of brain, liver, kidney and hematopoietic system, diabetes patients, cancer or mental patients, connective tissue disease and hemophilia, patients with bleeding tendency; patients with critical illness who were difficult to evaluate effectiveness and safety of treatment; patients who were treated with the corticosteroids or immunity inhibitor within one month.

2.2. General Information

All cases were come from the first affiliated hospital of Guangzhou university of Chinese traditional medicine,

Guangzhou hospital of traditional Chinese medicine, two Chinese medicine hospital in Guangdong Province, Chengdu Second People's Hospital, The affiliated hospital of Chengdu University of Traditional Chinese Medicine, traditional Chinese medicine research institute in Sichuan province and combining Chinese and Western Medicine Hospital of Wuhan at the time range from April 2007 to October 2009. A multicentric random trial(allocation concealment and central random are did in GCP center of Chengdu University of Traditional Chinese Medicine) was adopted, the 500 conforming cases who equally divided into five groups as follow: electroacupuncture (E); electroacupuncture + cotton-pave moxibustion (EC); electroacupuncture + fire acupuncture (EF); electroacupuncture + tapping combined with cupping (ET); control group (WM) with conventional western medicine therapy.

In E group, there were 45 male and 53 female cases included 4 cases with scab falling off, other 2 cases were eliminated; in EC group, there were 44 male and 56 female cases included 6 cases with scab falling off ; in EF group, there were 39 male and 58 female cases including 6 cases with scab falling off, and other 3 cases were eliminated; in ET group, there were 40 male and 56 female cases including only 1 case with scab falling off, and other 4 cases were rejected; in control group with conventional western medicine therapy group, there were 36 male and 62 female cases, including 3 dropping cases, and other 2 cases were eliminated. In five groups, the mean age was 43.76 ± 15.34, 46.98 ± 13.61, 45.20 ± 15.06, 44.33 ± 15.07 and 46.51 ± 15.30 years, respectively. Besides these, the time between feeling uncomfortable and medical consultation were 6.15 ± 4.11, 5.56 ± 3.14, 5.63 ± 2.70, 5.77 ± 3.05 and 5.24 ± 2.52 days, respectively. Meanwhile, the VAS scores of five groups were respectively 59.23 ± 25.71, 53.84 ± 25.95, 52.45 ± 28.11, 56.63 ± 25.44 and 57.20 ± 27.17 before treatment.

All indicators between the two as described above had no significant differences ($P > 0.05$), so, there was comparable between any two groups.

2.3. Treatment

All included patients kept the clean skin on parts of herpes zoster and protected skin lesions.

E: The main points included Ashi, Jiaji (on one side of sick), Zhigou and Houxi acupoints. The clients were adopted left and side-lying position, after routine disinfection, the Ashi acupoint was treated with acupuncture round pain; Jiaji point were treated with oblique insertion toward the spinal column; Zhigou and Houxi acupoints were dealt with coup droit. All points were inserted with needles at depths range from 0.8 to 1.0 cm, after result that patients suffered needling sensation response, the all cases were stimulated with Hans acupoint nerve stimulator (HANS; LH202H, China) which was operated in a standard method that adopted alternating current with frequency of 2/100 HZ and current of 2 ~ 5 mA, and a strength that all patients could bear.

EC: The cases were treated with cotton-pave moxibustion based on the E as described above. The clients were adopted lying position, then Ashi point was completely exposed to medical workers, after sterilization with iodine, the cotton wool that was tore into thin slices as cicada's wings (without a hole, 3×3 cm^2), was covered on the part of Ashi point, lit and burnt out rapidly. The acupuncture treatment was applied every 3 times.

EF: The patients were treated with fire acupuncture based on the E as described above. The clients were adopted lying position, then Ashi point was sterilized with iodine. Herpes central was penetrated with needle of moderate thickness that was heated until red and white, at depths range from 0.2 to 0.3 cm. Based on the number of herpes, early onset of herpes which selected numbers range from 3 to 5 were first pierced, and each was done 2 times. Postoperation, liquid of herpes zoster was drained then, the location was pressed for 30 s and coated with a flower oils.

ET: The cases were treated by combination tapping with cupping and E as described above. The clients were adopted sitting and side-lying position, after routine disinfection, the Ashi point was treated with plum blossom-needle tapping with slightly blooding. Cupping was pressed on the both ends of parts of collateral puncture and impairment. After bleeding by 3 to 5 ml and leaving the cupping for 5 to 10 min, the cupping was taken away and routinely sterilized.

Control: Valaciclovir and vitamin B1 were used through taken orally by 300 mg each with 2 times per day and 10 mg each with 2 times per day, respectively. The course of treatment consulted the E as described above.

2.4. Outcomes

Pain intensity (PI, VAS marking; mm): the tender spot was observed and noted in the 24 hours before the treatment. The interval range from 0 to 100 mm presented a level of pain intensity from indolence (0 mm) to maximum pain (100 mm) that patients could feel. We noted the pain intensity at first 10 days before treatment and at 11th day, respectively.

Duration of pain: we noted the time from pain presented to pain completely went away.

Incidence of postherpetic neuralgia PHN: we noted the postherpetic neuralgia PHN at 30th day.

2.5. Statistics

Values were shown mean ± SEM. The significance of differences between all groups was evaluated using one-way ANOVA with a post-hoc Student-Newman-Keuls multiple comparisons test. Chi-square test was used in enumeration data. Duration of pain analyses was adopted Log Rank test. Statistical analyses were performed using SPSS Software (V18.0, SPSS, USA), and a P-value < 0.05 was considered to be statistically significant.

3. Results

3.1. The Time of Staunch Bleb, Scab and Scab-Off

As shown in **Table 1**, the time of staunch bleb, scab and scab falling off had no statistical significance between any two groups (P > 0.05). So, five treatment methods showed a similar efficacy in time of staunch bleb, scab and scab falling off.

3.2. Aggregate Score of Herpes Zoster before and after Treatment

Before treatment, there were no statistical significance between five groups (P > 0.05), so it was comparability between the groups. However, at 5th days, the result (P < 0.01) was opposite compared to the pre-treatment, as described above. Compared to control group, the other four groups had statistical significance (P < 0.01), moreover, cotton-pave moxibustion group was superior to fire acupuncture group (P < 0.05). End-of-treatment, compared to control group, the other four groups had statistical significance (P < 0.01), the result as like as it as described above (P < 0.01 or P > 0.05), and there were statistical significance between pre-treatment and after 5 days treatment (P < 0.01). However, there was a difference between before and after treatment (P > 0.05). In summary, the five methods could reduce obviously the symptom of acute herpes zoster, and ameliorated the general symptoms. Within the first five days of treatment, compared to control, the other four methods could ameliorated more quickly the general symptom of herpes zoster, and fire acupuncture was superior to cotton-pave moxibustion (**Table 2**).

Table 1. The time of staunch bleb, scab and scab-off.

Group	Cases	Staunch vesicle (days)	Scab (days)	Scab-off (days)
E	94	5.02 ± 2.48	9.13 ± 3.90	21.49 ± 8.98
EC	94	4.54 ± 1.95	8.49 ± 3.47	20.87 ± 8.14
EF	91	4.87 ± 2.03	9.04 ± 4.57	20.13 ± 8.86
ET	95	5.05 ± 2.32	9.45 ± 4.90	21.06 ± 9.45
WM	95	4.83 ± 2.30	9.91 ± 3.63	24.27 ± 12.67

Table 2. Aggregate score of herpes zoster before and after treatment.

Group	Case (n)	pre-treatment	Treatment (within 5 days)	After treatment	Difference between treatment (5 days) and pre-treatment	Difference between before and after treatment
E	94	13.97 ± 3.31	8.27 ± 3.55	3.50 ± 2.79	5.70 ± 4.02	10.47 ± 3.79
EC	94	13.62 ± 3.50	8.77 ± 3.27	3.76 ± 2.56	4.85 ± 3.61	9.86 ± 3.82
EF	91	13.86 ± 3.69	7.44 ± 3.83	3.41 ± 2.80	6.42 ± 4.48	10.45 ± 4.44
ET	95	13.52 ± 3.94	8.11 ± 4.34	3.59 ± 3.03	5.41 ± 5.10	9.93 ± 4.51
WM	95	14.77 ± 3.30	10.23 ± 3.88	4.59 ± 3.02	4.54 ± 3.45	10.18 ± 3.36

3.3. Duration of Pain

As shown in **Table 3**, the pain lasting time had statistical significance between control and other four groups (P < 0.01). In addition, there was statistical significance between other three groups and ET group (P < 0.01 or P < 0.05). However, the pain lasting time had no statistical significance between any two groups for E, EC and EF groups as described above (P > 0.05). Therefore, the former four groups could obviously reduce the pain lasting time compared to western medicine group. However, the effects in three groups, including the E group, EC and EF group, were better compared to ET group.

3.4. VAS of Treatment

As shown in **Table 4**, there was no statistical significance between any two groups (P > 0.05). In addition, there was statistical significance between prior to the treatment and end-of-treatment between any two groups (P < 0.01). Meanwhile, at day 3, 5, 7 of their hospitalisation and end-of-treatment, there were significant difference between any two groups (P < 0.01). Besides that, there were statistical significance between former four groups and control group (P < 0.01). However, there were no statistical significance between any two groups of four groups included E, EC, EF and ET (P > 0.05). In summary, the five methods could reduce gradually the pain of nerve, the effects of former four methods was better compare to western medicine method. Moreover, at first 3 days of treatment, both the E, ET and EF had better therapeutical efficiency compared to EC, and the EF was superior to alone electroacupuncture.

3.5. Different VAS of Pre-treatment and Post-Treatment

After treatment for 5 days, there were statistical significance between the four groups and control group (P < 0.01). In addition, E, ET and EF were superior to EC (P < 0.01). Besides, E was better to ET and EF (P < 0.01). However, there was no statistical significance between pre-treatment and post-treatment. In short, the five methods could reduce gradually the pain of nerve, and former four methods had a better efficiency than control group. Furthermore, the three groups, including the E, ET and EF, which had better analgesic effect compared to EC, and E was superior to the EF and ET (**Table 5**).

3.6. VAS of during Follow-Up Period

As shown in **Table 6**, follow-up tests were applied at 22th, 30th, 60th and 90th day after treatments, respectively.

Table 3. Duration of pain.

Group	Case (n)	Duration of pain (days)
E	94	15.87 ± 11.86
EC	94	16.66 ± 8.80
EF	91	15.89 ± 12.00
ET	95	17.65 ± 13.53
WM	95	28.26 ± 19.69

Table 4. VAS of treatment.

Group	Case (n)	Pre-treatment	Treatment (3 days)	Treatment (5 days)	Treatment (7 days)	After treatment
E	94	58.88 ± 25.89	36.60 ± 24.18	22.88 ± 19.68	13.30 ± 17.52	4.03 ± 9.27
EC	94	54.09 ± 26.35	41.19 ± 24.61	27.30 ± 22.21	14.46 ± 16.76	6.05 ± 12.46
EF	91	52.67 ± 27.82	34.95 ± 23.98	23.63 ± 21.79	14.60 ± 16.65	5.01 ± 10.12
ET	95	56.17 ± 25.17	36.13 ± 23.17	25.96 ± 22.51	17.26 ± 19.49	5.16 ± 10.98
WM	95	58.01 ± 26.97	47.59 ± 23.96	34.73 ± 21.54	25.89 ± 19.43	14.30 ± 16.15

Table 5. Different VAS of pre-treatment and post-treatment.

Group	Case (n)	Difference between treatment (5 days) and pre-treatment	Difference between before and after treatment
E	94	36.00 ± 28.63	54.86 ± 25.84
EC	94	26.79 ± 23.26	48.03 ± 28.72
EF	91	29.04 ± 29.93	47.66 ± 27.73
ET	95	30.21 ± 25.18	51.01 ± 25.41
WM	95	23.28 ± 23.24	43.71 ± 27.55

Table 6. VAS of during follow-up period.

Group	Case (n)	22th day	39th day	60th day	90th day
E	94	1.44 ± 5.32	0.60 ± 3.52	0.27 ± 1.85	0.11 ± 1.03
EC	94	2.05 ± 7.03	1.04 ± 5.03	0.59 ± 4.01	0.53 ± 3.70
EF	91	2.33 ± 9.32	1.36 ± 7.40	0.22 ± 2.10	0 ± 0
ET	95	1.80 ± 8.22	1.13 ± 6.11	0.32 ± 2.28	0 ± 0
WM	95	8.18 ± 12.97	5.47 ± 10.72	2.21 ± 7.80	1.16 ± 6.03

There were statistical significance between the other four groups and control group ($P < 0.01$ or $P < 0.05$). Meanwhile, the E was superior to EF at 22th and 30th day ($P < 0.01$ or $P < 0.05$). In brief, levels of pain in E, ET, EF and EC groups were lighter compared to that in control group, and E was superior to EF group.

3.7. Incidence of Postherpetic Neuralgia

As shown in **Table 7**, Follow-up test were performed at 30th, 60th and 90th day after treatment, respectively ($P < 0.01$ or $P < 0.05$), in addition, postherpetic incidences in neuralgia E, ET, EF and EC groups were less compared to that in control ($P < 0.01$ or $P < 0.05$).

4. Discussion

Traditional Chinese medicine techniques such as acupuncture and moxibustion could be integrated with orthodox Western medicine therapies to fill the effectiveness gap in some pain problems included herpes zoster-associated pain to prevent or reduce pain with minimal adverse effects of treatment. The acute herpes zoster research is the first clinical study to investigate the effectiveness of an acupuncture treatment for acute herpes zoster pain in direct comparison to a standard analgesic treatment with gabapentine and to a sham laser acupuncture treatment in a three-armed, randomized controlled clinical trial. Compared to previous studies of acupuncture in the treatment of herpes zoster, this study has a more rigorous methodology and will include more patients.

In our study, for the time of staunch bleb, scab and scab falling off, there were no obvious statistical difference in E, EC, EF, ET and control groups, however, five methods could obviously reduce symptoms of herpes zoster and improved the general symptoms. At first five days of treatment, compared to control method, the other four methods could more quickly ameliorate the general symptoms of herpes zoster, and EF was superior to EC.

Acute herpes zoster is relieved during treatment; moreover, EC, EF and ET methods could reduce the neuralgia and shortened the duration of pain, which were superior to that treating with western medicine. In addition, at first 3 days of treatment, the efficacy of treatment with E, EF or ET was superior to that of EC, and EF method was better than E After the fifth day of treatment or end-of-treatment, the efficiency of relieve pain by treatment with EF, ET or EC was no more than alone E. The incidence of neurodynia was reduced after EC, EF or ET treatment at 30th, 60th and 90th day, and pain of postherpetic neuralgia was relived.

In my paper, base line of all cases in electro-acupuncture group was basically in compliance with the control

Table 7. Incidence of postherpetic neuralgia.

group	Case (n)	Follow-up (30th day)		Follow-up (60th day)		Follow-up (90th day)	
		No	Yes	No	Yes	No	Yes
E	94	90 (95.74)	4 (4.26)	92 (97.87)	2 (2.13)	93 (98.94)	1 (1.06)
EC	94	89 (94.68)	5 (5.32)	92 (97.87)	2 (2.13)	92 (97.87)	2 (2.13)
EF	91	87 (95.60)	4 (4.40)	90 (98.90)	1 (1.10)	91 (100.00)	0 (0.00)
ET	95	90 (94.74)	5 (5.26)	93 (97.89)	2 (2.11)	95 (100.00)	0 (0.00)
WM	95	63 (66.32)	32 (33.68)	86 (90.53)	9 (9.47)	90 (94.74)	5 (5.26)

group. Valaciclovir [18] was used in here, which had a bioavailability with 54.5%. So, it had a gender certainly as control.

In fact, the efficiency that local Ashi point was treated with stimulation of acupuncture which worked through a conducting system of cortex-meridians and collaterals-viscera. Varicella zoster viruses are almost lurked in spinal nerve root, namely locate in Du meridian and Jiaji points. In here, the partial skin lesions, painful place and relevant Jiaji points of ganglion are where pathogenic factors exist in, which could be thought as an Ashi point storing herpes zoster [19]. Jiaji point locates in between Du meridian and Sun meridians of foot, we can regulate the Yang-Heavy of Du meridian, Sun meridians of foot and the whole body, which makes it to reach the objective of regulation of meridians and collaterals and viscera.

5. Conclusion

In conclusion, it is a certain advantage for repairation of organism, abatement of neurodynia, and reduction of postherpetic neuralgia by acupuncture treatment, and the efficiency of combination electroacupuncture and fire acupuncture is better to that of the only electroacupuncture in the early days. However, at the end of the treatment period, the efficiency of electroacupuncture + cotton-pave moxibustion, electroacupuncture + fire acupuncture or electroacupuncture + tapping is no more than that of the only electroacupuncture. Further studies are required to determine the pre-clinical utility of this method.

References

[1] Burke, B.L., Steele, R.W., Beard, O.W., Wood, J.S., Cain, T.D. and Marmer, D.J. (1982) Immune Responses to Varicella-Zoster in the Aged. *Archives of Internal Medicine*, **142**, 291-293. http://dx.doi.org/10.1001/archinte.1982.00340150091017

[2] Meier, J.L. and Straus, S.E. (1992) Comparative Biology of Latent Varicella-Zoster Virus and Herpes Simplex Virus Infections. *The Journal of Infectious Diseases*, **166**, S13-S23. http://dx.doi.org/10.1093/infdis/166.Supplement_1.S13

[3] Gnann Jr., J.W. and Whitley, R.J. (2002) Herpes Zoster. *The New England Journal of Medicine*, **347**, 340-346. http://dx.doi.org/10.1056/NEJMcp013211

[4] Dworkin, R.H. and Portenoy, R.K. (1996) Pain and Its Persistence in Herpes Zoster. *Pain*, **67**, 241-251. http://dx.doi.org/10.1016/0304-3959(96)03122-3

[5] Gilden, D.H., Dueland, A.N., Cohrs, R., Martin, J.R., Kleinschmidt-DeMasters, B.K. and Mahalingam, R. (1991) Preherpetic Neuralgia. *Neurology*, **41**, 1215-1218. http://dx.doi.org/10.1212/WNL.41.8.1215

[6] Bowsher, D. (1995) Pathophysiology of Postherpetic Neuralgia: Towards a Rational Treatment. *Neurology*, **45**, S56-S57. http://dx.doi.org/10.1212/WNL.45.12_Suppl_8.S56

[7] Lydick, E., Epstein, R.S., Himmelberger, D. and White, C.J. (1995) Herpes Zoster and Quality of Life: A Self-Limited Disease with Severe Impact. *Neurology*, **45**, S52-S53. http://dx.doi.org/10.1212/WNL.45.12_Suppl_8.S52

[8] Graff-Radford, S.B., Kames, L.D. and Naliboff, B.D. (1986) Measure of Psychological Adjustment and Perception of Pain in Postherpetic Neuralgia and Trigeminal Neuralgia. *Clinical Journal of Pain*, **2**, 55. http://dx.doi.org/10.1097/00002508-198602010-00009

[9] Lancaster, T., Silagy, C. and Gray, S. (1995) Primary Care Management of Acute Herpes Zoster: Systematic Review of Evidence from Randomized Controlled Trials. *The British Journal of General Practice*, **45**, 39-45.

[10] Volmink, J., Lancaster, T., Gray, S. and Silagy, C. (1996) Treatments for Postherpetic Neuralgia—A Systematic Re-

view of Randomized Controlled Trials. *Family Practice*, **13**, 84-91. http://dx.doi.org/10.1093/fampra/13.1.84

[11] Alper, B.S. and Lewis, P.R. (2002) Treatment of Postherpetic Neuralgia: A Systematic Review of the Literature. *The Journal of Family Practice*, **51**, 121-128.

[12] Alper, B.S. and Lewis, P.R. (2000) Does Treatment of Acute Herpes Zoster Prevent or Shorten Postherpetic Neuralgia? *The Journal of Family Practice*, **49**, 255-264.

[13] Backonja, M. and Glanzman, R.L. (2003) Gabapentin Dosing for Neuropathic Pain: Evidence from Randomized, Placebo-Controlled Clinical Trials. *Clinical Therapeutics*, **25**, 81-104. http://dx.doi.org/10.1016/S0149-2918(03)90011-7

[14] Rice, A.S. and Maton, S. (2001) Gabapentin in Postherpetic Neuralgia: A Randomised, Double Blind, Placebo Controlled Study. *Pain*, **94**, 215-224. http://dx.doi.org/10.1016/S0304-3959(01)00407-9

[15] Owen, W. and Deadman, P. (1994) Treatment by Acupuncture for Herpes Zoster. *Journal of Chinese Medicine*, **45**, 1-2.

[16] Wu, J. and Guo, Z. (2000) Twenty-Three Cases of Postherpetic Neuralgia Treated by Acupuncture. *Journal of Traditional Chinese Medicine*, **20**, 36-37.

[17] Xuan, L. (2000) Treatment by Moxibustion for Herpes Zoster. *Journal of Chinese Medicine*, **64**, 17-18.

[18] Page, C.P., Curtis, M.J., Walker, M.J. and Hoffman, B.B. (2006) Integrated pharmacology. 3rd Edition, Elsevier (Mosby), Philadelphia, 87-160.

[19] Arora, A., Mendoza, N., Brantley, J., Yates, B., Dix, L. and Tyring, S. (2008) Double-Blind Study Comparing 2 Dosages of Valacyclovir Hydrochloride for the Treatment of Uncomplicated Herpes Zoster in Immunocompromised Patients 18 Years of Age and Older. *The Journal of Infectious Diseases*, **197**, 1289-1295. http://dx.doi.org/10.1086/586903

18

Acute and Long-Term Treatments with an Herbal Formula V-Vital Capsule Increase Exercise Endurance Capacity in Weight-Loaded Swimming Mice

Pou Kuan Leong[1], Hoi Yan Leung[1], Wing Man Chan[1], Ji Hang Chen[1], Hoi Shan Wong[1], Chung Wah Ma[2], Shi Yu Zou[2], Kam Ming Ko[1*]

[1]Division of Life Science, The Hong Kong University of Science & Technology, Hong Kong SAR, China
[2]Infinitus (China) Company Ltd., Guangzhou, China
Email: *bcrko@ust.hk

Abstract

Fatigue is a self-limiting response arising from physical and/or mental weariness, with a consequent personal and economic morbidity on work performance and social relationships. Anti-fatigue intervention is therefore urgently sought. "Qi-invigorating" Chinese tonic herbs, which can improve the energy status in the body according to the theory of traditional Chinese medicine, may produce beneficial effects in fatigue individuals. The herbal formula V-Vital capsule (VVC), which comprises 3 "Qi-invigorating" herbs, namely the root of *Rhodiola rosea*, *Eleutherococcus senticosus* and *Panax quinquefolium*, may produce anti-fatigue effect. In the present study, we investigated the effect of acute/long-term VVC treatment (acute: 0.75, 0.2 and 3.75 kg/day × 1 dose; long-term: 0.075 and 0.25 g/kg/day × 14 doses) on weight-loaded swimming female ICR mice. The weight-loaded swimming time until exhaustion, indicative of exercise endurance capacity, was recorded. Plasma levels of glucose, non-esterified fatty acid (NEFA), lactate and reactive oxygen metabolites (ROM) were measured in the exhausted mice. Glycogen levels in skeletal muscle and liver tissues were also measured. Mitochondrial function status [such as adenine nucleotide translocase (ANT) activity and coupling efficiency] was assayed. Results showed that acute VVC treatment increased the exercise endurance capacity in weight-loaded swimming mice. The ability of acute VVC treatment to enhance the exercise endurance was associated with increases in plasma glucose levels as well as glycogen levels in skeletal muscles and liver tissues, presumably due to the utilization of plasma lactate for gluconeogenesis and/or glycogen synthesis in the liver. While acute VVC treatment reduced the plasma ROM level in weight-loaded swimming mice, it increased the ANT activity. In this regard, the enhancement in exercise endurance afforded by acute

---

*Corresponding author.

VVC treatment might be due to an increase in the glucose supply to the skeletal muscle, the amelioration of systemic oxidative stress and the improvement in mitochondrial function of skeletal muscle. Consistent with the results obtained in acute VVC treatment experiment, the long-term VVC treatment enhances the exercise endurance in weight-loaded swimming mice. The ensemble of results suggests that VVC may offer a promising prospect for enhancing the exercise endurance and alleviating fatigue in humans.

Keywords

Fatigue, Exercise Endurance, *Rhodiola rosea*, *Eleutherococcus senticosus*, *Panax quinquefolium*

---

1. Introduction

Fatigue, which is a self-limiting response arising from physical and/or mental weariness, can be classified into three categories, namely secondary fatigue, physiologic fatigue and chronic fatigue [1]. Secondary fatigue refers to the weariness secondary to medical condition. While physiologic fatigue refers to an unbalance status of work and rest that can be recovered by taking rest, chronic fatigue is a pathological condition characterized by a persistent (or relapsing) debilitating and clinically unexplained fatigue that leads to a substantial impairment in functional status [2]. Chronic fatigue is a heterogeneous syndrome, characterized by a variety of pathophysiological features including neuroendocrine abnormalities, increased susceptibility to infections, obesity and chronic stress [2]. Despite the diversity of these pathophysiological anomalies, the disruption of structural and functional integrity of mitochondria has been shown to be crucially involved in the development of chronic fatigue, presumably due to an inadequate/inefficient energy supply to skeletal muscle [3] [4]. In order to sustain the energy demands in cytosol of muscle cells, the ATP synthesized in the mitochondria is exchanged with cytosolic ADP by adenine nucleotide translocase (ANT). In addition, the ANT-mediated ATP/ADP exchange was found to be critical for the maintenance of ATP synthase activity [5]. In view of the consequent personal and economic morbidity arising from the negative impacts of fatigue on work performance and social relationships [1], anti-fatigue intervention is urgently sought.

In an effort to develop safe interventions for fatigue, traditional Chinese medicine, which has a long history of use in safeguarding health, has attracted a lot of interest. In the realm of tradition Chinese medicine theories, Qi is a manifestation of energy status of the body [6]. In this connection, "Qi-invigorating" Chinese tonic herbs may produce beneficial effects in fatigue individuals. In support of this, recent studies have demonstrated that an extract of "Yang-invigorating" herb or a compound isolated from "Qi-invigorating" herb can enhance the mitochondrial ATP generation capacity in cultured cardiomyocytes as well as in mitochondria isolated from hearts of drug/herbal extract-treated rats [7] [8]. V-vital capsule (VVC) is an herbal formula comprising three "Qi-invigorating" herbs, namely, the root of *Rhodiola rosea*, the root of *Eleutherococcus senticosus* and the root of *Panax quinquefolium*. With respect to the increased capacity of mitochondrial ATP generation afforded by "Yang/Qi-invigorating" herbs [7] [8], VVC may offer a prospect for ameliorating physical and/or mental fatigue.

To evaluate the effectiveness of anti-fatigue intervention, force swimming test is a commonly adopted model for assessing the exercise endurance of mice [9] [10]. During the exercise, the supply of metabolic fuel molecules [such as glucose and non-esterified fatty acids (NEFA)] to skeletal muscle [11], the mobilization of energy reserves (such as glycogen in skeletal muscle and liver) [11] as well as the efficiency of mitochondrial respiration in skeletal muscle [12] determine the exercise endurance capacity. In the present study, we endeavored to examine the effect of acute and long treatment with VVC on exercise endurance and the associated changes in various biochemical parameters in mice using a weight-loaded forced swimming test. To assess the availability of fuel molecules, plasma levels of glucose and NEFA were measured. To examine the energy reserve, glycogen levels in skeletal muscle and liver tissues were also measured. In addition, various metabolites such as lactate (arising from the anaerobic glycolysis) and reactive oxygen metabolites (ROM, which is indicative of systemic oxidative stress) in plasma were measured. To assess the energy metabolic status of skeletal muscle, mitochondrial adenine nucleotide translocase (ANT) activity as well as state 3 and state 4 respiration rates of isolated mitochondria of skeletal muscle were assayed. The mitochondrial coupling efficiency was then estimated by computing the ratio of state 3 to state 4 mitochondrial respiratory rates.

2. Materials and Methods

2.1. Chemicals and Reagents

Lactate oxidase, horseradish peroxidase, bovine serum albumin (BSA) and 2,2'-azino-bis(3-ethylbenzothiazo-line-6-sulfonic acid) diammonium salt (ABST) were purchased from Sigma Chemical Co. (St. Louis, MO, USA). NEFA assay kits were purchased from Wako Pure Chemical Industries, Ltd. (Okasa, Japan). Glucose assay reagent was obtained from Sigma Chemical Co. The VVC were manufactured and supplied by Infinitus (China) Company Ltd. (Guangzhou, China). All other chemicals were of analytical grade.

2.2. Animal Care

Male ICR mice (8 - 10 weeks old, 30 - 25 g) were maintained under a 12-hour dark/light cycle at about 22°C, and allowed food and water *ad libitum* in the Animal and Plant Care Facility at the Hong Kong University of Science and Technology (HKUST). All experimental protocols were approved by the University Committee on Research Practice at HKUST.

2.3. Animal Treatment

In the acute VVC treatment, male ICR mice were randomly assigned to 4 groups, with 10 - 15 mice in each group: (1) control; (2) VVC (0.75 g/kg); (3) VVC (2.5 g/kg); (4) VVC (3.75 g/kg). Control mice received water (vehicle) only. Thirty min post-dosing, the mice were subjected to weight-loaded swimming test. Mice were sacrificed under phenobarbital anesthesia after the swimming test.

In the long-term VVC treatment, male ICR mice were randomly assigned to 6 groups, with 10 - 15 mice in each group: (1) non-swimming control; (2) non-swimming VVC (0.075 g/kg); (3) non-swimming VVC (0.25 g/kg); (4) swimming control; (5) swimming VVC (0.075 g/kg); (6) swimming VVC (0.25 g/kg). Immediately after the 1st weight-loaded swimming test (*i.e.* week 0), mice were intragastrically administered with VVC (0.075 and 0.25 g/kg/day) 5 days per week for 2 weeks (*i.e.* 10 doses) while control mice received water (vehicle) only. Mice were then subjected to weight-loaded swimming test once a week for 2 weeks (*i.e.* at week 1 and week 2), at 30 min post-dosing with VVC. Mice were sacrificed under phenobarbital anesthesia after the last swimming test.

2.4. Weight-Loaded Swimming Test

The exercise endurance capacity was assessed by weight-loaded swimming test. Swimming exercise was conducted with mice carrying a load of 6% of their body weight. The exhaustion time was defined as the inability of weight-loaded mice to rise to the water surface for 7 seconds. Swimming exercise was carried out in a tank (20 × 25 × 33 cm), which was filled with water to a depth of ~28 cm and maintained at 25°C ± 1°C. The tank was shaken at a speed of 40 rpm. To avoid the influence of circadian rhythm on physical activity, swimming exercise was done during 11:00 to 17:00, a period in which a minimal variation of endurance capacity has been reported in mice. Hairs of mice were wet with detergent water (1% w/v) to reduce surface tension. The swimming time (second) until exhaustion was recorded.

2.5. Preparation of Blood/Tissue Samples

Blood samples were drawn from phenobarbital-anesthetized mice by cardiac excision using syringes rinsed with 0.5% heparin in saline (w/v). Plasma samples were obtained by centrifuging whole blood samples at 1500 ×g for 10 min at 4°C. Plasma samples were then subjected to biochemical analysis.

Minced gastrocnemius muscle tissues were digested by collagenase solution [0.075% (w/v) in buffer] at 4°C for 20 min. After removing the collagenase solution by centrifugation, the digested muscle tissues were mixed with 20 mL of ice-cold homogenizing buffer (100 mM KCl, 50 mM MOPS, 10 mM EGTA, pH 7.2) and subjected to homogenization with a Teflon-glass homogenizer at 4,000 rpm for 25 - 30 complete strokes. Then the homogenates were centrifuged at 600 ×g for 10 min at 4°C. The resultant supernatant was nucleus-free fraction [13].

Mitochondrial pellets were prepared from nucleus-free fractions of muscle homogenates by centrifugation at 9200 ×g at 4°C for 30 min. The mitochondrial pellets were then resuspended in a buffer containing 250 mM sucrose, 50 mM Tris, pH 7.5 [13].

2.6. Biochemical Analysis

Plasma fuel molecules. Plasma glucose levels were measured using an assay kit utilizing the coupled hexoki-nase-catalyzed and glucose-6-phosphate dehydrogenase-catalyzed reactions, with a resultant NAD reduction. Absorbance changes at 340 nm of the assay mixture were monitored spectrophotometrically by Victor^3 Multi-label Counter (Perkin Elmer, Turku, Finland). Plasma NEFA level was measured using assay kit.

Glycogen levels in the liver and skeletal muscle. Liver and skeletal muscle tissues were weighed and then subjected to acidic hydrolysis with 2 M HCl at 100°C for 2 hours. The acidic hydrolyzed tissue samples were neutralized with 2 M NaOH and then centrifuged at 2150 ×g at 4°C for 10 min. The glucose level of the supernatant, which contained glucose releasing from glycogen hydrolysis, was measured using assay kit.

Plasma lactate level. Plasma lactate level was measured using a reaction cocktail made up of lactate oxidase, horseradish peroxidase and ABST in a buffer [0.1 M citric acid, 1 mg/mL BSA, 0.1% $CaCl_2$ (w/v), 0.02% sodium azide (w/v), pH 6.0]. Absorbances at 405 nm of the assay mixtures were measured spectrophotometrically by Victor^3 Multi-label Counter.

Plasma reactive oxygen metabolites (ROM) level. The extent of exercise-induced changes in systemic oxidative stress was assessed by the measurement of plasma ROM level. Aliquots (40 µL) of plasma samples were mixed with 20 µL of 100 mM N, N-dimethyl-p-phenylenediamine (DMPD) and 1.97 mL of incubation buffer (0.1 M sodium acetate, pH 4.8). The reaction mixtures were incubated at 37°C for 60 min in dark. Absorbances at 505 nm of the reaction mixtures were measured using Victor^3 Multi-Label Counter. The standard calibration curve was obtained by mixing 5 µL of *tert*-butylhydroperoxide (t-BHP) (up to 100 µM) with 20 µL phosphate-buffered saline, 5 µL of 2.52 mM $FeCl_2$ and 2 mL of DMPD. The amounts of hydroperoxyl compounds in plasma were estimated from the standard calibration curve and expressed in t-BHP equivalents [14].

Measurement of mitochondrial respiration. Mitochondrial respiratory rate was measured polarographically by a Clark-type oxygen electrode (Hansatech Instruments Ltd., Norfolk, UK) at 30°C. Mitochondrial fraction (~0.5 mg protein/mL) was incubated in a buffer containing 30 mM KCl, 6 mM $MgCl_2$, 75 mM sucrose, 1 mM EDTA, 20 mM KH_2PO_4 and 0.1% (w/v) fatty acid-free BSA, pH 7.0. Substrate solution containing 10 mM glutamate and 2.5 mM malate was added, and after a stable state 2 respiration had been established, state 3 respiration (coupling) was initiated by the addition of ADP (final concentration 0.6 mM). When all of the added ADP was used up for ATP generation, oligomycin (ATP synthase inhibitor) was added to induce the state 4 respiration (uncoupling). The mitochondrial coupling efficiency was estimated by calculating the ratio of state 3 to state 4 respirations [13].

Adenine nucleotide translocase (ANT) function. ANT function was assessed by noting the transportation of ATP (out) and ADP (in) through mitochondrial inner membrane [4]. The mitochondrial ATP level (**a**) was first measured. Secondly, the same mitochondrial fraction was mixed with a buffer (pH = 5.5 ± 0.2; serving as an artificial cytosol) containing ADP, which activates the ANT to transport ADP to the mitochondrial matrix. After 10 min of incubation, the mitochondrial ATP level (**b**) was measured again. The value of ANT_{in} was estimated by measuring the fractional increase in mitochondrial ATP as follow: $ANT_{in} = [(b - a)/a]$. Thirdly, the same mitochondrial fraction was mixed with a buffer (pH = 8.9 ± 0.2) containing no ADP, which activates the ANT to transport ATP from the mitochondrial matrix to the artificial cytosol. After 10 min of incubation, the mitochondrial ATP level was measured again (**c**). The value of ANT_{out} was estimated by measuring the fractional decrease in ATP as follows: $ANT_{out} = [(c - a)/a]$

2.7. Statistical Analysis

Data were analyzed by one-way Analysis of Variance (ANOVA), except the data of the swimming time in long-term VVC treatment, were analyzed by mixed ANOVA. Post-hoc multiple comparisons were performed using Least Significant Difference. P values < 0.05 were regarded as statistically significant.

3. Results

3.1. Effects of Acute VVC Treatment on Weight-Loaded Swimming Time in Mice

Acute VVC treatment (2.5 and 3.75 g/kg) 30 min prior to weight-loaded swimming increased the weight-loaded swimming time by ~1-fold (104% and 104%, respectively) until exhaustion in mice (**Figure 1**).

3.2. Effects of Acute VVC Treatment on Plasma Levels of Fuel Molecules in Non-Swimming and Weight-Loaded Swimming Mice

Acute VVC treatment (0.75, 2.5 and 3.75 g/kg) dose-dependently increased plasma glucose level (22%, 40% and 54%, respectively) in non-swimming mice (**Figure 2**). However, acute VVC treatment decreased the plasma NEFA level (29%, 33% and 47%, respectively) in a dose-dependent manner. Weight-loaded swimming until exhaustion decreased plasma levels of glucose (25%) and NEFA (32%) when compared with the non-swimming control. Acute VVC treatment increased plasma glucose level (44%, 46% and 31%, respectively) and decreased plasma NEFA level (21% and 25% at 2.5 and 3.75 g/kg, respectively) in weight-loaded swimming mice.

3.3. Effects of Acute VVC Treatment on Skeletal/Hepatic Glycogen Levels in Non-Swimming and Weight-Loaded Swimming Mice

Acute VVC treatment did not produce any detectable changes in hepatic/skeletal muscle glycogen in

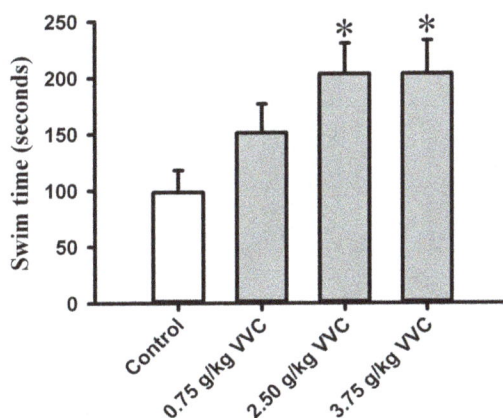

Figure 1. Effects of acute VVC treatment on weight-loaded swimming time in mice. Mice were intragastrically administered with VVC (0.75, 2.5 and 3.75 g/kg). At 30 minutes post-dosing, the mice were subjected to weight-loaded swimming test, as described in Materials and Methods. The swimming times of mice until exhaustion were recorded. Data were expressed as swimming time (second). Value given are means ± SEM, with n = 10 - 15. * Significantly different from drug-untreated control.

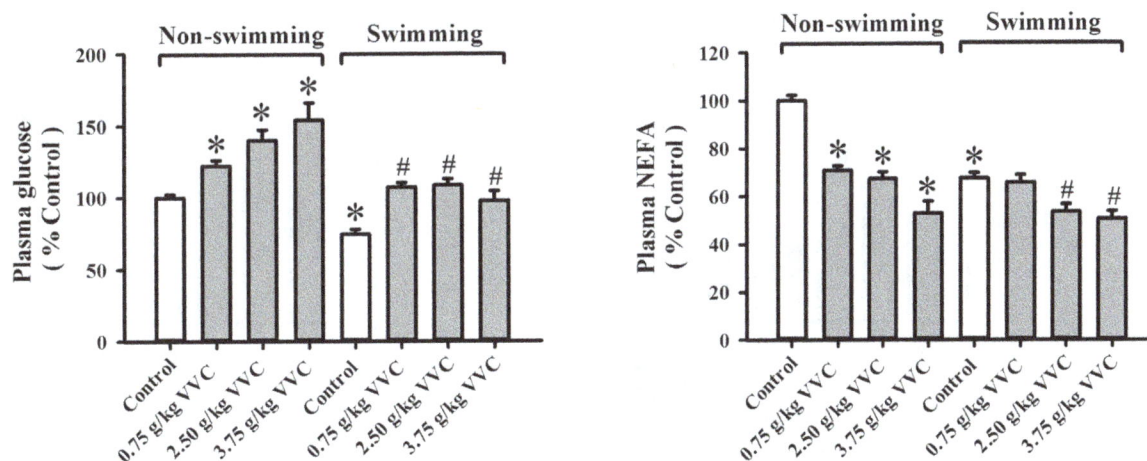

Figure 2. Effects of acute VVC treatment on plasma levels of fuel molecules in non-swimming and weight-loaded swimming mice. Mice were sacrificed after weight-loaded swimming until exhaustion. Plasma glucose level (Non-swimming control = 71.62 ± 2.61 mg/mL) and plasma non-esterified fatty acid (NEFA) level (Non-swimming control = 1.44 ± 0.05 mEq/L) were measured, as described in Materials and Methods. Data were expressed as % control, by normalizing with the value of non-swimming control. Value given are means ± SEM, with n = 10 - 15. * Significantly different from non-swimming control; # Significantly different from swimming control.

non-swimming mice. Weight-loaded swimming until exhaustion depleted skeletal muscle (49%) but not hepatic glycogen level in mice (**Figure 3**). Acute VVC treatment caused increases in skeletal muscle and hepatic glycogen levels in weight-loaded swimming mice, with maximal stimulation being 60% and 87% at the doses of 2.5 and 3.75 g/kg, respectively.

3.4. Effects of Acute VVC Treatment on Plasma Levels of Metabolites in Non-Swimming and Weight-Loaded Swimming Mice

Acute VVC treatment did not change plasma lactate levels in non-swimming mice. Weight-loaded swimming until exhaustion increased plasma lactate level (45%) (**Figure 4**), which was associated with the decrease in

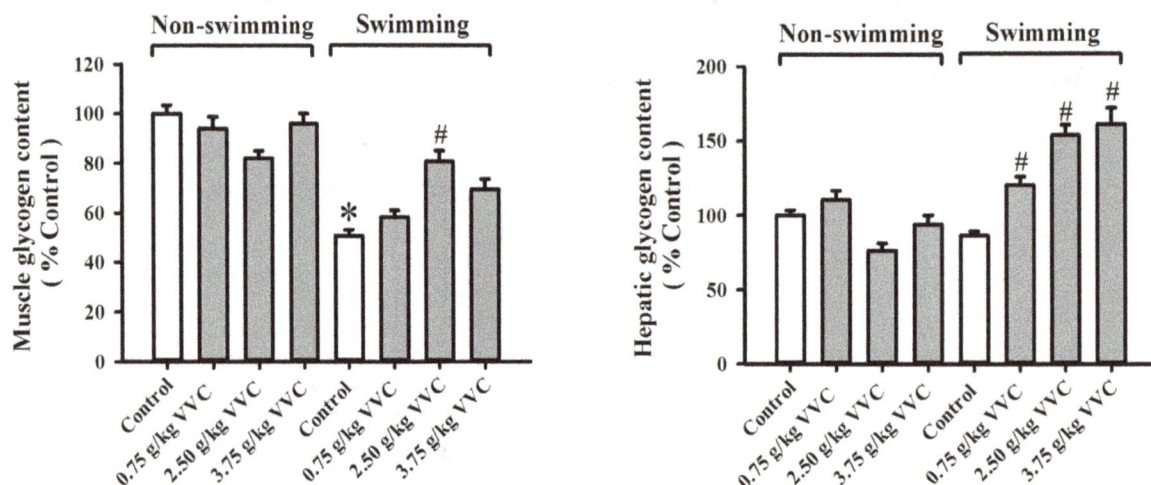

Figure 3. Effects of acute VVC treatment on skeletal/hepatic glycogen levels in non-swimming and weight-loaded swimming mice. Mice were sacrificed after weight-loaded swimming until exhaustion. Skeletal glycogen level (Non-swimming control = 0.52 ± 0.03 µmol glucosyl unit/unit g tissue) and hepatic glycogen level (Non-swimming control = 5.95 ± 0.41 µmol glucosyl unit/unit g tissue) were measured, as described in Materials and Methods. Data were expressed as % control, by normalizing with the value of non-swimming control. Value given are means $\pm$ SEM, with n = 10 - 15. * Significantly different from non-swimming control; # Significantly different from swimming control.

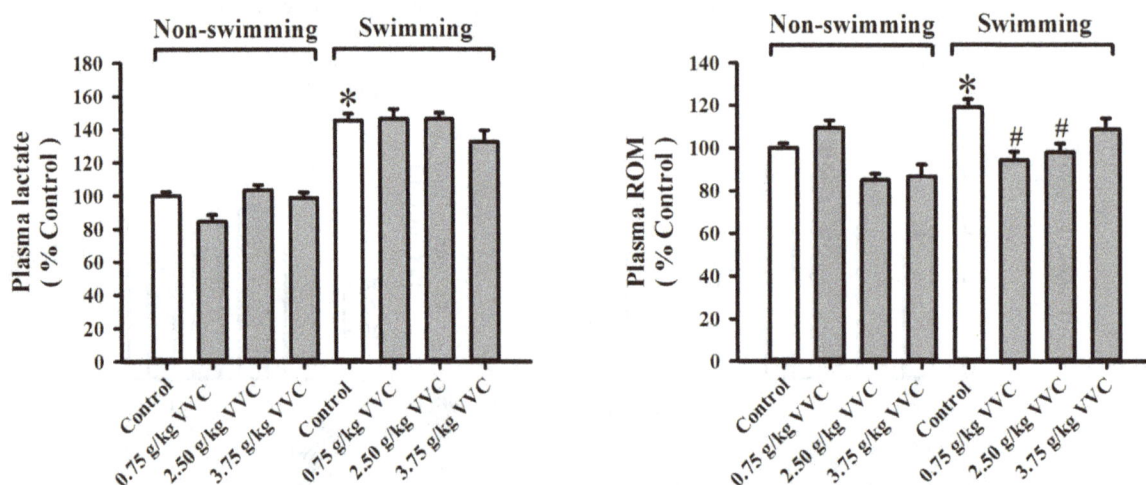

Figure 4. Effects of acute VVC treatment on plasma levels of metabolites in non-swimming and weight-loaded swimming mice. Mice were sacrificed after weight-loaded swimming until exhaustion. Plasma lactate level (Non-swimming control = 4.33 ± 0.24 mM) and plasma reactive oxygen metabolites (ROM) level (Non-swimming control = 105 ± 4.39 µmol tBHP equivalent) were measured, as described in Materials and Methods. Data were expressed as % control, by normalizing with the value of non-swimming control. Value given are means $\pm$ SEM, with n = 10 - 15. * Significantly different from non-swimming control; # Significantly different from swimming control.

plasma glucose level in weight-loaded swimming. Despite the fact that acute VVC treatment increased in plasma glucose level in weight-loaded swimming mice, plasma lactate levels were not affected. Acute VVC treatment also did not alter plasma ROM level in non-swimming mice. Weight-loaded swimming until exhaustion increased plasma ROM level (19%) in mice which was found to be reduced by acute VVC treatment (21% and 18% at 0.75 and 2.5 g/kg, respectively).

3.5. Effects of Acute VVC Treatment on Mitochondrial Functional Status of Skeletal Muscle in Non-Swimming and Weight-Loaded Swimming Mice

Acute VVC treatment did not produce any detectable change in the mitochondrial coupling efficiency of skeletal muscle in non-swimming mice (**Figure 5**). Weight-loaded swimming until exhaustion decreased mitochondrial coupling efficiency (24%) in mouse skeletal muscle. Acute VVC treatment at 0.75 g/kg significantly increased mitochondrial coupling efficiency (37%) in weight-loaded swimming mice. Acute VVC treatment (0.75, 2.5 and

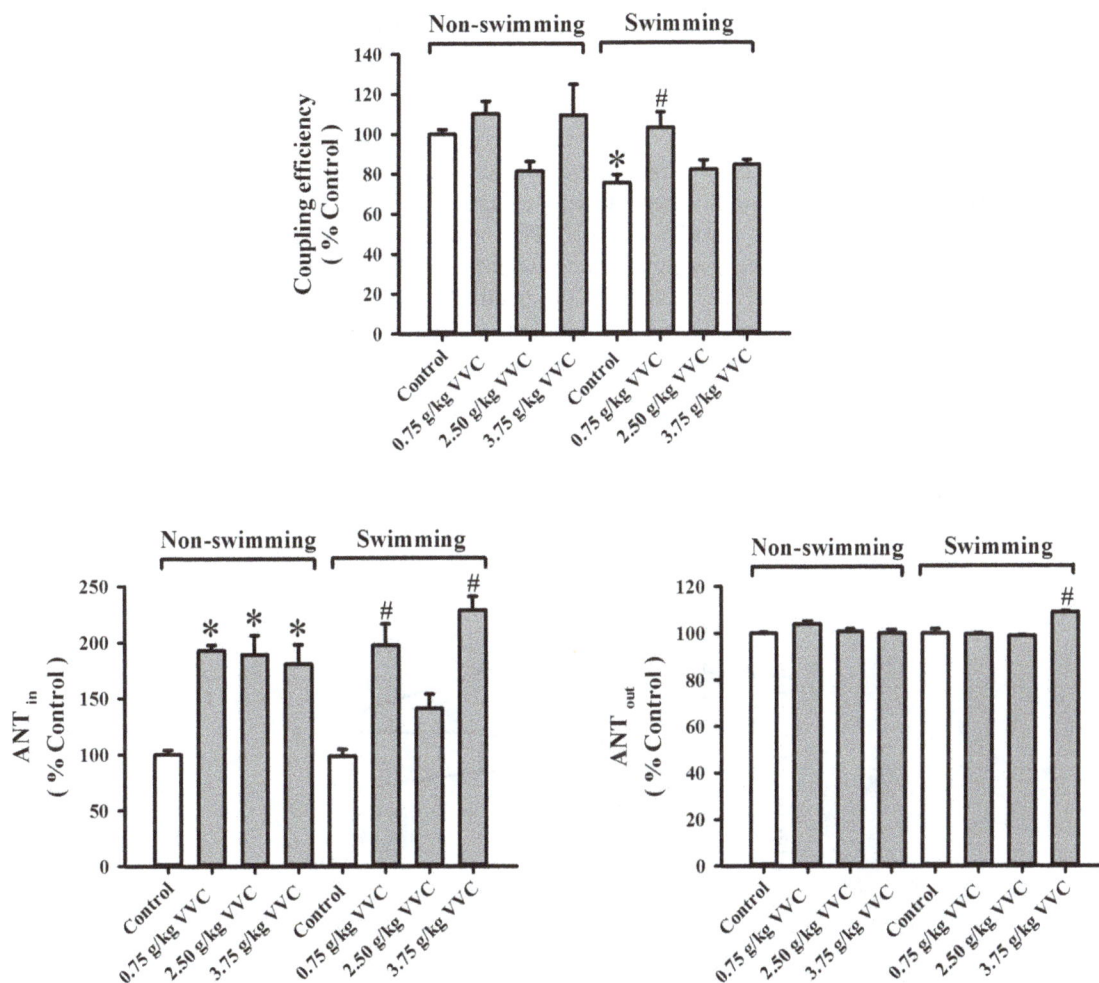

Figure 5. Effects of acute VVC treatment on mitochondrial functional status of skeletal muscle in non-swimming and weight-loaded swimming mice. Mice were sacrificed after weight-loaded swimming until exhaustion. Mitochondrial respiratory rates of skeletal muscle was measured polarographically by a Clark-type oxygen electrode at 30°C. The coupling efficiency was estimated by calculating the ratio of state 3 to state 4 respirations (Non-swimming control = 2.51 ± 0.07). The effectiveness of adenosine nucleotide translocase (ANT) of skeletal muscle was also assessed, as described in Materials and Methods. ANT_{in} (which indicates the effectiveness of ADP influx in mitochondria; Non-swimming control = 9.02 ± 1.00) and ANT_{out} (which indicates the effectiveness of ATP outflux from mitochondria; Non-swimming control = 0.94 ± 0.01) were measured. Data were expressed as % control, by normalizing with the value of non-swimming control. Values given are means $\pm$ SEM, with n = 5 - 10. *Significantly different from non- swimming control; # Significantly different from swimming control.

3.75 g/kg) significantly increased mitochondrial ANT_{in} activity (93%, 89% and 81%, respectively) in skeletal muscle of non-swimming mice, but it did not affect the ANT_{out} activity. While weight-loaded swimming until exhaustion did not alter mitochondrial $ANT_{in/out}$ activities, acute VVC treatment increased the ANT_{in} activity (101% and 92% at 0.75 and 3.75 g/kg, respectively) in weight-loaded swimming mice. The ANT_{out} activity seemed to be slightly but significantly increased (9%) in acute VVC-treated (3.75 g/kg) and weight-loaded swimming mice.

3.6. Effects of Long-Term VVC Treatment on the Weight-Loaded Swimming Time of Mice

Long-term treatment (0.075 and 0.25 g/kg) for 2 weeks progressively increased the weight-loaded swimming time of mice, with the effect produced by the low dose of VVC being more prominent at 1 week post-treatment and the extent of prolongation in weight-loaded swimming time being 35.6% for both doses at 2 weeks post-treatment (**Figure 6**).

3.7. Effects of Long-Term VVC Treatment on Various Biochemical Parameters in Non-Swimming and Weight-Loaded Swimming Mice

Long-term VVC treatment did not produce any significant changes in the levels of plasma glucose, muscle glycogen, plasma metabolites as well as mitochondrial coupling efficiency in skeletal muscle of non-swimming mice, except a decrease in plasma NEFA (15% at 0.25 g/kg), increases in hepatic glycogen (29% and 25% at 0.075 and 0.25 g/kg, respectively) as well as a dose-dependent increase in mitochondrial ANT_{in} activity in skeletal muscle (95% and 115% at 0.075 and 0.25 g/kg, respectively) (**Table 1**). Consistent with the results obtained from acute VVC treatment, weight-loaded swimming until exhaustion significantly decreased the plasma glucose as well as NEFA levels (25% and 32%, respectively), skeletal muscle glycogen level (46%) and hepatic glycogen level (37%). The weight-loaded swimming-induced depletions in plasma fuel molecules and energy reserves were associated with increases in plasma levels of metabolites, such as lactate (30%) and ROM (39%). While the long-term VVC treatment at low dose increased the mitochondrial ANT_{in} activity (79% vs. swimming control) in skeletal muscle of weight-loaded swimming mice, the long-term VVC treatment at high dose further increased the glycogen level (44% vs. swimming control) as well as mitochondrial coupling efficiency (83% vs swimming control) in skeletal muscle. The plasma ROM level was reduced (19% vs. swimming control) in VVC-treated (0.25 g/kg) weight-loaded swimming mice.

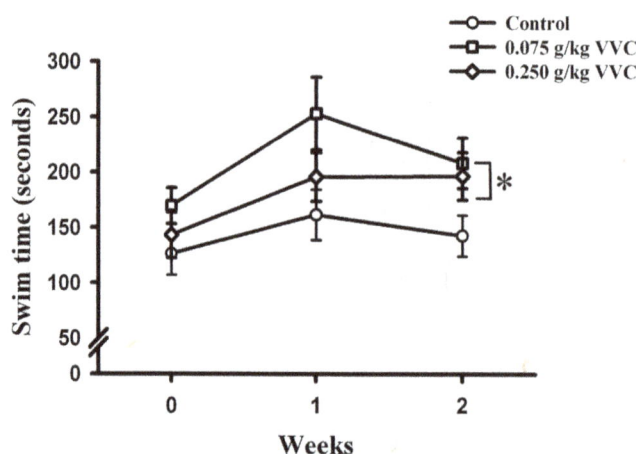

Figure 6. Effects of long-term VVC treatment on the weight-loaded swimming time of mice. Mice were subjected to weight-loaded swimming test every week (including the week 0) during the 2-week period of experiment, as described in Materials and Methods. The swimming times of mice until exhaustion were recorded. Immediately after the 1st weight-loaded swimming test (*i.e.* week 0), mice were intragastrically administered with VVC (0.075 and 0.25 g/kg/day) 5 days per week for 2 weeks (*i.e.* 10 doses), while control mice received water (vehicle) only. Data were expressed as swim time (second). Value given are means ± SEM, with n = 10 - 15. * Significantly different from drug-untreated control.

Table 1. Effects of long-term VVC treatment on various biochemical parameters in non-swimming and weight-loaded swimming mice.

	Non-Swim			Swim		
	Control	VVC		Control	VVC	
		0.075 g/kg	0.25 g/kg		0.075 g/kg	0.25 g/kg
Fuel molecules						
Plasma glucose	100 ± 2.4	108 ± 4.9	107 ± 3.2	74.5 ± 3.3[a]	61.0 ± 2.1	68.0 ± 3.5
Plasma NEFAs	100 ± 2.4	98.1 ± 3.0	84.8 ± 2.2[a]	68.2 ± 3.3[a]	65.8 ± 209	74.3 ± 3.2
Energy reserves						
Muscle glycogen	100 ± 2.2	93.3 ± 2.5	99.5 ± 2.7	53.8 ± 2.1[a]	65.5 ± 4.1	77.6 ± 4.4[b]
Hepatic glycogen	100 ± 2.3	129 ± 5.7 [a]	125 ± 3.9[a]	62.6 ± 2.4[a]	74.7 ± 3.8	84.1 ± 4.5
Metabolites						
Plasma lactate	100 ± 1.7	91.0 ± 4.0	90.9 ± 3.7	130 ± 4.1[a]	123 ± 3.4	115 ± 2.8
ROM	100 ± 2.8	95.9 ± 2.9	90.1 ± 3.3	139 ± 5.2[a]	126 ± 2.9	113 ± 2.9[b]
Mitochondrial functional status in skeletal muscle						
Coupling efficiency	100 ± 2.7	88.1 ± 14.7	87.7 ± 5.4	67.1 ± 10.2	90.9 ± 5.1	123 ± 17.8[b]
ANT_{in}	100 ± 4.5	195 ± 15.6[a]	215 ± 22.0[a]	144 ± 14.2	258 ± 32.8[b]	110 ± 7.7
ANT_{out}	100 ± 0.4	101 ± 0.2	102 ± 0.8	99.8 ± 0.2	100 ± 0.1	101 ± 0.3

a. significantly different from non-swimming control; b. significantly different from swimming control.

4. Discussion

Acute VVC treatment increased the exercise endurance capacity in mice, as indicated by the increase in the swimming time of weight-loaded swimming mice. The ability of VVC to enhance exercise endurance is consistent with the experimental observations that all component herbs of VVC (*i.e.*, the root of *Rhodiola rosea*, *Eleutherococcus senticosus* and *Panax quinquefolium*) independently increased the exercise endurance capacity in rodents. In this regard, the treatment with *Rhodiola rosea* extract was found to increase the swimming performance in both weight-unloaded and loaded rats [15] [16]. While the *Eleutherococcus senticosus* extract could increase the swimming time in forced swimming mice [17], the treatment with a protein fraction (containing proteins ranging from 8 - 66 kDa) isolated from *Panax quinquefolium* was able to increase the exercise endurance in weight-loaded swimming mice [18].

Force swimming-induced exhaustion, as observed in the present and other studies [9] [10], was found to be accompanied by depletions in plasma fuel molecules, suggestive of their involvement in muscle fatigue. In the present study, acute VVC treatment was found to increase the plasma level of glucose, with a concomitant decrease in plasma NEFA level, in both non-swimming and swimming mice. While the adipose tissue-derived NEFA is the major oxidative fuel molecule in skeletal muscle during low intensity exercise (such as weight-unloaded swimming) [19], plasma glucose is the major fuel molecule in skeletal muscle during high intensity exercise (such as weight-loaded swimming) [20]. As such, the enhancement in exercise endurance, as assessed by weight-loaded swimming, afforded by VVC may be due to the increase in plasma glucose supply to skeletal muscle for the anaerobic glycolysis. The lactate arising from anaerobic glycolysis then can undergo Cori cycle in the liver, with a resultant synthesis of glucose or glycogen. Given that high intensity exercise was found to time-dependently increase the plasma lactate level in rodents [21], VVC-treated mice, of which the swimming time is longer than those of VVC-untreated mice, should be expected to exhibit a higher plasma lactate level. However, VVC treatment did not increase the plasma lactate level in swimming mice, suggesting that plasma lactate may be utilized for gluconeogenesis and/or glycogen synthesis in the liver. This postulation is further strengthened by the observation that the glycogen levels in skeletal muscle and liver were elevated in VVC-treated weight-loaded swimming mice.

The increased production of metabolites [e.g. H^+ ion, lactate and reactive oxygen species (ROS)] during high intensity exercise was also found to be associated with muscle fatigue [22]. High plasma levels of H^+/lactate were conventionally considered as the major cause of muscle fatigue [23]. As mentioned earlier, VVC may facilitate the metabolism of lactate in the liver, leading to a postponed increase in plasma lactate level, which in turn enhances the exercise endurance. Recent studies have shown that low pH [24] [25] and high lactate level [26] [27] may have less inhibitory effect on the muscle contraction than that of previously assumed. The muscle fatigue may be mainly caused by the reduction of sarcoplasmic reticulum (SR) Ca^{2+} release [28]. With this notion in mind, ROS, which could reduce the maximum Ca^{2+}-activated force in skeletal muscle, the SR Ca^{2+} release and the Ca^{2+} sensitivity of contractile proteins [28], are hypothesized to play a critical role in muscle fatigue. In this connection, the acute VVC treatment-induced amelioration of systemic oxidative stress in swimming mice, as evidenced by a reduction of plasma ROM, may also contribute to the enhancement on exercise endurance. In support of this, a constituent of VVC, *Rhodiola rosea*, was also found to reduce swimming-enhanced oxidative stress in rat, possibly via its ROS scavenging capability and induction of the antioxidant defense system [15].

Acute VVC treatment improved the mitochondrial function in swimming mice, as indicated by increases in mitochondrial coupling efficiency and $ANT_{in/out}$ activities. An earlier study suggested that the mitochondrial function in skeletal muscle was positively correlated with the physical exercise performance in humans [29]. In this regard, the VVC-induced enhancement in exercise endurance may also be attributed to the improvement of mitochondrial function in skeletal muscle of swimming mice. In addition, a recent study showed that the PGC-1α-mediated activation of ANT reduced the production of mitochondrial ROS in cultured endothelial cells, with a resultant protection against oxidant-induced apoptosis [30]. Therefore, the activation of ANT by VVC may also be involved in the attenuation of systemic oxidative stress.

Consistent with the results obtained in acute VVC treatment, we further demonstrated that a long-term and low dose VVC treatment enhanced the exercise endurance in weight-loaded swimming mice, with an associated increase in ANT_{in} activity at a low dose of treatment. However, varied effects on plasma fuel molecules, plasma metabolites, glycogen levels in skeletal muscle and liver, as well as mitochondrial functional status were observed between the acute and long-term treatment, which may possibly be related to the differences in the dose and duration of VVC treatment.

5. Conclusion

In conclusion, both acute and long-term VVC treatments were found to enhance the exercise endurance in weight-loaded swimming mice. The enhancement in exercise endurance afforded by acute VVC treatment was associated with the increase in plasma fuel molecule, the amelioration of systemic oxidative stress, and the improvement in mitochondrial function of skeletal muscle. The ensemble of results suggests that VVC may offer a promising prospect for enhancing the exercise endurance and alleviating fatigue in humans.

References

[1]   Rosenthal, T.C., Majeroni, B.A., Pretorius, R. and Malik, K. (2008) Fatigue: An Overview. *American Family Physician*, **78**, 1173-1179.

[2]   Afari, N. and Buchwald, D. (2003) Chronic Fatigue Syndrome: A Review. *The American Journal of Psychiatry*, **160**, 221-236. http://dx.doi.org/10.1176/appi.ajp.160.2.221

[3]   Plioplys, A.V. and Plioplys, S. (1995) Electron-Microscopic Investigation of Muscle Mitochondria in Chronic Fatigue Syndrome. *Neuropsychobiology*, **32**, 175-181. http://dx.doi.org/10.1159/000119233

[4]   Myhill, S., Booth, N.E. and McLaren-Howard, J. (2009) Chronic Fatigue Syndrome and Mitochondrial Dysfunction. *International Journal of Clinical and Experimental Medicine*, **2**, 1-6.

[5]   Vander Heiden, M.G., Chandel, N.S., Schumacker, P.T. and Thompson, C.B. (1999) Bcl-xL Prevents Cell Death Following Growth Factor Withdrawal by Facilitating Mitochondrial ATP/ADP Exchange. *Molecular Cell*, **3**, 159-167. http://dx.doi.org/10.1016/S1097-2765(00)80307-X

[6]   Zhang, D. and Wu, X. (1991) Chapter 5 Qi, Blood, Body Fluid, Essence of Life and Spirit. In: Liu, Y., Ed., *The Basic Knowledge of Traditional Chinese Medicine*, Hai Feng Publishing Co., Hong Kong, 49-53.

[7]   Wong, H.S., Chen, N., Leong, P.K. and Ko, K.M. (2013) β-Sitosterol Enhances Cellular Glutathione Redox Cycling by Reactive Oxygen Species Generated From Mitochondrial Respiration: Protection Against Oxidant Injury in H9c2 Cells

and Rat Hearts. *Phytotherapy Research*, **28**, 999-1006. http://dx.doi.org/10.1002/ptr.5087

[8]   Chiu, P.Y. and Ko, K.M. (2003) Time-Dependent Enhancement in Mitochondrial Glutathione Status and ATP Generation Capacity by Schisandrin B Treatment Decreases the Susceptibility of Rat Hearts to Ischemia-Reperfusion Injury. *Biofactors*, **19**, 43-51. http://dx.doi.org/10.1002/biof.5520190106

[9]   Su, K.Y., Yu, C.Y., Chen, Y.W., Huang, Y.T., Chen, C.T., Wu, H.F. and Chen, Y.L. (2014) Rutin, a Flavonoid and Principal Component of Saussurea Involucrata, Attenuates Physical Fatigue in a Forced Swimming Mouse Model. *International Journal of Medical Sciences*, **11**, 528-537. http://dx.doi.org/10.7150/ijms.8220

[10] Chen, J.C., Hsiang, C.Y., Lin, Y.C. and Ho, T.Y. (2014) Deer Antler Extract Improves Fatigue Effect through Altering the Expression of Genes Related to Muscle Strength in Skeletal Muscle of Mice. *Evidence-Based Complementary and Alternative Medicine*, **2014**, Article ID: 540580. http://dx.doi.org/10.1155/2014/540580

[11]   Holloszy, J.O. and Kohrt, W.M. (1996) Regulation of Carbohydrate and Fat Metabolism during and after Exercise. *Annual Review of Nutrition*, **16**, 121-138. http://dx.doi.org/10.1146/annurev.nu.16.070196.001005

[12]   Conley, K.E., Jubrias, S.A., Cress, M.E. and Esselman, P.C. (2013) Elevated Energy Coupling and Aerobic Capacity Improves Exercise Performance in Endurance-Trained Elderly Subjects. *Experimental Physiology*, **98**, 899-907. http://dx.doi.org/10.1113/expphysiol.2012.069633

[13]   Leong, P.K., Leung, H.Y., Wong, H.S., Chen, J.H., Chan, W.M., Ma, C.W., Yang, Y.T. and Ko, K.M. (2014) Long-Term Treatment with an Herbal Formula MCC Ameliorates Obesity-Associated Metabolic Dysfunction in High Fat Diet-Induced Obese Mice: A Comparative Study among MCC and Various Combinations of Its Constituents. *Chinese Medicine*, **5**, 34-46. http://dx.doi.org/10.4236/cm.2014.51005

[14]   Leong, P.K., Chen, N., Chiu, P.Y., Leung, H.Y., Ma, C.W., Tang, Q.T. and Ko, K.M. (2010) Long-Term Treatment with Shengmai San-Derived Herbal Supplement (Wei Kang Su) Enhances Antioxidant Response in Various Tissues of Rats with Protection against Carbon Tetrachloride Hepatotoxicity. *Journal of Medicinal Food*, **13**, 427-438. http://dx.doi.org/10.1089/jmf.2009.1296

[15]   Huang, S.C., Lee, F.T., Kuo, T.Y., Yang, J.H. and Chien, C.T. (2009) Attenuation of Long-Term *Rhodiola rosea* Supplementation on Exhaustive Swimming-Evoked Oxidative Stress in the Rat. *Chinese Journal of Physiology*, **52**, 316-324. http://dx.doi.org/10.4077/CJP.2009.AMH029

[16]   Lee, F.T., Kuo, T.Y., Liou, S.Y. and Chien, C.T. (2009) Chronic *Rhodiola rosea* Extract Supplementation Enforces Exhaustive Swimming Tolerance. *The American Journal of Chinese Medicine*, **37**, 557-572. http://dx.doi.org/10.1142/S0192415X09007053

[17]   Kimura, Y. and Sumiyoshi, M. (2004) Effects of Various *Eleutherococcus senticosus* Cortex on Swimming Time, Natural Killer Activity and Corticosterone Level in Forced Swimming Stressed Mice. *Journal of Ethnopharmacology*, **95**, 447-453. http://dx.doi.org/10.1016/j.jep.2004.08.027

[18]   Qi, B., Liu, L., Zhang, H., Zhou, G.X., Wang, S., Duan, X.Z., Bai, X.Y., Wang, S.M. and Zhao, D.Q. (2014) Anti-Fatigue Effects of Proteins Isolated from *Panax quinquefolium*. *Journal of Ethnopharmacology*, **153**, 430-434. http://dx.doi.org/10.1016/j.jep.2014.02.045

[19]   Frayn, K.N. (2010) Fat as a Fuel: Emerging Understanding of the Adipose Tissue-Skeletal Muscle Axis. *Acta Physiologica*, **199**, 509-518. http://dx.doi.org/10.1111/j.1748-1716.2010.02128.x

[20]   Jeppesen, J. and Kiens, B. (2012) Regulation and Limitations to Fatty Acid Oxidation during Exercise. *Journal of Physiology*, **590**, 1059-1068.

[21]   Kato, M., Kurakane, S., Nishina, A., Park, J. and Chang H. (2013) The Blood Lactate Increase in High Intensity Exercise Is Depressed by *Acanthopanax sieboldianus*. *Nutrients*, **5**, 4134-4144. http://dx.doi.org/10.3390/nu5104134

[22]   Green, H.J. (1997) Mechanisms of Muscle Fatigue in Intense Exercise. *Journal of Sports Sciences*, **15**, 247-256. http://dx.doi.org/10.1080/026404197367254

[23]   Fitts, R.H. (1994) Cellular Mechanisms of Muscle Fatigue. *Physiological Reviews*, **74**, 49-94.

[24]   Cady, E.B., Jones, D.A., Lynn, J. and Newham, D.J. (1989) Changes in Force and Intracellular Metabolites during Fatigue of Human Skeletal Muscle. *Journal of Physiology*, **418**, 311-325.

[25]   Stary, C.M. and Hogan, M.C. (2005) Intracellular pH during Sequential, Fatiguing Contractile Periods in Isolated Single *Xenopus* Skeletal Muscle Fibers. *Journal of Applied Physiology*, **99**, 308-312. http://dx.doi.org/10.1152/japplphysiol.01361.2004

[26]   Karlsson, J., Funderburk, C.F., Essen, B. and Lind, A.R. (1975) Constituents of Human Muscle in Isometric Fatigue. *Journal of Applied Physiology*, **38**, 208-211.

[27]   Van Beekvelt, M.C., Drost, G., Rongen, G., Stegeman, D.F., Van Engelen, B.G. and Zwarts, M.J. (2006) Na^+-K^+-ATPase Is Not Involved in the Warming-Up Phenomenon in Generalized Myotonia. *Muscle & Nerve*, **33**, 514-523. http://dx.doi.org/10.1002/mus.20483

[28] Allen, D.G., Lamb, G.D. and Westerblad, H. (2008) Skeletal Muscle Fatigue: Cellular Mechanisms. *Physiological Reviews*, **88**, 287-332. http://dx.doi.org/10.1152/physrev.00015.2007

[29] Jacobs, R.A., Flück, D., Bonne, T.C., Bürgi, S., Christensen, P.M., Toigo, M. and Lundby C. (1985) Improvements in Exercise Performance with High-Intensity Interval Training Coincide with an Increase in Skeletal Muscle Mitochondrial Content and Function. *Journal of Applied Physiology*, **115**, 785-793. http://dx.doi.org/10.1152/japplphysiol.00445.2013

[30] Won, J.C., Park, J.Y., Kim, Y.M., Koh, E.H., Seol, S., Jeon, B.H., Han, J., Kim, J.R., Park, T.S., Choi, C.S., Lee, W.J., Kim, M.S., Lee, I.K., Youn, J.H. and Lee, K.U. (2010) Peroxisome Proliferator-Activated Receptor-γ Coactivator 1-α Overexpression Prevents Endothelial Apoptosis by Increasing ATP/ADP Translocase Activity. *Thrombosis, and Vascular Biology*, **30**, 290-297. http://dx.doi.org/10.1161/ATVBAHA.109.198721

List of Abbreviations

Adenine nucleotide translocase (ANT); Analysis of Variance (ANOVA); 2,2'-azino-bis(3-ethylbenzothiazoline-6-sulfonic acid) diammonium salt (ABST); Bovine serum albumin (BSA); tert-Butylhydroperoxide (t-BHP); N, N-dimethyl-p-phenylenediamine (DMPD); Non-esterified fatty acid (NEFA); Reactive oxygen metabolites (ROM); Reactive oxygen species (ROS); Sarcoplasmic reticulum (SR); V-vital capsule (VVC).

19

Effects of mRNA, Protein Expression and Activity for Myocardial SOD2 by a Single Bout of or Long-Term Strenuous Endurance Exercise in Rats

Simao Xu*, Weichun Liu, Minhua Li

Department of Physical Education, Guangxi Normal University, Guilin, China
Email: *xusimao666@163.com

Abstract

Objective: To explore the effects of myocardial SOD2 by strenuous endurance exercise. Methods: 27 grown male SD rats were randomly divided into control group (C), a single bout of strenuous endurance exercise group (E1) and seventh-week strenuous endurance exercise group (E2). Real-time PCR was used to observe the changes of mRNA expression for myocardial SOD2. Western bolt was used to observe the changes of SOD2 protein expression. In addition, SOD2, T-SOD and SOD1 activity changes were observed. Results: Myocardial SOD2 expression level at mRNA and protein of Group E1, E2 was significantly higher than that in group C, and SOD2 and T-SOD activity in group E2 were significantly higher than those in group C. Those changes were more obvious in group E2. Conclusions: Strenuous endurance exercise can improve level of myocardial SOD2 expression at mRNA and protein, and enhance the activity for SOD2, thus increasing the activity for T-SOD. Effect of long-term strenuous endurance exercise was better than a single bout of one.

Keywords

SOD2, Strenuous Endurance Exercise, Myocardia

1. Introduction

In recent years, with the development of economy and society, people's diet and lifestyle change, and heart

---

*Corresponding author.

health is also seriously threatened, *i.e.*, the incidence of ischemic heart disease was on the rise "year by year". Therefore, heart health maintenance has always been an important issue. According to the researches, the damage of Reactive Oxygen Species (ROS) plays a considerable role in the process of myocardial pathological changes. It is of great significance to maintain the heart health, such as the prevention of ischemic cardiomyopathy, to increase the ability of heart's antioxidant as well as to effectively remove ROS. Numerous studies have indicated that appropriate exercises can promote heart health and resist to myocardial ischemia-reperfusion injury [1]-[4]. What's more, according to powers and other researchers, the effect of exercise on heart health is closely related to the improved myocardial antioxidant capacity [5]. However, it has yet to explore the improved myocardial antioxidant capacity caused by exercise and cardioprotective effects.

As it's known to all, enzymatic defensive system acts as a considerable part in body issue's antioxidant and ROS removal, among which Superoxide Dismutase (SOD) is regarded as the first protective barrier to defense ROS. Therefore, the improvement of SOD activity marks the myocardial antioxidant capacity enhancement. A great number of researches have shown that exercise can improve the activity of myocardial Total Superoxide Dismutase (T-SOD). However it is not difficult to find that exercise models in studies concerned focus on the high-intensity intermittent exercise or moderate-intensity endurance exercise model; other possibly existed and targeted suitable exercise models needed further exploration. On the other hand, SOD has two types in higher animal vivo, one being Cu, Zn Superoxide Dismutase (SOD1) existed in cytoplasm, another Manganese Superoxide Dismutase (SOD2) in mitochondria; therefore, strengthening in-depth study of SOD types will contribute a further understanding of protective effects of exercise on the heart and its possible mechanisms. Since mitochondria play a crucial role in the maintenance of cardiomyocytes normal function and structural integrity. In addition, they are main sites of ROS production. Theoretically, the increase of SOD2 function has a significant effect on ROS removal as well as myocardial protection. Taking the above reasons into consideration, this study is to observe whether strenuous endurance exercise can accelerate the improvement of myocardial SOD2 expression at mRNA and protein as well as their activity level or not, trying to prove that this effect can be enhanced by long-term endurance exercise. It's also expected to rich the theory of exercise's protective effect on the heart, and to improve practical applications of sports and fitness on cardioprotective effects.

2. Materials and Methods

2.1. Research Objects

27 grown male Sprague Dawley (SD) rats (SPF grade), weighting 146 ± 15 g, are bought from Guangxi Medical University Laboratory Animal Center. They are raised in standard rodent cages, feeding freely. Favorable ventilated conditions, controlling room temperature at about 27°C and natural light are provided.

2.2. Experiment Methods

2.2.1. Groups and Exercise Modes
After one week adaptive feeding, 27 grown male SD rats were randomly divided into control group (group C, n = 9), a single bout of strenuous endurance exercise group (group E1, n = 9) and seventh-week strenuous endurance exercise group (group E2, n = 9). Group E1 and E2 trained endurance running on treadmills (Type DSPT 202 made by Hangzhou Litai S & T Co. Ltd.). Before formal training, the both groups firstly conducted three-day adaptive treadmill exercise (0°, 15 m/min), and then strenuous endurance running at a speed of 22 m/min and gradient of +10° (85% VO2$_{max}$) for 30 min daily referred to Bedford and other researchers standards [6]. Group E1 only exercised one day while group E2 exercised 6 days/week (Sunday off) for continuous 7 weeks.

2.2.2. Drawing Materials
Intraperitoneal anesthesia with urethane (1.2 g/kg) were performed when group E1 after exercise within 24 h - 48 h, group E2 after the last exercise within 24 h - 48 h together with group C, and then hearts were quickly taken and ventricular myocardia were cut, washing with PBS. Ventricular myocardia were cut into small pieces during an ice-bath. Most ventricular myocardial pieces, placed immediately into the −80°C ultra-low temperature refrigerator after liquid nitrogen flash freeze, were used for determining SOD2 expression at mRNA and protein; that remaining small portion was used for the observation of SOD activity after weighing (about 100 mg) and recording.

2.2.3. Real-Time Fluorescent Quantitative PCR

SYBR Green I method was adopted, with necessary reagent provided by American Life Technologies Co. Ltd. Real-time PCR primers were synthesized by Invitrogen Corporation Shanghai Representative Office.

Upstream of SOD2: AAGGAGAGTTGCTGGAGGCTATC

Downstream: CTCCTTATTGAAGCCAAGCCAG

Upstream of β-actin: CATTGTCACCAACTGGGACGATA

Downstream: GGATGGCTACGTACATGGCTG

1) RNA extraction

A portion of frozen myocardial tissue was taken, weighted (100 mg) and recorded. Grind into powder after adding liquid nitrogen, and then the total myocardial RNA were immediately extracted under the guidance of Trizol kit instructions after the liquid nitrogen were evaporated.

2) Synthesize cDNA by Reverse Transcription (RT)

5 µl (5 µg) of extracted myocardial RNA samples, together with 0.5 µl of Oligo (dt) primer (50 uM), 0.5 µl of random primer, 1 µl of dNTP Mix (10 mM), and 5 µl of DEPC-treated water added one after another, gets a Mix I of 12 µl, 5 min warm bath at 65°C and then 1 min ice bath at once. Afterwards, 20 µl of Mix II, received by adding 4 µl of 5× First-Strand buffer, 2 µl of 0.1 M dTT, 1 µl of RNaseout (40 U/µl), and 1 µl of SuperScrip III RT (200 U/µl) into Mix I, was treated with 5 min bath at 25°C, 60 min bath at 50°C and 15 min bath at 70°C. The resulting cDNA was placed on ice immediately.

3) Real-time PCR

PCR solution was carried out PCR amplification reaction in real-time PCR instrument (Type 7500 Fast, Life technologies' product). The real-time PCR reaction system is: 14 µl of ultrapure water, 2 µl of 10× PCR buffer solution, 1 µl of magnesian ion (50 mM), 0.5 µl of upstream primer (10 uM), 0.3 µl of SYBR (20×) fluorescent dye, 0.5 µl of downstream primer (10 uM), 0.2 µl of Taq DNA Polymerase, 1 µl of template, accounting for 20 µl. Reaction parameters are: initial denaturation for 2 min at 95°C; 40 PCR cycles (95°C, 10 S; 60°C, 30 S; 70°C, 45 S). During this course, Ct values (cycled threshold values) of tested products were recorded when fluorescence signal intensity was significantly enhanced; three wells were made in each test sample, calculating the average of each sample's Ct value. Continue to slowly heat from 70°C to 95°C after completion, and then melting curves of PCR products were established in order to observe the specificity of amplified products.

After that, the Relative Expression (RE) of target gene SOD2 mRNA was calculated by the $2^{-\Delta\Delta Ct}$ Method [7], using housekeeping gene β-actin as reference gene. Average value of each sample was taken as Ct,

$\Delta Ct = (Ct_{target\ gene} - Ct_{reference\ gene})$, $\Delta\Delta Ct = (Ct_{experimental\ group} - Ct_{control\ group})$, $2^{-\Delta\Delta Ct}$ was RE of mRNA for SOD2.

2.2.4. Western Bolt for Myocardia SOD2

The remaining frozen myocardial tissues, weighted and recorded, were speedily ground into powder with liquid nitrogen. They were immediately placed in EP tube after evaporation, and then RIPA lysate (a concentration of 1 mM) formulated from PMSF buffer was added to fully lyse in the proportion of 20 mg of myocardial tissues to 200 µl of lysate (protein extraction reagent); supernatant was collected by hypothermic centrifugal machine (centrifugal force 10,000 - 14,000 ×g, 3 - 5 min). BSA (Bicinchonininc acid) Method was adopted to determine the total protein concentration.

50 µg of myocardial total protein, using prestained maker as protein molecular weight marker, were carried out 12% SDS-PAGE protein electrophoresis (constant pressure electrophoresis with separating gel at 80 V and stacking gel at 100 V) until the front edge of color marker-bromophenol blue stopped electrophoresis when went down to the end of gel. The separated protein bands (0.20 µm of SOD2 and 0.45 µm of i-actin) were transferred to a PVDF membrane by wet cell transmembrane method (250 mA constant current for 1 h). 5% BSA buffer was closed at room temperature for 2 h. After that, SOD2 primary antibodies (diluted rabbit anti-human polyclonal antibody at the ratio of 1 to 1000) and β-actin primary antibodies (diluted mouse anti-human monoclonal antibody at the ratio of 1 to 1000) were added into these two membranes correspondingly. Incubate them overnight at 4°C, and then wash the membrane with TBST three times (10 min/time). Secondary antibodies marked by rabbit anti-horseradish peroxidase (dilute at the ratio of 1 to 2000) and by mouse anti-horseradish peroxidase (dilute at the ratio of 1 to 2000) were mixed in correspondingly. The two mixtures were incubated on the shaking table at room temperature for 1 h, and then washed with TBST three times (10 min/time) as well as developed with chemiluminescence. Electrophoretic bands were treated by Gel-pro analyzer software to analyze the gray value of each band area, the ratio of target band (SOD2)'s grey value to reference band (β-actin)'s grey

value representing the expression level at target protein.

For the main reagents used in experiments, RIRA lysate, BCA kit as well as ECL kit were bought from Shanghai Beyotime Biotechnology Co., Ltd., PMSF buffer is provided by Amresco Company, BSA by Sigma-Aldrich Co. LLC; β-actin primary antibodies, secondary antibodies labeled rabbit anti-horseradish peroxidase as well as secondary antibodies labeled mouse anti-horseradish peroxidase were bought from Beijing Zhongshan Golden Bridge Biotechnology Co., Ltd. while SOD2 primary antibodies from Epitomics Biotechnology Co., Ltd.; TBST from Beijing Solarbio Science & Technology Co., Ltd. Electrophoresis was Powerpac Basic Electrophoresis bought from American Bio-Rad Laboratories, Inc.

2.2.5. Determination of Myocardial SOD2 Activity

10% homogenates were made and then supernatant was collected by centrifuge (4000 rpm, 30 min). SOD1 and T-SOD activity were detected with hydroxylamine method, and finally SOD2 activity was obtained by T-SOD activity minus SOD1 activity. SOD kits were bought from Nanjing Jiancheng Biotechnology Co., Ltd.

2.2.6. Statistical Analysis

Experimental data were presented as "mean ± standard deviation" ($\overline{X} \pm S$). Statistical analysis was completed by SPSS for windows version 17.0 software. The experimental results were all analyzed with One-Way Analysis of Variance (ANOVA). After-effect test was conducted by Least-Significant Difference (LSD) Method in the case of homogeneity of variance, otherwise by Tamhane's T2 Method. $P < 0.05$ was regarded as the standard of significant differences.

3. Results

3.1. Comparisons of RE of mRNA for Myocardia SOD2 in Rats

Melting curve of amplification products in SYBR Green I real-time PCR reflects that solubility changes with temperature, with temperatures as ordinate against solubility as abscissa. In this study, melting curve of both myocardia SOD2 gene and myocardia β-actin gene in rats only appeared a single peak; besides, the melting temperature (Tm) were about 85.35°C and 88.43°C respectively, approximately nearing to the annealing temperature of the corresponding products: amplification products were in preferable specificity.

Real-time PCR amplification curve was used cycles as ordinate against real-time fluorescence intensity as abscissa during PCR. According to statistics, RE of mRNA for myocardia SOD2 in group E1 and E2 was obviously higher than that in group C (control group), marking significant differences; RE in group E2 were more distinct than those in group E1, marking significant differences (**Table 1**; **Figure 1**).

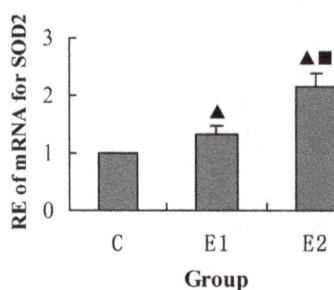

Figure 1. Diagram of changes in RE of mRNA for myocardia SOD2 in rats. [▲]Compared with group C, p < 0.05; [■]Compared with group E1, p < 0.05.

Table 1. Changes in RE of mRNA for myocardia SOD2 in rats.

Group	N	SOD2 mRNA
C	9	1.00 ± 0.00
E1	9	1.32 ± 0.16^{a}
E2	9	2.16 ± 0.23^{ab}

[a]Compared with group C, p < 0.05; [b]Compared with group E1, p < 0.05.

3.2. Changes in RE of Protein for Myocardia SOD2 in Rats

Group E1 and E2 myocardia SOD2 expression level at protein was clearly improved compared with group C, marking meaningful differences; levels in group E2 were more distinct than those in group E1, marking meaningful differences (**Figure 2**; **Table 2**; **Figure 3**).

3.3. Changes of Activity Level for Myocardia SOD2 in Rats

SOD2 activity was gotten by T-SOD activity subtracting the SOD1. The activity of myocardia SOD2 and T-SOD in group E1 and E2 was clearly improved compared with group C, marking significant differences; improvements in group E2 were more distinct than those in group E1, marking significant differences (**Table 3**; **Figure 4**).

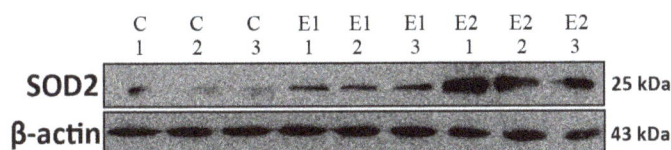

Figure 2. Diagram of western blotting for myocardia SOD2 in rats. 1, 2, 3, three different individual samples in each group rats for C, E1, E2.

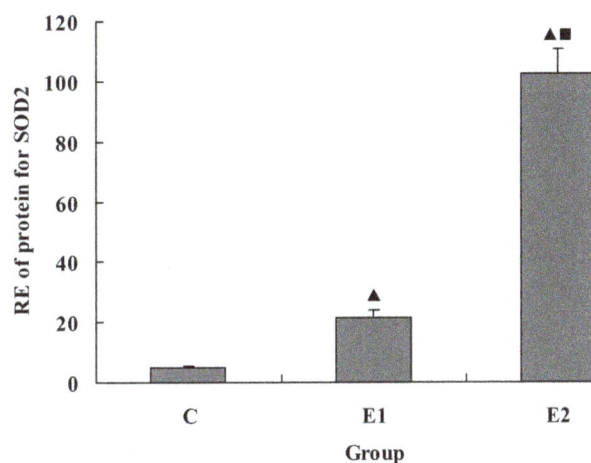

Figure 3. Diagram of changes in RE of protein for myocardia SOD2 in rats. ▲Compared with group C, p < 0.05; ■Compared with group E1, p < 0.05.

Table 2. Changes in RE of protein for myocardia SOD2 in rats.

Group	n	SOD2
C	9	4.743 ± 0.652
E1	9	21.367 ± 2.787[a]
E2	9	102.424 ± 8.336[ab]

[a]Compared with group C, p < 0.05; [b]Compared with group E1, p < 0.05.

Table 3. Changes in activity of myocardia SOD2, T-SOD in rats (U/mg·prot).

Group	n	SOD1	SOD2	T-SOD
C	9	77.820 ± 8.955	39.653 ± 6.032	117.473 ± 13.852
E1	9	76.674 ± 9.743	54.274 ± 7.257[a]	131.948 ± 14.285[a]
E2	9	77.221 ± 9.724	79.314 ± 8.456[ab]	156.535 ± 15.755[ab]

[a]Compared with group C, p < 0.05; [b]Compared with group E1, p < 0.05.

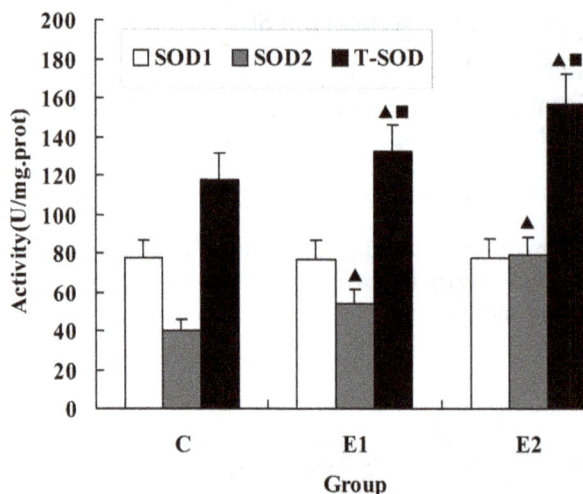

Figure 4. Diagram of changes in activity of myocardia SOD2, T-SOD in rats. ▲Compared with group C, $p < 0.05$; ■Compared with group E1, $p < 0.05$.

4. Discussion

Studies on the impact of exercise on the heart earliest started in an anatomy find, Robinson, an Englishman, pointed out that relative weight of heart in high-intensity physical activity animal was heavier than that in low-intensity physical activity animal in 1748. As humans, Henschen, a Swedish scholar, first discovered the enlargement of skier's heart by percussion in 1899, and then put forward the term of "Athlete's Heart". Afterwards, the field of sports medicine had committed to the study of "effect of exercises on cardiac structure and function", and gradually penetrated into the field of molecular biology. Up to now, it's generally viewed that the exercise is a "double-edged sword" for excessive exercises may be harmful to heart health while moderate exercises are beneficial to it, being able to pre-treat various cardiovascular diseases. In the past reports about "exercise and heart health", most intervention models were moderate-intensity endurance exercise. In recent years, some researches had been conducted by using high-intensity intermittent exercise as intervention model at home, e.g. some references pointed out that intermittent high-intensity exercise can protect the heart and improve myocardial tolerance of ischemia [8] [9]. However, it still needed to build more sports models for reference how to enhance heart health by rationally using physical exercise with targets, such as the improvement of myocardial antioxidant capacity. What's more, this study suggested that excessive exercise, such as intermittent high-intensity exercise, may not be practical for the old and infirm as well as for the crowd urgently needing for sports and fitness, and was somewhat difficult to popularize. That is why endurance exercise was more widespread in physical exercise at present. Taking these conditions into consideration, this study chose the model of "a single bout of or seven-week strenuous endurance exercise" to investigate the effects of myocardial antioxidase SOD by strenuous endurance exercise. It's clear that there were two kinds of SOD in myocardial tissue, namely SOD1 and SOD2.

According to this study, a single bout of or seven-week strenuous endurance exercise can outstandingly improve the level of myocardial SOD2 expression at mRNA and protein. SOD's main function was to remove ROS in vivo, which was mainly produced in mitochondria, where also lay SOD2, a type of SOD. In this study, the increase of myocardial SOD2 expression level may be adaptive changes of ROS increase and oxidative stress stimulate made by mitochondrial. It was found that a single bout of long-term high-intensity endurance exercise can give rise to the increase of myocardial malondialdehyde (MDA) content [10], suggesting the increase of myocardial oxidative stress level. The author considered that the improving myocardial oxidative stress level after exercise resulted from exercise-induced myocardial ischemia and hypoxia. In one recent study, rats were carried out a single bout of strenuous endurance exercise at a speed of 19 - 21 m/min and gradient of $+10°$ (80% $VO2_{max}$) to "exhaustion" [11]. And then they found that rats' ECG presented characteristic changes of myocardial ischemia and myocardial stunning, and myocardia had ischemic necrosis, both of which showing that exercise can induce myocardial ischemia [11]. In addition, other similar studies showed that a single bout of exhaustive strenuous endurance exercise can induce myocardial ischemia in rats [12]. The model of a single bout of "exhaustive" strenuous endurance exercise in the above references, differing from that of a single bout of or long-term strenuous endurance exercise with quantitative loads in the present study, still suggested the existence of myocardial ischemia phenomenon by strenuous endurance exercise. Great amount of studies had proved that effects of exercise-induced myocardial ischemia and hypoxia on myocardial structure and function were bitterly similar to the clinical pathological myocardial ischemia; Large quantity of ROS were generated and oxidative stress levels were significantly increased in myocardium in the process of exercise-induced myocardial ischemia (hypoxia) and reperfusion. Distinguished from clinical pathological myocardial ischemia, exercise-induced myocardial ischemia was relative myocardial ischemia and hypoxia due to the high level of myocardial metabolic as well as initiative ischemia and hypoxia occurred under the protective monitoring system [13]. When cannot tolerate hypoxia, the body will reduce the degree of ischemia and hypoxia by reducing exercise intensity or stopping exercise, thus avoiding myocardial irreversible damage resulted from excessive ischemia and hypoxia [13]. Therefore, combined this study's results and analyses, the author held that relative myocardial ischemia and hypoxia of reasonable duration caused by strenuous endurance exercise gave impetus to a certain amount of ROS and some degree of oxidative stress in mitochondria, which were extremely sensitive to ischemia, as long as exercise will not be too durative. Adaptive changes, occurring after mitochondria were stimulated by oxidative stress, manifested as increased expression at SOD2 mRNA as well as at protein. Their heighten guarantees the increase of activity with the consequences of enhanced mitochondrial elimination ability of ROS. Furthermore, from the comparisons of changes in a single bout of strenuous endurance exercise group (group E1) and seven-week strenuous endurance exercise group (group E2), those changes were more obvious in group E2, which demonstrated that the improving amount of SOD2 mRNA and protein expression of long-term endurance exercise was clearly more than that of a single bout of exercise.

Yamashita and other researchers certified that long-term moderate-intensity endurance exercise increased the activity of myocardial SOD2 by antisense oligonucleotides technology [14]. Hou and other scholars detected that myocardial SOD2 activity in rats can be improved by swimming without load, 1 h per day for three days while SOD1 activity was unchanged [15]. In this study, a single bout of or seven-week strenuous endurance exercise gave rise to distinguished improvement of SOD2 and T-SOD activity; meanwhile, SOD1 activity showed no significant change. Some references discovered that endurance exercise stepped up muscle SOD2 protein expression and activity [16] [17]. Moreover, in this study, myocardial SOD2 activity trends were consistent with those of SOD2 mRNA and protein expression. Therefore, exercise can increase myocardial SOD2 protein expression, enhance its activity as well as improve T-SOD activity by stimulating SOD2 mRNA expression in this study. Moreover, it was found that both the increasing level of myocardial mRNA and protein expression and improvement level of SOD2 and T-SOD activity after seven-week strenuous endurance exercise were much better than those after a single bout of strenuous endurance exercise, which revealed that long-term endurance exercise can improve exercise effects.

5. Conclusions

Strenuous endurance exercise can stimulate myocardial SOD2 expression at mRNA and protein and enhance the activity for SOD2, thus increasing the activity for T-SOD.

The improvements of myocardial mRNA and protein expression as well as the activity for SOD2 by seven-week strenuous endurance exercise were all more obvious than those by a single bout of strenuous endurance exercise, demonstrating that long-term endurance exercise can improve exercise effects.

Research Support

Guangxi Natural Science Foundation of China (Project Number: 2013GXNSFBA019146).

References

[1] Ascensao, A., Ferrira, R. and Magalhaes, J. (2007) Exercise-Induced Cardioprotection-Biochemical, Morpho-Logical and Functional Evidence in Whole Tissue and Isolated Mitochondria. *International Journal of Cardiology*, **117**, 16-30. http://dx.doi.org/10.1016/j.ijcard.2006.04.076

[2] Brown, D.A., Chicco, A.J., Jew, K.N., Johnson, M.S., Lynch, J.M., Watson, P.A. and Moore, R.L. (2005) Cardioprotection Afforded by Chronic Exercise Is Mediated by the Sarcolemmal, and Not the Mitochondrial, Isoform of the KATP Channel in the Rat. *The Journal of Physiology*, **569**, 913-924. http://dx.doi.org/10.1113/jphysiol.2005.095729

[3]   Budiono, B.P., Hoe, L.E.S., Peart, J.N., Sabapathy, S., Ashton, K.J., Haseler, L.J. and Headrick, J.P. (2012) Voluntary Running in Mice Beneficially Modulates Myocardial Ischemic Tolerance, Signaling Kinases, and Gene Expression Patterns. *American Journal of Physiology-Regulatory Integrative and Comparative Physiology*, **302**, R1091-R1100. http://dx.doi.org/10.1152/ajpregu.00406.2011

[4]   French, J.P., Quindry, J.C., Falk, D.J., Staib, J.L., Lee, Y., Wang, K.K.W. and Powers, S.K. (2006) Ischemia-Reperfusion-Induced Calpain Activation and SERCA2a Degradation Are Attenuated by Exercise Training and Calpain Inhibition. *American Journal of Physiology. Heart and Circulatory Physiology*, **290**, H128-H136. http://dx.doi.org/10.1152/ajpheart.00739.2005

[5]   Powers, S.K., Sollanek, K.J., Wiggs, M.P., Demirel, H.A. and Smuder, A.J. (2014) Exercise-Induced Improvements in Myocardial Antioxidant Capacity: The Antioxidant Players and Cardioprotection. *Free Radical Research*, **48**, 43-51. http://dx.doi.org/10.3109/10715762.2013.825371

[6]   Bedford, T.G., Tipton, C.M., Wilson, N.C., Oppliger, R.A. and Gisolfi, C.V. (1979) Maximum Oxygen Consumption of Rats and Its Changes with Various Experimental Procedures. *Journal of Applied Physiology: Respiratory, Environmental and Exercise Physiology*, **47**, 1278-1283.

[7]   Pfaffl, M.W. (2001) A New Mathematical Model for Relative Quantification in Real-Time PT-PCR. *Nucleic Acids Research*, **29**, e45. http://dx.doi.org/10.1093/nar/29.9.e45

[8]   Peng, F.L., Lu, Y.L., Zhang, L., Chen, D.Q. and Deng, S.X. (2009) The Cardioprotective Effect of Intermittent Exercises on Ischemia-Reperfusion Rats' Myocardium. *Chinese Journal of Rehabilitation Medicine*, **24**, 910-913.

[9]   Peng, F.L., Guo, Y.J. and Zhang, L. (2010) The Effects of Interval Training and Acute Interval Exercise on Ischemia-Reperfusion Rats' ECG and Serum Myocardial Enzymes. *China Sport Science and Technology*, **46**, 102-105.

[10]   Xu, S.M., Liu, T.B. and Su, Q.S. (2011) Study on Heavy Load Training-Induced Cardiac Contractility Changes of Rats, and the Relationship between This Changes and the Levels of Cardiac Free Radical, Calcium Ions. *China Sport Science*, **31**, 73-78.

[11]   Li, S.C., Duan, Y.M. and Su, Q.S. (2012) The Establishment of Exercise-Induced Myocardial Stunning Model of Rat with Repeated Exhaustive Exercise on Treadmills. *China Sport Science*, **32**, 49-54.

[12]   Xu, S.M, Zhou, Y. and Wang, J. (2014) Abnormal ECG Changes and Energy Metabolic Disturbance after an Exhaustive Exercises in Rats. *Journal of Tianjin University of Sport*, **29**, 132-135.

[13]   Su, Q.S. (2004) Effect on the Structure of Heart during Re-Oxygen Process. *Journal of Chengdu Physical Education Institute*, **30**, 61-64.

[14]   Yamashita, N., Hoshida, S., Otsu, K., Asahi, M., Kuzuya, T. and Hori, M. (1999) Exercise Provides Direct Biphasic Cardioprotection via Manganese Superoxide Dismutase Activation. *The Journal of Experimental Medicine*, **189**, 1699-1706. http://dx.doi.org/10.1084/jem.189.11.1699

[15]   Hou, Y.Y, Ma, Z.Y. and Fan, X.Z. (2010) Protective Effect of Short-Term Exercise on Rat Ischemic/Reperfused Myocardium and Its Mechanism. *Suzhou University Journal of Medical Science*, **30**, 50-53.

[16]   Wenz, T., Diaz, F., Hernandez, D. and Moraes, C.T. (2009) Endurance Exercise Is Protective for Mice with Mitochondrial Myopathy. *Journal of Applied Physiology*, **106**, 1712-1719. http://dx.doi.org/10.1152/japplphysiol.91571.2008

[17]   Smuder, A.J., Min, K., Hudson, M.B., Kavazis, A.N., Kwon, O., Nelson, W.B. and Powers, S.K. (2012) Endurance Exercise Attenuates Ventilator-Induced Diaphragm Dysfunction. *Journal of Applied Physiology*, **112**, 501-510. http://dx.doi.org/10.1152/japplphysiol.01086.2011

List of Abbreviations

Reactive Oxygen Species (ROS); Superoxide Dismutase (SOD); Total Superoxide Dismutase (T-SOD); Cu, Zn Superoxide Dismutase (SOD1); Manganese Superoxide Dismutase (SOD2); Sprague Dawley (SD); Reverse Transcription (RT); Relative Expression (RE); Analysis of Variance (ANOVA); Least-Significant Difference (LSD); Temperature (Tm); Malondialdehyde (MDA).

20

Effects of Qing'E Formula on the Expression of Bone Metabolic Markers and VDR mRNA in Postmenopausal Osteoporosis Patients

Bo Shuai, Yanping Yang[*], Lin Shen[#], Hui Ke

Department of Integrated Traditional Chinese and Western Medicine, Union Hospital, Tongji Medical College, Huazhong University of Science and Technology, Wuhan, China
Email: [#]bobo3137@126.com

Abstract

Objectives: To study the partial mechanism of treating postmenopausal osteoporosis patients (POPs) using the ancient recipe of Qing'E Formula (QEF) by observing its effects on bone metabolic markers and VDR mRNA expression in primary POPs. Methods: Analysis was performed on 120 outpatient and inpatient POPs treated in our hospital between January and October 2013, where the patients were randomly divided into Qing'E group (QEF + Caltrate), Calcitriol group (Caltrate + Calcitriol soft capsules), and Compare group (Caltrate), each with a follow-up period of 1 year. Statistical analysis was then performed on bone mineral density, blood bone metabolic markers (β-CTX, N-MID, T-PINP) and changes in VDR mRNA expressions in the POPs before and after the treatments. Results: Prior to the treatments, bone mineral density and blood β-CTX, N-MID, T-PINP and VDR mRNA expression in the 3 groups of POPs exhibited no statistically significant differences, and the blood β-CTX, N-MID, T-PINP and VDR mRNA expression in the control group showed no statistically significant differences before and after the treatments. There were no significant differences in bone mineral density in the Qing'E group and the Calcitriol group before and after the treatments whereas the bone mineral density decreased in the control group after the treatments. As for blood β-CTX, N-MID, T-PINP and VDR mRNA expression, the measurements in POPs in the Qing'E group and the Calcitriol group were significantly higher than that of the control group. Conclusion: By adjusting the VDR mRNA expression, the QEF, a kidney-invigorating Chinese herbal formula, is capable of activating bone metabolism to prohibit further losses of bone mass, thereby preventing the deterioration of osteoporosis.

Keywords

Qing'E Formula, VDR mRNA, Osteoporosis, Bone Metabolism, Bone Density

[*]This author contributed equally to this work.
[#]Corresponding author.

1. Introduction

With the aging of population in our society, osteoporosis and other metabolic bone diseases and their complications have become one of the key factors affecting the healthy living of the elderly population and increasing the society's economic burdens. The QEF, a Chinese herbal formula, has the efficacy of "nourishing livers and kidneys", "increasing energy and blood" and "regenerating bone marrows". Preliminary studies by the research team showed that QEF could effectively raise $1,25(OH)_2D_3$ and mRNA expression in the blood of ovariectomized rats, thereby effectively controlling osteoporosis. This study proposes the further study on the partial mechanism of treating POPs using ancient recipe QEF by studying its effects on the special sequence of β collagen in blood markers of bone metabolism (β-Crosslaps, β-CTX), N-terminal osteocalcin (N-MID), total N-terminal propeptide of type I procollagen (T-PINP) and VDR mRNA expression in POPs.

2. Materials and Methods

2.1. Research Objects and Grouping

The research objects were 120 primary POPs, with an average age of 53 ± 6 years old. The subjects, comprising of either inpatient or outpatient patients of the hospital, were randomly segregated into three groups, *i.e.* the Qing'E group, who were given the treatment combination of Caltrate and QEF; the Calcitriol group, who were given the treatment combination of Caltrate and Calcitriol soft capsules; and the compare group, who were only given Caltrate treatments. The groups, consisting of 40 POPs each, were given treatments for the period of 1 year. The administering method of medicine is in the "Experiment Medicine" section. This study has been approved by the ethics committee of Wuhan Union Hospital Research Center, along with endorsement from all personnel participating in the study. The participating POPs had also refrained from taking any medicine that affects bone metabolism and coagulation functions two weeks prior to the determination.

2.2. Experiment Medicine

The making process of experiment medicine—ancient herbal formula QEF: The ingredients include the following: *Eucommia* (fried with salt) 480 g, Psoralen (fried with salt) 240 g, walnut (fried) 150 g, Salvia 240 g and garlic 120 g. Garlic was steamed, dried, crushed into fine powder with *Eucommia*, Salvia and Psoralen and then sifted. Walnut was then mashed and grinded with the above powder before the mixture was further sifted and mixed. For every 100 grams of the powder, 50 - 70 grams of refining honey was added for producing the Qing'E pill. The experiment objects were then allocated randomly and received treatments under the experiment medicine or the control medicine. QEF were administered three times daily with warm water whereas Calcitriol soft capsules were administered twice a day, with 1 pill for each intake. In addition to the experiment medicine, the experiment groups and the control group were also given 1 piece of Caltrate daily to ensure patients' compliance and facilitate better treatments. Any traditional Chinese medicine or modern western medicine that affects bone metabolism and coagulation functions were prohibited during the course of the observation period.

2.3. Experiment Methods

2.3.1. Information Collection and Bone Density Testing

Physical examination and survey results of all patients were recorded in detail before and after the treatments. The U.S. made Hologic 2000 Plus Dual-energy X-ray Bone Densitometer and conventional standard software were used to measure bone density at the lumbar spine, the proximal femur, Ward', and greater trochanter. Patients were placed in the position according to requirements, followed by analysis of the images and the results were reported with reference to the WHO diagnostic criteria (g/cm^2). The results were automatically printed and exported from the equipment's supporting printer. The bone density of all patients was measured by one single person using the same equipment to minimize variations in statistical analysis.

2.3.2. Measurement of Blood Bone Metabolic Markers in Patients

Blood samples were drawn from the cubital vein in patients at approximately 10 a.m. every day. Part of the collected blood sample was then centrifuged for 15 minutes (speed: 1000 ×g, temperature 2°C - 8°C) and stored in refrigerator at −70°C while bone metabolic markers β-CTX, N-MID, T-PINP in blood were collected, all the blood were delivered to the same central biochemical lab for tests following the collection, and the tests were conducted strictly according to the instructions listed on the test kits.

2.3.4. Measurement of Blood Adiponectin mRNA in Patients

VDR mRNA expression was measured in the other portion of the blood samples, the VDR primer: under the role of reverse transcriptase M-MLV, the m RNA reverse transcribed into c-DNA molecules. The reaction system was as follows: H_2O 5.5 μl, Oligo (dT18) 1.0 μl, TRNA 6.0 μl, RNasin 0.5 μl, 5 × buffer 4.0 μl, 10 mM dNTP 2.0 μl, RTase 1.0 μl; the reaction conditions: 42 Celsius for 60 minutes, and 95 Celsius for 5 minutes. Quantitative PCR reaction system as follows: cDNA 1 μl, Buffer 10 × 5 μl, $MgCl_2$ (25 mM) 7 μl, dNTP 10 mM 1 μl, F (20 pmol/μl) 0.8 μl, R (20 pmol/μl) 0.8 μl, SYBR GreenI 1 μl, Taq enzyme (5 U/μl) 0.5 μl; the reaction conditions: 94 Celsius for 30 minutes, 53 Celsius for 30 minutes, and 72 degree for 30 minutes for 50 cycles. Ct values were calculated and analyzed: the sample relative value = $2^{-(\Delta Ct\beta\text{-actin} - \Delta Ct\,\text{test sample})}$, ΔCt = Ct negative control − Ct sample, $\Delta\Delta Ct = \Delta Ct\beta$-actin − ΔCt sample = Ct sample − Ctβ-actin.

2.4. Statistical Methods

Statistical Methods: Test results were represented by $\bar{x} \pm S$, statistical methods such as analysis of variance, paired sample t test and t-test for independent samples were used for testing and analysis, $p < 0.05$ represented statistical significance and data was analyzed using the SPSS13.0 software.

3. Results

3.1. BMD Changes in the 3 Groups of Patients before and after Treatments

There was no statistically significant difference in BMD among the three groups of patients before the treatments. After the treatments, the Qing'E group of patients saw slight increases in the BMD in lumbar spine, femoral neck, ward and the greater trochanter when compared with the measurements before the treatment; however, the difference was not statistically significant. There was no difference in the BMD in lumbar spine, femoral neck, ward and the greater trochanter in the Calcitriol group before and after the treatments whilst the BMD in these same parts saw significant decrease in the control group. There was no difference in BMD in lumbar spine, femoral neck, ward and the greater trochanter between the Qing'E group and the Calcitriol group, whilst, the measurements in the control group were significantly lower than the above 2 groups (**Figure 1**).

3.2. Changes in Bone Metabolic Markers β-CTX, N-MID and T-PINP Expression in the 3 Groups of Patients before and after the Treatments

The β-CTX, N-MID and T-PINP expression in the blood of the 3 groups of patients had no statistical significance before the treatments. After the treatments, there was no difference in the content of β-CTX, N-MID and T-PINP between the Qing'E and Calcitriol groups, however, the post-treatment contents were lower after treatments in both groups. There was no statistically significant difference in β-CTX, N-MID and T-PINP in the control group before and after the treatments, and the content in this group were significantly higher than that of the Qing'E and Calcitriol groups (**Figure 2**).

3.3. Difference in VDR mRNA Expression in the 3 Groups of Patients before and after the Treatments

There was no significant difference in VDR mRNA expression among the 3 groups of patients before the treatments. The post-treatment VDR mRNA expression in the Qing'E and Calcitriol groups were higher after treatments, but there was no significant difference between the 2 groups. There was no difference in VDR mRNA expression in the control group before and after treatments (**Figures 3(a)-3(c)**).

4. Discussion

Due to the withering of ovary, older women experience sharp decrease in estrogen in the body, which leads to significant negative balance of bone metabolism where the rate of bone resorption becomes faster than bone formation, resulting in osteoporosis. Postmenopausal women experience significant reduction in estrogen, which

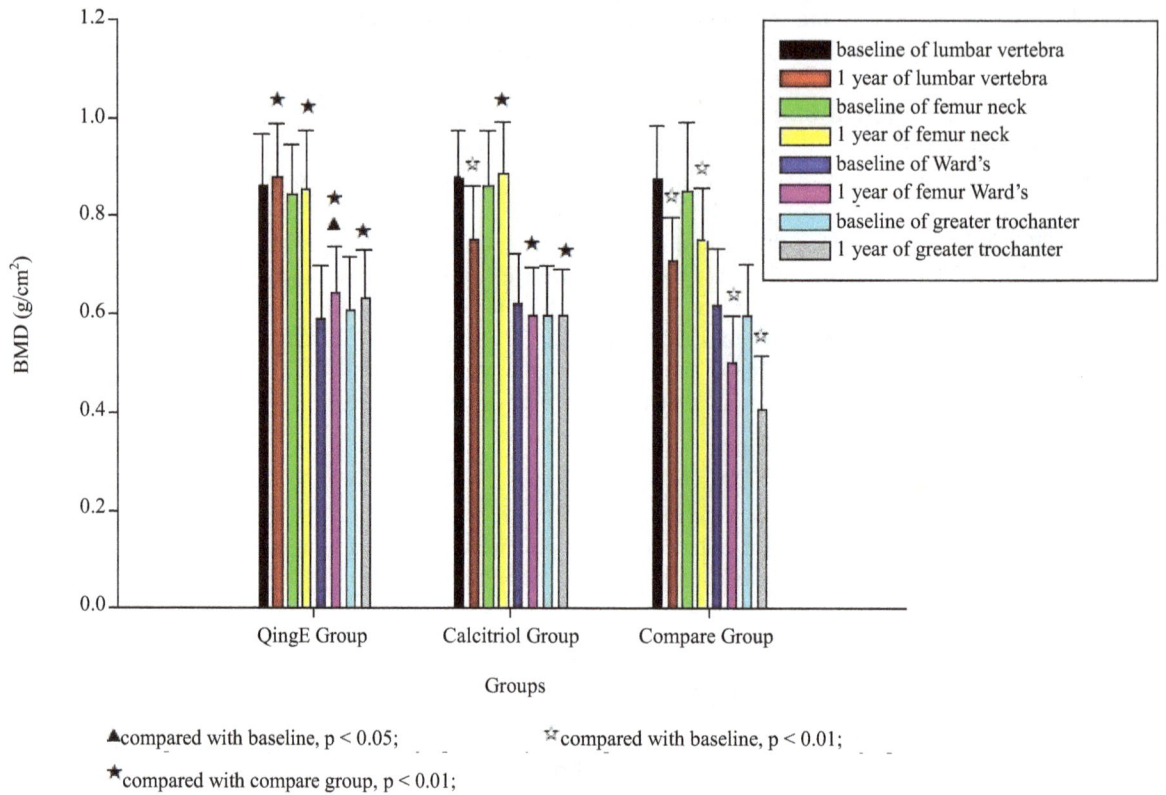

▲compared with baseline, p < 0.05; ☆compared with baseline, p < 0.01;

★compared with compare group, p < 0.01;

Figure 1. BMD changes in the 3 groups of patients before and after treatments.

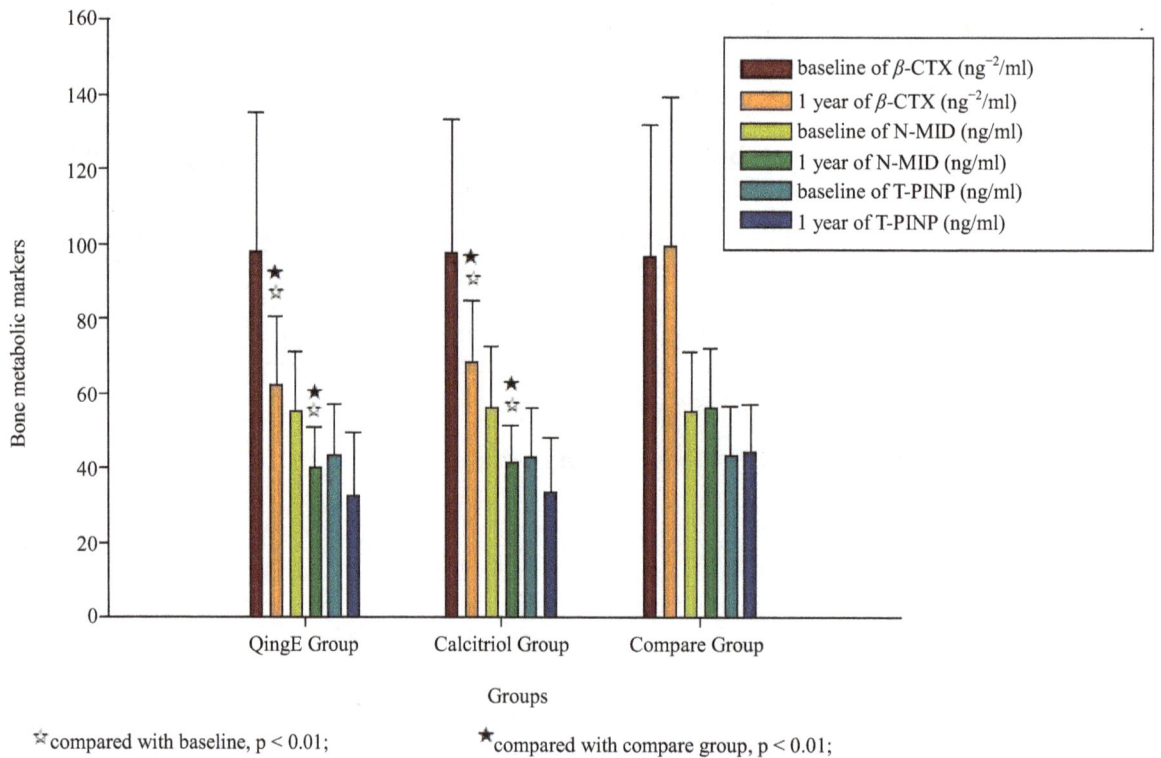

☆compared with baseline, p < 0.01; ★compared with compare group, p < 0.01;

Figure 2. Changes in bone metabolic markers β-CTX, N-MID and T-PINP expression in the 3 groups of patients before and after the treatments.

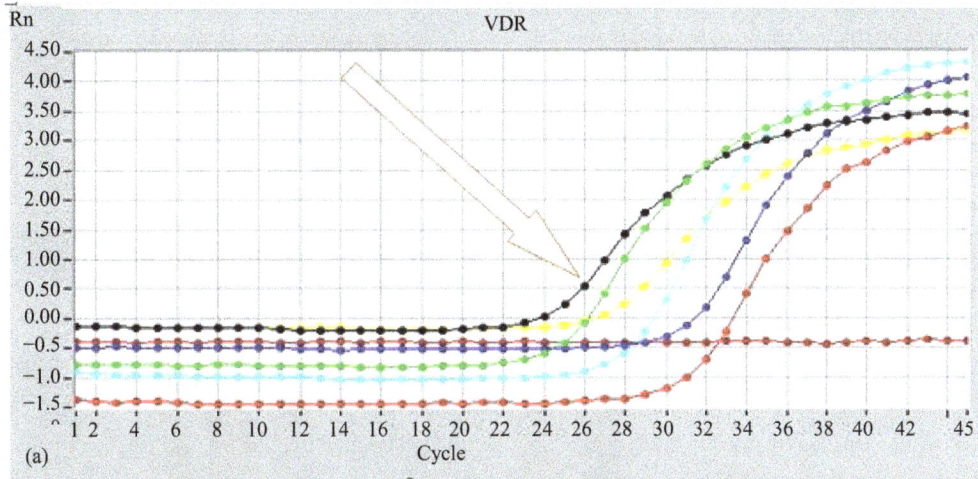

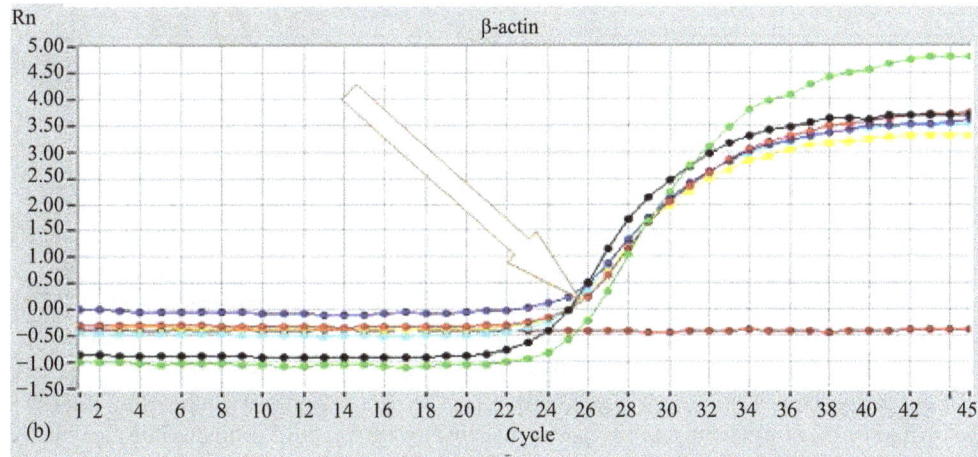

(a)

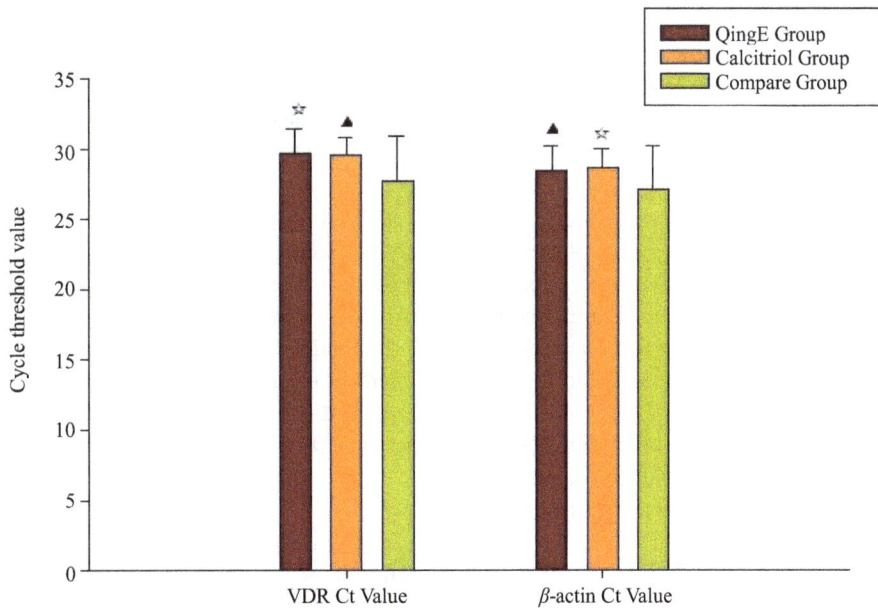

▲compared with compare group, p < 0.05;   ☆compared with compare group, p < 0.01;

(b)

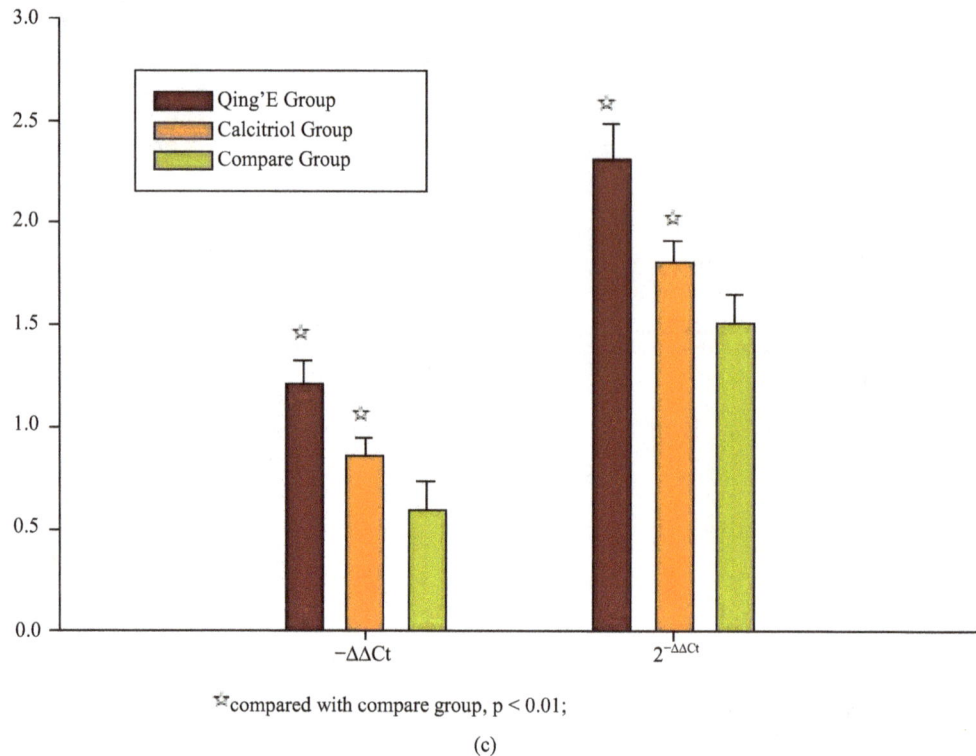

☆compared with compare group, p < 0.01;

(c)

Figure 3. Difference in VDR mRNA expression in the 3 groups of patients before and after the treatments.

inhibits the secretion of parathyroid hormone (PTH) and the reduction of PTH creates barriers to the activation of 1α-hydroxylase in livers, which would in turn lead to decrease in the synthesis of $1,25(OH)_2D_3$. Addition of active vitamin D_3 in the treatment for postmenopausal women could promote intestinal absorption of calcium and enhance the cellular activity of osteoclasts and osteoblasts, thereby promoting the mineralization of bones, bone formation and the absorption of the old bones. $1,25(OH)_2D_3$ is the active form of the most bioactive vitamin D in the body. The biological activity of vitamin D is mainly the result of the interaction of $1,25(OH)$ and the VDR of the nucleus in target organs. The combination of $1,25(OH)_2D_3$ and VDR forms a hormone-receptor complex, which would combine with the hormone response elements in the VDR gene to regulate VDR expression through the interaction with other regulatory factors [1] [2]. Researches have shown that vitamin D receptor gene polymorphism is closely associated with bone density of Han race in Guangxi, Beijing, Wuhan, Fujian and Guangzhou and other racial groups [3]-[5]. Preliminary studies by the research team showed that QEF could effectively suppress VDR mRNA expression in the kidney of ovariectomized rats to promote the expression of vitamin D and the absorption of calcium, thereby effectively controlling postmenopausal osteoporosis [6] [7]. Research has shown that the relative expression of VDR mRNA in the kidney of ovariectomized rats is significantly lower than the normal control group, which is consistent with the findings of this study [8]. VDR mRNA expression in the figure has significantly strengthened in the blood of active vitamin D_3 treatment group (Calcitriol group). This might be attributable to the direct supplement of active vitamin D_3, which has led to the significant increase in the content of "exogenous" $1,25(OH)_2D_3$ in the blood, which in turn leads to the increase in VDR mRNA expression. There is no significant difference in VDR mRNA between QEF and Calcitriol groups, suggesting the possibility of including "kidney essence", etc. in QEF to increase VDR mRNA expression, thereby achieving the same effects as Calcitriol soft capsules.

In "Qing'E Pill" prescription, *Eucommia ulmoides* oliv is warm-natured, with the effect of making kidney and bones strong, so in the book "Ben Cao Ji Yan", there was such a description, "*Eucommia ulmoides* oliv is only herb to strengthen lower energizer, remove pains of foots and legs, and fix knees and loins." Also in another ancient book named "Ben Cao Jing Shu", it was said "*Psoralea corylifolia* can warm the kidney, raise 'Yang' from 'Yin', raise 'fire' from 'soil', can cure kidney weakness and difficulties in sitting up." In "Ju Fang Qing'E Pill", it described that "*Juglans regia* can invigorate the kidney and promote blood circulation, garlic bulb can make the retention pass and dredge collaterals... The combination of these four kinds of herb is called 'Qing'E Pill', which can not only cure kidney weakness and difficulties in sitting up, but also strengthen bone and musculature, promote blood circulation, make hair dark, and bring a good look." After thousands years of clinical validation, Qing'E Pill was effective, safe and economical, however, there was a lack of specific mechanism research.

The β-CTX, N-MID and T-PINP are three types of bone metabolic markers recommended by the International Osteoporosis Foundation (IOF). The β-CTX is the organic component of bone matrix, of which 90% are type I collagen synthesized in bones, but are also decomposed into degradation products that are released into the blood. The β-CTX is a typical product of collagen degradation of type I collagen. The examination of β-CTX can be used for monitoring the anti-resorptive treatment for osteoporosis or other bone diseases, and the efficacy can be reflected within several weeks. The N-MID are produced by osteoblasts during bone synthesis. Both complete osteocalcin and large N-MID fragments are present in the blood; however, the former is unstable and may split and degrade into the latter. The N-MID osteocalcin is regarded as a marker of bone synthesis, which can be used in conjunction with β-CTX for monitoring the treatment of diseases such as osteoporosis. The determination of the concentration of total PINP in the blood is one of the test items of bone markers, which can be used for monitoring the treatment of osteoporosis in postmenopausal women clinically.

The biological activity of vitamin D is mainly the result of the interaction of 1,25(OH) and the VDR of the nucleus in target organs. Vitamin D can enhance osteoblast activity in bone metabolism and promote the formation of bone mineralization. In addition, it also has positive effects on relatively mature osteoblasts, such as increasing the expression of OC and ALP, promoting the mRNA expression of type I collagen of osteoblast in the late maturity stage and the secretion of type I collagen, promoting the synthesis and secretion of osteoblasts and the mineralization of bone matrix, as well as improving the quality and quantity of bones.

The results of this study show that QEF can reduce bone resorption through the adjustment of VDR mRNA expression. This experiment uses stable and effective active vitamin D_3 reported in literatures as the reference drug for the control study [9]-[11]. Data shows similar drug efficacy between QEF and active vitamin D_3, as both are able to increase VDR mRNA expression in the body in reducing bone resorption and strengthening the quality and quantity of bones. The results suggest that the ancient recipe QEF has comparable efficacy in the prevention and treatment of postmenopausal osteoporosis as appropriate supplement of active vitamin D_3.

Acknowledgements

The authors would like to thank LV Lin for his expertise and assistance in performing the blood collection, and Wang Quanshen for his technical assistance.

Research Support

Innovation Fund of Huazhong University of Science and Technology (Item Number: 2013QN235); National Natural Science Foundation of China (Project Number: 81273907 and 81072493).

References

[1] Fan, L.Y., Tu, X.Q., Zhu, Y., Zhou, L., Pfeiffer, T., Feltens, R., Stoecker, W. and Zhong, R. (2005) Genetic Association of Vitamin D Receptor Polymorphisms with Autoimmune Hepatitis and Primary Biliary Cirrhosis in the Chinese. *Journal of Gastroenterology and Hepatology*, **20**, 249-255. http://dx.doi.org/10.1111/j.1440-1746.2005.03532.x

[2] Van Etten, E. and Mathieu, C. (2005) Immunoregulation by 1,25-Dihydroxyvitamin D_3: Basic Concepts. *The Journal of Steroid Biochemistry and Molecular Biology*, **97**, 93-101. http://dx.doi.org/10.1016/j.jsbmb.2005.06.002

[3] Zhou, Y., Zhang H. and Cai D.H. (2005) Influence of Estrogen and Progesteron on Bone Metabolism and Renal Expression of 1,25-Dihydroxyvitamin D_3 Receptors mRNA in Ovariectomized Rats. *Academic Journal of Second Military Medical University*, **26**, 1270-1273.

[4] Municio, M.J. and Traba, M.L. (2004) Effects of 24, 25-$(OH)_2D_3$, 1,25-$(OH)_2D_3$ and 25$(OH)D_3$ on Alkaline and Tartrate-Resistant Acid Phosphatase Activities in Fetal Rat Calvaria. *Journal of Physiology and Biochemistry*, **60**, 219-224. http://dx.doi.org/10.1007/BF03167032

[5] Uchida, M., Shima, M., Chikazu, D., Fujieda, A., Obara, K., Suzuki, H., Nagai, Y., Yamato, H. and Kawaguchi, H. (2001) Transcriptional Induction of Matrix Metalloproteinase-13 (Collagenase-3) by 1 Alpha,25-Dihydroxyvitamin D_3 in Mouse Osteoblastic MC3T3-E1 Cells. *Journal of Bone and Mineral Research*, **16**, 221-230.

http://dx.doi.org/10.1359/jbmr.2001.16.2.221

[6]   Shuai, B., Shen, L., Yang, Y.P., Xie, J., Zhou P.Q., Xu X.J., Li, C.G. and Wu, M.X. (2012) Effect of Bushenhuoxue Decoction on the Osteogenic Differentiation of Bone Marrow Stromal Cells in the Steroid Induced Osteonecrosis of the Femoral Head. *Research of Integrated Traditional Chinese and Western Medicine*, **4**, 297-301.

[7]   Shuai, B., Shen, L., Yang, Y.P., Xie, J., Shou, Z.X. and Wei, B. (2010) Low Plasma Adiponectin as a Potential Biomarker for Osteonecrosis of the Femoral Head. *The Journal of Rheumatology*, **37**, 2151-2155. http://dx.doi.org/10.3899/jrheum.100342

[8]   Guo, L.J., Luo, X.H., Xie, H., Zhou, H.D. and Liao, E.Y. (2005) The Effects of 1Alpha,25-Dihydroxyvitamin D_3 in Regulation Matrix Metalloproteinase and Tissue Metalloproteinase Inhibitors in Human Osteoblasts. *Zhonghua Nei Ke Za Zhi*, **44**, 125-128.

[9]   Xue, Z.W., Shang, X.M., Lv, S.H., Xu, H., Zhang, Q. and Wang, C. (2013) Effects of Shenshao Decoction on the Inflammatory Response in The aorta of a Rat Atherosclerotic Model. *Chinese Journal of Integrative Medicine*, **19**, 347-352. http://dx.doi.org/10.1007/s11655-013-1457-z

[10] Yao, F.A., Dobs, A.S. and Brown, T.T. (2006) Alternative Therapies for Osteoporosis. *The American Journal of Chinese Medicine*, **34**, 721. http://dx.doi.org/10.1142/S0192415X06004235

[11] Ling, J.Y., Shen, L., Liu, Q., Xue, S., Ma, W., Wu, H., Li, Z.X. and Zhu, R. (2013) Changes in Platelet GPIbα and ADAM17 during the Acute Stage of Atherosclerotic Ischemic Stroke among Chinese. *Journal of Huazhong University of Science and Technology* (*Medical Sciences*), **33**, 438-442.

21

Key Plants in Fighting Cancer in the Middle East

Aref Abu-Rabia

Ben-Gurion University of the Negev, Beersheba, Israel
Email: arefabu@gmail.com

Abstract

This article is derived from a broader study of ethno-botany, medical anthropology and alternative medicine in Middle Eastern countries, which has been conducted during the past two decades. It presents examples of different edible and medicinal plants and their uses by different communities (urban, peasant and Bedouin) in the treatment of diseases and various medical disorders. Alongside, the article reviews current knowledge concerning plants and cancer prevention and treatment. The article shows that people of these countries use various parts of the plant in a host of manners-fresh and soft, cooked or dried, as both food and medicine. These plants—part of the natural fauna of the Middle Eastern countries—grow in the wild and are cultivated. The author found that the most significant plants used were in the following families: Compositae, Gramineae, Labiatae, Lamiaceae, Liliaceae, Malvaceae, Oleaceae, Ranunculaceae, Umbelliferae, and Urticaceae.

Keywords

Medicinal Plants, Alternative Medicine, Cancer, Middle East

1. Background

Ancient Arab medicine was greatly influenced by medicinal practices in Persia, Mesopotamia, India, Greece, and Rome. The Greco-Roman system of medicine was based primarily on the writing of Hippocrates, Dioscorides, and Galen. The Arab system grew and developed during the rule of the Umayyad (661-750) and the Abbasids (750-1258). Ibn Sina (Avicenna 980-1037), who compiled the *Canon of Medicine*, and al-Razi (Rhazes 865-923), who compiled the *Comprehensive Book on Medicine*, were the most renowned Islamic physicians [1] [2].

Notably, the works of Ibn Sina and al-Razi were translated into Latin, and continued to influence medical work until as late as the nineteenth century [3] [4].

Most physicians in the Andalus (Islamic Spain) were herbalists. Among them was Ibn al-Baytar (1197-1248) whose *Compendium of Simple Drugs and Food* described more than 1400 medicinal drugs, including 300 not previously covered by other works [5]. The Arab medical tradition was established in the tenth century, developed in the eleventh and twelfth centuries, reached its peak from the thirteenth to the sixteenth centuries, and declined in the seventeenth to nineteenth centuries [6] [7]. Medical literature and healing methods that had been at the focus of traditional medicine for over a thousand years were marginalized by the advent of western medicine in the nineteenth and twentieth centuries, becoming the exclusive domain of traditional medicine and folk healers [7] [8]. Yet, the use of traditional medicine, particularly herbal medicine, was still widespread throughout the Middle East in the twentieth century, and remains so today [9] [10]. Most of the herbs used in herbal medicine serve both as food and as medications [11] [12].

2. Introduction

A famous Arab saying claims that "prevention is better than a cure", much like the old [Western] saying "an ounce of prevention is worth a pound of cure". Hippocrates, the father of medicine, recognizing the link between food and health, advised that "let your food be your medicine, and let your medicine be your food". The connection between diet and the risk of illness is apparent in the case of cancer. Cancer risk factors fall into two main categories: inherited and environmental. The considerable variation in dietary habits from culture to culture is widely accepted as a factor that underlies differences in cancer incidences in different populations around the globe [13] [14]. Inherited genetic defects are responsible for only about 15 percent of all cancers. This means that approximately 85 percent of all cancers result from environmental risk factors such as diet, lifestyle, and exposure to harmful substances [14]. The majority of cancers in humans are induced by carcinogenic factors present in our environment, including our diet.

Dietary influences have frequently been invoked to explain the marked variation in breast cancer incidence among racial and geographic groups [15]. The incidence of cancer overall in Mediterranean countries is lower than in Scandinavian countries and the United States, perhaps due to differences in diet. This difference is accounted for mainly by the lower incidence in Mediterranean countries of cancer of the large intestine, breast, endometrium, and prostate. Research shows that approximately one third of all cancer deaths are related to dietary factors and lack of physical activity in adulthood. There is increasing evidence that monounsaturated oils are associated with a lower risk of some cancers. This evidence is in line with the composition of olive oil and the potential role of monounsaturated fatty acids and minor compounds that are protective against reactive oxygen species [16].

The traditional Mediterranean diet is characterized by high consumption of plant foods, relatively low consumption of red meat, and high consumption of olive oil. The findings of studies in Italy, Spain, and Greece, suggest that olive oil may provide some protection against the development of breast cancer. Incidence rates of breast cancer in Mediterranean countries are relatively low compared with those in most other Western countries [17]. In a study assessing changes in diet and cancer mortality in Mediterranean countries, it was found that Greece and Spain had the lowest rates of ovarian cancer, the lowest intakes of animal fat and the highest consumption of olive oil [18]. It was reported that prostate cancer mortality in 32 countries was correlated with total fat consumption, although the association was not as strong as it was for breast cancer and appeared to be limited to animal fats. On the other hand, death rates from prostate cancer have been lower in areas with high olive oil consumption, such as Greece and Italy [19] [20]. A number of studies conducted in Mediterranean countries have reported inverse associations between olive oil consumption, on the one hand, and cancers of the stomach [21], lung [22], bladder [23], or urinary tract [24] on the other, even without controlling for energy intake.

Poor diet is a major cause of cancers in the United States. When diet is poor, the immune system is less able to defend the body against foreign invaders that can trigger the onset of cancer. In countries where people eat a Western diet, the rate of colorectal cancer is up to 10 times higher than that in countries where people follow an Asian diet [14].

The human body is designed to function efficiently by obtaining most of its energy and nutrition from plant sources [25]. In the absence of the important vitamins and minerals available in plant foods, the risk of cancer increases. Vegetables and fruits contain the anti-carcinogenic cocktail to which we are adapted [26].

The fact that many conventional drugs used in chemotherapy come from plants supports the use of natural medicines in treating cancers. Among these are vincristine and vinblastine from the periwinkle plant (*Vinca mi-*

nor) and paclitaxel from the Pacific yew tree (*Taxus brevifolin/Taxus brevifolia*) [14].

Interestingly, some studies find that several herbs used in conjunction with conventional medicine can control and improve certain symptoms, such as fear and anxiety, better than medication alone and can support the social and psychological wellbeing of cancer patients and others [27].

3. Methodology

The data for this paper are derived from a broad study of ethno-botany and traditional medicine in the Middle East that took place over the course of two decades (in Palestine, Israel, Jordan, Sinai, and Egypt). The paper is based on interviews with healers and patients that were conducted using semi-structured questionnaires. All the data were recorded in field logs, and some were tape-recorded. The study included men and women of different ages and from a variety of groups. Plant samples were collected and identified by healers, elderly people, and university botanists. The samples were identified and classified according to the plants' leaves, flowers, barks, stems, stalks, roots, rhizomes, bulbs, tubers, fruits, corns, shells, seeds, stones/pits, soft seed pods, grain buds, shoots, twigs, oils, resins and gums, taste, and color.

4. Results

This article is derived from a broader study of ethno-botany, medical anthropology and alternative medicine in Middle Eastern countries. It presents examples of different edible and medicinal plants and their uses by different communities (urban, peasant and Bedouin) in the treatment of diseases and various medical disorders, as well as cancer prevention and treatment.

The article shows that peoples of these countries use various parts of the plant in a host of manners as both food and medicine. These plants parts are used fresh and soft, or cooked or dried. Toxic plants/bulbs are dried, boiled several times in water, or placed in hot ashes and then used for medicines or foods. The dosages for patients with the same diseases or disorders may vary, according to the ages and the structures of the patients' bodies.

Analysis of the findings shows that the Middle East is the geographic origin of both wild and cultivated medicinal plants. These plants may be picked in the wild or bought in specialty shops as well as from herbalists ('*attarin*).

The rich variety of approaches employed by different healers to treat or prevent cancer is indicative of the depth and breadth of indigenous medicine practiced among the Arab in the twentieth and twenty first centuries. It should be noted that wild desert plants also contain a host of other biologically active compounds besides nutrients. The physiological effects of these other compounds in relation to plant nutrients are not well known, but could affect nutrient and medical utilization or other functions. These topics are of relevance for future research in terms of improving our understanding of human nutritional and medical requirements of the people in the Middle East, especially with reference to cancer prevention and treatment.

Interviews results of the healers and patients are titled after Abu-Rabia 1993-2013, fieldwork notes.

The author found that the most significant plants that used are found in the following ten families as described below:

Compositae, Gramineae, Labiatae, Lamiaceae, Liliaceae, Malvaceae, Oleaceae, Ranunculaceae, Umbelliferae, and Urticaceae.

Plants

Warning: It is extremely important to note that in order to avoid side-effects, toxicity, or possible herb-drug interactions, caution should be exercised and all herbs should be taken only after consulting a physician or clinical herbalist.

5. Compositae

Taraxacum cyprium H. Lind

Arabic: *salatat al-ruhban, handaba.*
English: common dandelion.
Plant parts: whole herb, flowers, leaves, stems, and roots.

Preparation: eat raw as a salad.

Active constituents: latex, bitter principles, alkaloids [28], vitamins A, B1, B2, B complex, and E, calcium, sodium, iron, potassium, phosphorus, chloride compound, and magnesium. The roots contain enzymes [29].

Properties and ethno-botanical uses: digestive, diuretic, tonic. It stimulates bile secretion and is used in the treatment of hepatic disorders, venereal diseases, herpes and other simple lip lesions, and piles. The flowers and leaves are eaten as a raw salad daily for one month to treat urinary retention and infections, renal stones, and hepatic disorders [11] [28]. The nuns and monks in Palestine's monasteries use the leaves and roots in green salad. It is also used to treat digestion problems and liver diseases, and may be pounded and boiled in water to treat cancerous tumors, anemia, acne, furuncles, and other skin conditions and tumors [30] [31]. Additionally, it is used to strengthen the bodies of infants and elderly people during and after recovery from disease [31]. The dandelion works against cancer by inducing apoptosis and differentiation, enhancing the immune system, inhibiting angiogenesis, and reversing multidrug resistance, and improves survival, increases tumor response and quality of life, and reduces chemotherapy toxicity [32].

6. Gramineae

Avena sterilis L.

Arabic: *khafour, shufan, sha'ir al-hsayni.*
English: oats.
Plant parts: seeds, hay and bran.
Active constituents: soluble fibers, proteins, unsaturated fatty acids, vitamins, niacin, and phytochemicals. Oat bran contains B complex vitamins, protein, fat, minerals, and heart-healthy soluble fiber called β-glucan, as well as magnesium, iron, copper, potassium, and selenium [33].

Properties and ethno-botanical uses: nutrient, diuretic, laxative, sedative, calmative, antispasmodic, and tonic. Water in which the seeds have been boiled is administered orally, to strengthen women after childbirth and to increase milk during breastfeeding. Seeds soaked in water are used as a cosmetic [30]. Oat seeds and hay are soaked in water to prepare a drink for the treatment of genitourinary tract infections, abdominal disorders, constipation, and diabetes, and to increase sexual desire. Oats are used to treat skin diseases, tumors, and cancer [11]. They also act as an antiseptic for the sexual organs of men and women and are used to treat prostate problems [31].

Various studies have shown that oats have the potential to prevent the appearance and progression of various conditions such as cancer, bowel malfunction, obesity, and celiac disease. Avena sativa has been reported as an antispasmodic and stimulant. It is used mainly for its nutritional value and is particularly beneficial in special diets for convalescents or for patients with illness such as gastroenteritis and dyspepsia [33]. Its dietary fiber complex, with its antioxidants and other phytochemicals, is effective against cardiovascular disease and some types of cancer [34]. Oats, like other grains and vegetables, contain hundreds of phytochemicals (plant chemicals), some of which are thought to possess cancer-preventive properties. Lignans, phytoestrogen compounds that are present   in oats, have been linked to decreased risk of hormone-related diseases such as breast cancer [35], and similar effects are expected to be found regarding other hormone-related cancers such as prostate, endometrial, and ovarian cancers. International research has shown that women with a relatively high intake of dietary fiber have lower circulating estrogen levels, a factor associated with a reduced risk of breast cancer. The insoluble fibers in oats are also thought to reduce carcinogens in the gastrointestinal tract [36].

7. Labiatae

7.1. Salvia officinalis L.

Arabic: *miramia, na'ema.*
English: white sage.
Plant parts: leaves, seeds.
Active constituents: essential oil, tannin, camphor, cineol, borneol, pinene, resin [28], vitamin B complex, sulfur and steroid substances [29].

Ethno-botanical uses: antiseptic, astringent, antispasmodic, anti-inflammatory, gargle, emmenagogue, diuretic, cholagogue, infusion stimulant, tonic. Midwives used it to strengthen the uterus [28] [37]. *Salvia officinalis* essential oils and some identified terpenes inhibit human tumor cell growth [38]. Saliva officinalis oils inhibit human head and neck squamous cell carcinoma growth [39].

7.2. *Salvia fruticosa* Mill

Arabic: *marmarya, miramia.*
English: three-lobed sage, sage.
Plant parts: leaves and flowers.
Active constituents: essential oil, tannin, camphor cineol, borneol, pinene, resin [28], vitamin B complex [29]. The leaves contain essential oil, phenols, and thujone [10].

Properties and ethno-botanical uses: carminative, sedative. It is used to treat genitourinary tract infections, stomachache, diarrhea, open wounds, and nausea, and to regulate menstruation and ease menstrual pain [11] [31] [28]. It is also employed in the treatment of tumors, and stomach disturbances and administered to help women recover from miscarriage and after childbirth [31]. Other uses include the regulation of menstruation and treatment of urinary tract disorders [10]. It is also used to treat cancer [40]. Foods enriched with bioactive compounds, such as *Salvia fruticosa* Mill, have significant effects on health and represent a promising adjuvant treatment in patients with advanced breast cancer, due to their contribution in lowering the high oxidative stress present in these patients [41] [42].

8. Lamiaceae

Origanum majorana L.

Arabic: *mardaddoush, mardaqoush, rayhan dawoud, za'ater.*
English: sweet marjoram, knotted marjoram.
Plant parts: leaves.
Active constituents: ethanolic essential oil, linalool, and terpinen [43] [44].

Properties and ethno-botanical uses: *Origanum majorana* is used as an aphrodisiac, emmenagogue, tonic, hemorrhoid treatment, carminative, diuretic, and stimulant [37]. It is also used in the treatment of kidney stones, genitourinary tract infections, skin diseases, prostate, tumors and cancer as well as to strengthen the body and act as an appetizer [11] [40]. Among Arabs, marjoram (origanum) with olive oil is a favorite condiment [11]. Marjoram has been found to have potential anti-cancer (breast, colon, lung, pancreas, and prostate) effects [24] [45]. A comparative study between Arabs and Jews in Israel reveals that the striking differences in cancer prevalence are the result of different dietary patterns, which may include nutritional factors (like marjoram and olive oil) that serve as cancer-inducing or cancer-protective mechanisms [11]. Steam-distilled volatile oil from marjoram has been evaluated for its antibacterial and antifungal activities [46].

9. Liliaceae

9.1. *Allium cepa* L.

Arabic: *basal.*
English: onion.
Plant parts: leaves, bulb.
Preparation: fresh, dried, or cooked.
Active constituents: quercetin, glucokinin, pectin, essential oil [28]; vitamin C, potassium, phosphorus, sulfur, iron [29]; steroidal saponins and sapogenins [47] [48].

Properties and ethno-botanical uses: carminative, emmenagogue, aphrodisiac, hypoglycemic, appetizer [28]; antiseptic, and diuretic.

Onion may be squeezed onto the hands or into the mouth and nose to prevent influenza, colds, and other epidemic diseases. Fresh green onion leaves are eaten as salad or with other food. Eating leaves and bulbs is believed to treat genitourinary infections, increase sexual desire, and treat and prevent cancer [11] [49]. Onion is used to treat cancer in Palestinian traditional medicine [40]. Breast cancer risk was shown to decrease as consumption of onion increased, and consumption of onions is a risk reduction factor for prostate cancer mortality [50]. Onion is used to treat breast cancer [51], colorectal adenoma [52], gastric cancer [53], prostate [54], stomach, esophageal [55] and endometrial cancers [56].

9.2. *Allium sativum*

Arabic: *thoum, thum.*
English: garlic.
Plant parts: leaves and cloves.
Preparation: eat fresh leaves and cloves, or dried cloves.
Active constituents: alliin, essential oil, vitamins A, C, minerals [28], phosphorus, sulfur [29], alliin, allicin, garlic oil [57]-[60].
Properties and ethno-botanical uses: carminative, cholagogue, aphrodisiac, diuretic, and purgative [28]. Fresh green leaves/bulbs are eaten with salad. It is used to treat hemorrhoids, skin diseases, ulcers, kidney infections, intestinal worms, genitourinary infections, prostate and skin cancer, furuncles, and cancerous tumors [11] [40] [49].
Allium sativum (*thoum*) is added to the plants reported to augment natural killer (NK) cell activities, explaining and justifying the treatment of cancer patients with mixtures of these plant extracts. In many cases, there is marked improvement and, in some, complete cure [61]. *Allium sativum* was found to have several antimicrobial compounds, as well as active antitumor elements such allicin and ajoene [62] [63]. It has been reported that *Allium sativum* enhances the anti-tumor activity of immune cells [64]. Tumor cells cover themselves with proteins rich in SH groups, thus preventing their destruction by the immune system. Ingestion of *Allium sativum* facilitates the destruction of tumor cells by blocking and/or oxidizing these SH groups [61].

10. Malvaceae

Malva sylvestris L

Arabic: *khubiza, khubaizih.*
English: blue mallow.
Plant parts: leaves, seeds and flowers.
Preparation: eat as raw salad, cook, or boil in water and drink.
Active constituents: malvine, tannin, mucilage [28], sterols, terpenes [65].
Properties and ethno-botanical uses: the flowers are used as an expectorant and antitussive. The leaves are used as a laxative and emollient for the intestinal mucosa, totreat urinary tract diseases and vaginal infections, urinary retention and prostate illnesses, and skin irritation [28] [30].
The leaves have laxative properties and are used to treat night blindness. They are also used to treat tumors and cancer [11] [40]. The leaves and seeds increase breast milk production following childbirth. Blue mallow has nutritional value and is used as a tonic to increase sexual desire, mainly in the elderly. It is also used in the treatment of colds, cough, piles, and prostate problems (*masour*) [31].

11. Oleaceae

Olea europaea L.

Arabic: *zaytun, zayt.*
English: olive tree, olive oil.
Plant parts: olive oil, fruit, and leaves.
Preparation: oil made from olives, olives cured for eating.
Active constituents: the composition of olive oil depends on the geographic location of the tree. Its components include olein, stearin, fixed oil, acids (palmitic and stearic) [28], vitamin E, and iron [29]. Olive leaves contain the glycoside oleuropein [10]. The oil of the fruit contains triglycerides (oleic, palmitic, linoleic, stearic and myristic acids; iridoid glycosides, oleuropein, and ligstroside). Olive stems containkaempferol, quercetin, esculentin, and esculin. The bark contains phenolic glucosides [58] [66].
Properties and ethno-botanical uses: The oil has nutritional value and is used as a laxative, tonic, lubricant, an emollient for skin and hair, a food, antiseptic, astringent, and febrifuge. Olive oil and a little salt may be rubbed over a baby's body to strengthen his bones and muscles and to prevent diaper rash [11] [40]. It is also used to treat venereal diseases, diabetes, prostate problems, kidney stones and infections [11] [40], and in cases of con-

stipation, trachoma, gonorrhea, kidney stones, impaired virility, urinary retention, and urinary tract infection [28] [30].

Olive oil represents an important component of the Mediterranean diet [67] [68], which has been associated with some of the lower overall mortality patterns observed in large human populations. In Greece and Spain, long-time consumption of olive oil is associated with a decreased risk of breast cancer [69] [70]. It has been suggested that olive oil or olive oil-derived monounsaturated fat may have some absolute or relative protective effect on risk for breast and possibly other cancers [71] [17]. In Italy, the consumption of salad and vegetables containing olive oil is associated with a significantly reduced (34% - 35%) incidence of breast cancer compared to groups where olive oil is not consumed). These findings suggest that a diet rich in raw vegetables and olive oil protects against breast cancer [72]. Studies in Mediterranean countries revealed an inverse relation between consumption of olive oil and cancers of the bladder [23], stomach [21], urinary tract [24], and lung [22] [73].

Olive oil is the most widely used oil in Arab cuisine, and in several studies has been reported to offer some of its own protection against cancer compared to other forms of added lipids [14] [24]. In Italy, Buiatti *et al.* [21] found an inverse relation between gastric cancer and olive oil consumption; they suggest that vitamin E might contribute to this protective effect [74].

12. Ranunculaceae

Nigella sativa L.

Arabic: *habbit al-barakah, habbih suda, qazhih.*
English: Nigella, black cumin.
Plant parts: seeds or extracted oil.
Preparation: boil the seeds in water and drink, or drink the oil.
Active constituents: essential oil, fixed oil, nigellin, saponin [28], nigellimine N-oxide, and isoquinoline alkaloid [58] [75].
Properties and ethno-botanical uses: digestive, diuretic, emmenagogue, galactogogue, carminative [28] [37]. Black cumin is also used as a spice and to treat urinary tract infections and urinary retention, blood in the urine, diabetes, impotence, infertility, nausea and vomiting, prostate problems, tumors, ulcers, and furuncles. The oil extracted from the seeds is used to treat and prevent cancer and skin tumors [11] [30] [40] [49]). According to the Prophet Muhammad, it heals every illness. Its oil is beneficial for ophiasis, warts, and moles [76]. *Nigella sativum* is one of several plants reported to augment natural killer cell activities [77], so it has a potential role in cancer care [78]-[80].

13. Umbelliferae

13.1. *Coriandrum sativum* L.

Arabic: *kuzbarah, kusbara.*
English: coriander.
Plant parts: seeds and leaves.
Preparation: boil in water and drink.
Active constituents: essential oil, linalool, terpinene, corinadrol [28], and Vitamin C [29]. The essential oil of the fruit contains a high concentration (55% - 74%) of linalool, a material used in the production of vitamin A. The leaves of the plant are a source of vitamin A and vitamin C as well as coriander oil [10]. The fruit and leaves contain fats, proteins, and volatile oil [81]. The leaves contain caffeic acid, ferulic acid, gallic acid, and chlorogenic acid [82].
Properties and Ethno-botanical uses: stomachic, stimulant, pectoral, diuretic, antispasmodic, aphrodisiac [28]. Coriander is used by women after childbirth to strengthen the body and to increase milk production. It is also used to increase sexual desire and to treat urinary infections and prostate problems [11].

13.2. *Foeniculum vulgare* Mill

Arabic: *shawmar.*
English: fennel.
Plant parts: stems, leaves, and seeds.

Preparation: boil leaves in water and drink two cups a day for three weeks. The green leaves of fennel are also eaten raw as a green salad and added to cooked food or to tea.

Active constituents: Essential oils including anethole, anisic acid, and fixed oil [28], potassium, and sulfur [29]. Fennel oil, anethole, enol, liquorice, and senna are produced from the fruit [10]. The seeds contain volatile oil; phenolic anethole, and fenchone, a ketone [61].

Properties and ethno-botanical uses: bronchodilator, antitussive, stimulant, diuretic, galactogogue, aphrodisiac, tonic and emmenagogue [28] [30]. It is also used to increase sexual passions and treatrenal infections [11] [40] and swollen breasts. Fennel is also used in the treatment of asthma, dizziness, nausea, vomiting, diarrhea, swelling of the stomach and abdomen, tonsillitis, sore throat, and oral infections. It is used to dissolve kidney stones and is employed in the treatment of constipation, obstructions of the urinary tract, trachoma, and infections of the sexual organs [31]. The seeds have nutritional value and are used as an appetizer and a sedative as well as to sweeten the breath. *Foeniculum vulgare* is among other medicinal herbs used in traditional Uighur medicine for the treatment and prevention of cancer, diabetes and cardiovascular diseases [83].

14. Urticaceae

14.1. *Urtica pilulifera* L.

Arabic: *qurrais, hurriqi.*
English: Roman nettle.
Plant parts: leaves, seeds, and roots.
Preparation: boil in water and drink.
Active constituents: glycoquinine, histamine, acids (silicic and formic), and tannin [28]; vitamins A and C, calcium, potassium, sulfur, and iron [29].

Properties and ethno-botanical uses: aphrodisiac, and diuretic. Fresh young leaves/roots are eaten to treat kidney stones and infections, rheumatism, female sterility, bleeding and cancer, intestinal pain and inflammation, liver disease, and bed wetting [11] [49], urinary tract infection and retention. It causes dermatitis upon contact [28]. It is supposed to be effective against cancer and prostate disorders [9] [40]. A diuretic is made by boiling the leaves drinking the liquid. This liquid is used to treat uterine bleeding [10] [30] [37].

14.2. *Urtica urens* L.

Arabic: *qurrais, hurriqi.*
English: large nettle.
Plant parts: young leaves.
Preparation: eat the fresh, young leaves.
Active constituents: glycoquinine, histamine, acids (silicic and formic), and tannin [28].

Properties and ethno-botanical uses: aphrodisiac, diuretic, styptic, antihemorrhagic, and galactogogue. It is used to treat kidney stones and infections, urinary retention, impotence, female sterility, sexual problems, rheumatism, and bleeding (to stop nose-bleed) [28] [37]. It causes dermatitis.

It has an antiproliferative effect on human prostate cancer cells [84], and induces adenosine deaminase inhibition in prostate tissue from cancer patients [85]. It may cause potential drug-herb interactions (including interaction with chemotherapy) [86].

References

[1]   Hitti, P. (1952) History of the Arabs, from the Earliest Times to the Present. Macmillan & Co. LTD, London.

[2]   Ullmann, M. (1978) Islamic Surveys: Islamic Medicine. University Press, Edinburgh.

[3]   Murad, A. (1966) Lamhat min tarikh al-tibb al-qadim = Glimpses from the History of Early Medicine. Maktabat al-Nasr al-Haditha, al-Qahira. (In Arabic)

[4]   Al-Shatti, A. (1970) Al-'Arab waal-tibb = The Arabs and Medicine. Manshurat Wazarat al-Thaqafa, Dimashq. (In Arabic)

[5]   Al-Najjar, A. (1994) Fi Tarikh al-Ttib fi al-Dawlah al-lslamyya: History of Medicine in the Islamic Empire. Dar al-Ma'aref, Al-Qahira. (In Arabic)

[6]   Hamarneh, S. (1991) Ibn al-Quff's Contribution to Arab-Islamic Medical Sciences. *Hamdard Medicines*, **34**, 27-36.

[7]   Lev, E. (2002) Reconstructed *material medica* of the Medieval and Ottoman al-Sham. *Journal of Ethnopharmacology*, **80**, 167-179. http://dx.doi.org/10.1016/S0378-8741(02)00029-6

[8]   Lev, E. and Ammar, Z. (2000) Ethnopharmacological Survey of Traditional Drugs Sold in Israel at the End of the 20th Century. *Journal of Ethnopharmacology*, **72**, 191-205. http://dx.doi.org/10.1016/S0378-8741(00)00230-0

[9]   Ali-Shtayeh, M.S., Yaniv, Z. and Mahajna, J. (2000) Ethnobotanical Survey in the Palestinian Area: A Classification of the Healing Potential of Medicinal Plants. *Journal of Ethnopharmacology*, **73**, 221-232. http://dx.doi.org/10.1016/S0378-8741(00)00316-0

[10]   Palevitch, D. and Yaniv, Z. (2000) Medicinal Plants of the Holy Land. Modan Publishing House, Tel-Aviv, 104, 122, 205, 266-269.

[11]   Abu-Rabia, A. (2005) Herbs as a Food and Medicine Source in Palestine. *Asian Pacific Journal of Cancer Prevention*, **6**, 404-407.

[12]   Abu-Rabia, A. (2014) Ethnobotany among Bedouin Tribes in the Middle East. In: Yaniv-Bachrach, Z. and Dudai, N., Eds., *Medicinal and Aromatic Plants of the Middle East*, Springer, Berlin, 27-36. http://dx.doi.org/10.1007/978-94-017-9276-9_3

[13]   World Cancer Research/American Association for Cancer Research (1997).

[14]   Murray, M., Birdsall, T., Pizzorno, J. and Reilly, P. (2002) How to Prevent and Treat Cancer with Natural Medicine. The Berkley Publishing Group, New York, 3-23, 89-99, 165.

[15]   Lipworth, L., Martínez, M.E., Angell, J., Hsieh, C.C. and Trichopoulos, D. (1997) Olive Oil and Human Cancer: An Assessment of the Evidence. *Preventive Medicine*, **26**, 181-190. http://dx.doi.org/10.1006/pmed.1996.9977

[16]   Sergio, L., Yolanda M., P., Beatriz, B., *et al.* (2004) Olive Oil and Cancer. *Grasas y Aceites*, **55**, 33-41.

[17]   Cohen, L.A. and Wynder, E.I. (1990) Do Dietary Monounsaturated Fatty Acids Play a Protective Role in Carcinogenesis and Cardiovascular Disease? *Medical Hypotheses*, **31**, 83-89. http://dx.doi.org/10.1016/0306-9877(90)90002-V

[18]   Serra-Majem, L., La Vecchia, C., Ribas-Barba, L., *et al.* (1993) Changes in Diet and Mortality from Selected Cancers in Southern Mediterranean Countries, 1960-1989. *European Journal of Clinical Nutrition*, **47**, S25-S34.

[19]   Rose, D.P. and Connolly, J.M. (1992) Dietary Fat, Fatty Acids and Prostate Cancer. *Lipids*, **27**, 798-803. http://dx.doi.org/10.1007/BF02535853

[20]   Kushi, L.H., Lenart, E.B. and Willet, W. (1995) Health Implications of Mediterranean Diets in Light of Contemporary Knowledge. Meat, Wine, Fats and Oils. *The American Journal of Clinical Nutrition*, **61**, 1416-1427.

[21]   Buiati, E., Palli, D., Decarli, A., Amadori, D., Avellini, C. and Bianchi, S. (1989) A Case-Control Study of Gastric Cancer in Italy. *International Journal of Cancer*, **44**, 611-616. http://dx.doi.org/10.1002/ijc.2910440409

[22]   Fortes, C., Forastiere, F., Anatra, F. and Schmid, G. (1995) Consumption of Olive Oil and Specific Groups in Relation to Breast Cancer Risk in Greece. *Journal of the National Cancer Institute*, **87**, 1020-1021. http://dx.doi.org/10.1093/jnci/87.13.1020-a

[23]   Gonzalez, C.A., Torrent, M. and Agudo, A. (1990) Dietary Habits in Spain: An Approximation. *Tumori*, **76**, 311-314.

[24]   Bitterman, W.A., Farhadian, H., Abu Samra, C., Lerner, D., Amoun, H., Krapf, D. and Makov, UE. (1991) Environmental and Nutritional Factors Significantly Associated with Cancer of the Urinary Tract Among Different Ethnic Groups. *The Urologic Clinics of North America*, **18**, 501-508.

[25]   Ryde, D. (1984) What Should Humans Eat? *Practitioner*, **232**, 415-418.

[26]   Steinmetz, K. and Potter, J. (1996) Vegetables, Fruit, and Cancer Prevention. *Journal of the Academy of Nutrition and Dietetic*, **96**, 1027-1039. http://dx.doi.org/10.1016/S0002-8223(96)00273-8

[27]   Gilbar, O., Iron, G. and Goren, A. (2001) Adjustment to Illness of Cancer Patients Treated by Complementary Therapy along with Conventional Therapy. *Patient Education & Counseling*, **44**, 243-249. http://dx.doi.org/10.1016/S0738-3991(00)00194-4

[28]   Karim, F. and Qura'an, S. (1986) Medicinal Plants of Jordan. Yarmouk University, Irbid, 45, 68.

[29]   Lust, J. (1980) The Herb Book. Bantam Books, Toronto & New York, 501-508.

[30]   Krispil, N. (2000) Medicinal Plants in Israel and throughout the World: The Complete Guide. Hed Arzi Publishing House, Or Yehuda, 226, 239.

[31]   Abu-Rabia, A. (2013) Fieldwork Notes and Interviews with Healers, 1993-2013.

[32]   Ruan, W., Mao-de, L. and Zhou, J. (2006) Anticancer Effects of Chinese Herbal Medicine, Science or Myth? *Journal of Zhejiang University SCIENCE B*, **7**, 1006-1014.

[33]   Chatuevedi, N., Yadav, S. and Shukla, K. (2011) Diversified Therapeutic Potential of Avena Sativa: An Exhaustive

Review. *Asian Journal of Plant Science and Research*, **1**, 103-114.

[34] Slavin, J., Marquart, L. and Jacobs, D.J. (2000) Cereal Food World. **45**, 54-58.

[35] Limer, J.L. and Speirs, V., (2004) Phyto-Oestrogens and Breast Cancer Chemoprevention. *Breast Cancer Research*, **6**, 119-127. http://dx.doi.org/10.1186/bcr781

[36] Guo, W., Nie, L., Wu, D., Wise, M., Collins, W., Meydani, S. and Meydani, M. (2010) Avenanthramides Inhibit Proliferation of Human Colon Cancer Cell Lines *in Vitro*. *Nutrition and Cancer*, **62**, 1007-1016.

[37] Boulos, L. (1983) Medicinal Plants of North Africa. Reference Publications, Algonac, 110.

[38] Loizzo, M.R., Tundis, R., Menichini, F., *et al.*, (2007) Cytotoxic Activity of Essential Oils from Labiatae and Lauraceae Families Against *in Vitro* Human Tumor Models. *Anticancer Research*, **27**, 3293-3299.

[39] Sertel, S., Eichhorn, T., Plinkert, P.K. and Efferth, T. (2012) [Anticancer Activity of Saliva Officinalis Essential Oil against HNSCC Cell Line (UMSCC1)]. *HNO*, **59**, 1203-1208.

[40] Ali-Shtayeh, M., Jamous, R. and Jamous, R. (2011) Herbal Preparation Use by Patients Suffering from Cancer in Palestine. *Complementary Therapies in Clinical Practice*, **17**, 235-240. http://dx.doi.org/10.1016/j.ctcp.2011.06.002

[41] Drăgan, S., Nicola, T., Ilina, R., *et al.* (2007) Role of Multi-Component Functional Foods in the Complex Treatment of Patients with Advanced Breast Cancer. *Revista Medico-Chirurgicală a Societăţii de Medici şI Naturalişti din Iaşi*, **111**, 877-884.

[42] Duggan, C., Gannon, J. and Walker, W.A. (2002) Protective Nutrients and Functional Foods for the Gastrointestinal Tract. *The American Journal of Clinical Nutrition*, **75**, 789-808.

[43] Charai, M., Mosaddak, M. and Faid, M. (1996) Chemical Composition and Antimicrobial Activities of Two Aromatic Plants: *Origanum majorana* L. and *O. compactum* Benth. *Journal of Essential Oil Research*, **8**, 657-664. http://dx.doi.org/10.1080/10412905.1996.9701036

[44] Vági, E., Simándi, B., Suhajda, Á. and Héthelyi, É. (2005) Essential Oil Composition and Antimicrobial Activity of *Origanum majorana* L. Extracts Obtained with Ethyl Alcohol and Supercritical Carbon Dioxide. *Food Research International*, **38**, 51-57. http://dx.doi.org/10.1016/j.foodres.2004.07.006

[45] Dursun, E., Otles, S. and Akcicek, E. (2004) Herbs as a Food Source in Turkey. *Asian Pacific Journal of Cancer Prevention*, **5**, 334-339.

[46] Deans, S. and Svoboda, K. (2006) The Antimicrobial Properties of Marjoram (*Origanum majorana* L.) Volatile Oil. *Flavour and Fragrance Journal*, **5**, 187-190.

[47] Salveron, M. and Cantonia, M. (1989) Phillipine-Grown Cultivars of *Allium cepa*. *Planta Medica*, **55**, 662. http://dx.doi.org/10.1055/s-2006-962255

[48] Vollerner, Y., Abdullaev, N., Gorovits, M. and Abubakkirov, N. (1983) Steroidal Saponins and Sapogenins of *Allium* XVIII. The Structure of Karatavioside B. *Khimiya Prirodnykh Soedinii*, **2**, 197-201.

[49] Zaid, H., Rayan, A., Said, O. and Saad, B. (2010) Cancer Treatment by Greco-Arab and Islamic Herbal Medicine. *The Open Nutraceuticals Journal*, **3**, 203-212.

[50] Ben-Arye, E., Schiff, E., Hassan, E., *et al.* (2011) Integrative Oncology in the Middle East: From Traditional Herbal Knowledge to Contemporary Cancer Care. *Annals of Oncology*, **23**, 211-221. http://dx.doi.org/10.1093/annonc/mdr054

[51] Challier, B., Perarnau, J.M. and Viel, J.F. (1998) Garlic, Onion and Cereal Fibre as Protective Factors for Breast Cancer: A French Case-Control Study. *European Journal of Epidemiology*, **14**, 737-747. http://dx.doi.org/10.1023/A:1007512825851

[52] Millen, A.E., Subar, A.F., Graubard, B.I., *et al.* (2007) Fruit and Vegetable Intake and Prevalence of Colorectal Adenoma in a Cancer Screening Trial. *The American Journal of Clinical Nutrition*, **86**, 1754-1764.

[53] Boeing, H., Jedrychowski, W., Wahrendorf, J., *et al.* (1991) Dietary Risk Factors in Intestinal and Diffuse Types of Stomach Cancer: A Multicenter Case-Control Study in Poland. *Cancer Causes & Control*, **2**, 227-233. http://dx.doi.org/10.1007/BF00052138

[54] Grant, W.B. (2004) A Multicountry Ecologic Study of Risk and Risk Reduction Factors for Prostate Cancer Mortality. *European Urology*, **45**, 271-279. http://dx.doi.org/10.1016/j.eururo.2003.08.018

[55] Gonzalez , C.A., Pera, G., Agudo, A., *et al.* (2006) Fruit and Vegetable Intake and the Risk of Stomach and Oesophagus Adenocarcinoma in the European Prospective Investigation into Cancer and Nutrition (EPIC-EURGAST). *International Journal of Cancer*, **118**, 2559-2566. http://dx.doi.org/10.1002/ijc.21678

[56] Galeone, C., Pelucchi, C., Dal Maso, L., *et al.* (2009) *Allium* Vegetables Intake and Endometrial Cancer Risk. *Public Health Nutrition*, **12**, 1576-1579. http://dx.doi.org/10.1017/S1368980008003820

[57] Block, E., Saleem, A., Mahendra, J., Crecely, R., Apitz-Castro, R. and Cruz, M. (1984) The Chemistry of Alkyl Thio-

sulphate Esters. 8. (E,Z)-Ajoene: A Potent Antithrombotic Agent from Garlic. *Journal of the American Chemical Society*, **106**, 8295-8296. http://dx.doi.org/10.1021/ja00338a049

[58] Ghazanfar, S. and Al-Sabahi, A. (1993) Medicinal Plants of Northern and Central Oman. *Economic Botany*, **47**, 89-98. http://dx.doi.org/10.1007/BF02862209

[59] McElnay, J.C. and Po, A.L.W. (1991) Dietary Supplements. 8. Garlic. *Pharmaceutical Journal*, **246**, 324-326.

[60] Muller, B. (1990) Garlic (*Allium sativum*): Quantitative Analysis of the Tracer Substances Alliin and Allicin. *Planta Medica*, **56**, 589-599. http://dx.doi.org/10.1055/s-2006-961198

[61] Abulafatih, H.A. (1987) Medicinal Plant of Southwestern Saudi Arabia. *Economic Botany*, **41**, 354-360. http://dx.doi.org/10.1007/BF02859051

[62] Dirsch, V.M., Kiemer, A.K., Wagner, H. and Vollmar, A.M. (1988) The Effect of Allicin and Ajoene, Two Compounds of Garlic, on Inducible Nitric Oxide Synthase. *Atherosclerosis*, **139**, 333-335. http://dx.doi.org/10.1016/S0021-9150(98)00094-X

[63] Singh, A. and Shukla, Y. (1998) Antitumor Activity of Diallyl Sulfide in Two-Stage Skin Model of Carcinogenesis. *Biomedical and Environmental Sciences*, **11**, 258-263.

[64] Lipinski, B. and Egyud, L. (1992) Thiole Induced Cross-Linking of Human Blood Proteins: Implications for Tumor Immunity. *Bioorganic & Medicinal Chemistry Letters*, **2**, 919-924. http://dx.doi.org/10.1016/S0960-894X(00)80588-0

[65] Abbas, J.A., El-Oqlah, A.A. and Mahasneh, A.M. (1992) Herbal Plants in the Traditional Medicine of Bahrain. *Economic Botany*, **46**, 158-163. http://dx.doi.org/10.1007/BF02930630

[66] Gariboldi, P., Jommi, G. and Verotta, L. (1986) Two New Secoiridoids from *Olea europaea*. *Phytochemistry*, **25**, 865-869. http://dx.doi.org/10.1016/0031-9422(86)80018-8

[67] Ferro-Luzzi, A. and Sette, S. (1989) The Mediterranean Diet: An Attempt to Define Its Present and Past Composition. *European Journal of Clinical Nutrition*, **43**, 13-29.

[68] Trichopoulou, A. (1992) Composition of Greek Foods and Dishes (in Greek and English). Athens School of Public Health, Athens.

[69] Martin-Moreno, J.M., Willet, W.C., Gorgojo, L., Banegas, J.R., Rodriguez-Artalejo, F., Fernandez-Rodriguez, J.C., Maisonneuve, P. and Boyle, P. (1994) Dietary Fat, Olive Oil Intake and Breast Cancer Risk. *International Journal of Cancer*, **58**, 774-780. http://dx.doi.org/10.1002/ijc.2910580604

[70] Trichopoulou, A., Katsouyanni, K., Stuver, S., Tzala, L., Gnardellis, C., Rimm, E. and Trichopoulous, D. (1995) Consumption of Olive Oil and Specific Food Groups in Relation to Breast Cancer Risk in Greece. *Journal of the National Cancer Institute*, **87**, 110-116. http://dx.doi.org/10.1093/jnci/87.2.110

[71] Rose, D.P., Boyar, A.P. and Wynder, E.L. (1986) International Comparisons of Mortality Rates for Cancer of the Breast, Ovary, Prostate, and Colon and Per Capita Food Consumption. *Cancer*, **58**, 1986, 2363-2371. http://dx.doi.org/10.1002/1097-0142(19861201)58:11<2363::AID-CNCR2820581102>3.0.CO;2-#

[72] Sieri, S., Krogh, V., Pala, V., Muti, P., Micheli, A., Evangelista, A., Tagliabue, G. and Berrino, F. (2004) Dietary Patterns and Risk of Breast Cancer in the ORDET Cohort. *Cancer Epidemiology, Biomarkers & Prevention*, **13**, 567-572.

[73] Fortes, C., Forastiere, F., Farchi, S., Mallone, S., Trequattrinni, T., Anatra, F., Schmid, G. and Perucci, C.A. (2003) The Protective Effect of the Mediterranean Diet on Lung Cancer. *Nutrition and Cancer*, **46**, 30-37. http://dx.doi.org/10.1207/S15327914NC4601_04

[74] Passmore, R. and Eastwood, M.A. (1986) Fats. In: Passmore, R. and Eastwood, M.A., Eds., *Davidson and Passmore: Human Nutrition and Dietetics*, Churchill Livingstone, Edinburgh, 55-58.

[75] Atta-ur-Rehman, M., Sohail, M., Jon, C., *et al.* (1985) Isolation and Structure Determination of Nigellicine, a Novel Alkaloid from the Seeds of *Nigella sativa*. *Tetrahedron Letters*, **26**, 2759-2762. http://dx.doi.org/10.1016/S0040-4039(00)94904-9

[76] al-Jawziyya, I.Q. (1998) Medicine of the Prophet. The Islamic Texts Society, Cambridge. (Translated and Edited by Penelope Johnstone)

[77] Shen, R.N., Lu, L., Jia, X.Q., Wong, M.L. and Kaiser, H.E. (1996) Naturin: A Potent Bio-Immunomodifier in Experimental Studies and Clinical Trials. *In Vivo*, **10**, 201-209.

[78] El-Obeid, A., Al-Harbi, S., Al-Jomah, N. and Hassib, A. (2006) Herbal Melanin Modulates Tumor Necrosis Factor Alpha (TNF-Alpha), Interleukin 6 (IL-6) and Vascular Endothelial Growth Factor (VEGF) Production. *Phytomedicine*, **13**, 324-333.

[79] Abuharfeil, N.M., Maraqa, A. and Von Kleist, S. (2000) Augmentation of Natural Killer Cell Activity *in Vitro* against Tumor Cells by Wild Plants from Jordan. *Journal of Ethnopharmacology*, **71**, 55-63. http://dx.doi.org/10.1016/S0378-8741(99)00176-2

[80] Salim, E.I. and Fukushima, S. (2003) Chemo Preventive Potential of Volatile Oil from Black Cumin (*Nigella sativa* L.) Seeds against Rat Colon Carcinogenesis. *Nutrition and Cancer*, **45**, 195-202. http://dx.doi.org/10.1207/S15327914NC4502_09

[81] Potter, T. and Fagerson, I. (1990) Composition of Coriander Leaf Volatiles. *Journal of Agriculture and Food Chemistry*, **38**, 2054-2056. http://dx.doi.org/10.1021/jf00101a011

[82] Papai, *et al.* (2005) Encyclopedia of Agriculture and Food Systems. e-book, 473-481.

[83] Kizaibek, M., Kopp, B., Prinz, S., Popescu, R. and Upur, H. (2009) Antiproliferative Activity of Individual Herbs of Abnormal Savda Munziq on HL-60 Cells. *Science & Technology Review*, **19**, 94-98.

[84] Konrad, L., Muller, H.H., Lenz, C., *et al.* (2000) Antiproliferative Effect on Human Prostate Cancer Cells by a Stinging Nettle Root (*Urtica dioica*) Extract. *Planta Medica*, **66**, 44-47. http://dx.doi.org/10.1055/s-2000-11117

[85] Durak, I., Biri, H., Devrim, E., *et al.* (2004) Aqueous Extract of Urtica Dioica Makes Significant Inhibition on Adenosine Deaminase Activity in Prostate Tissue from Patients with Prostate Cancer. *Cancer Biology & Therapy*, **3**, 855-857. http://dx.doi.org/10.4161/cbt.3.9.1038

[86] Agus, H.H., Tekin, P., Bayav, M. and Semiz, A.S. (2009) A Drug Interaction Potential of the Seed Extract of *Urtica urens* L. (Dwarf Nettle). *Phytotherapy Research*, **23**, 1763-1770. http://dx.doi.org/10.1002/ptr.2848

22

Expert Survey on the Prevention and Treatment Situation of Traditional Chinese Medicine for Coronary Artery Disease

Ying-Fei Bi, Jing-Yuan Mao, Xian-Liang Wang, Zhi-Qiang Zhao, Bin Li, Ya-Zhu Hou

Cardiovascular Department, First Teaching Hospital of Tianjin University of Chinese Medicine, Tianjin, China
Email: yingfei1981@126.com

Abstract

Objective: To grasp the current situation of Traditional Chinese Medicine (TCM) on prevention and treatment for coronary artery disease (CAD) and the possible advantages and disadvantages. Method: Using a survey in the form of questionnaire among 60 cardiovascular disease experts, to grasp current situation of TCM on prevention and treatment of CAD and the possible advantages and disadvantages. Results: In most areas of China, CAD is common, and angina is the most common clinical type. More than 91% experts choose to integrate traditional and western medicine for treatment and prevention of CAD. TCM proprietary medicine, traditional herbal decoction and intravenous TCM are widely used in the clinical work. Clinical advantages of TCM in the prevention of CAD that are listed in the questionnaire include improving symptoms, enhancing quality of life, increasing exercise tolerance, improving cardiac function, relieving angina, secondary prevention of myocardial infarction, etc. The shortcomings include troublesome brewing of herbal medicine, unpleasant taste of decoction, minimal clinical evidence, slow onset of effects and non-standardized prescription of medicine, etc. Conclusion: The survey reflects the present situation of clinical diagnosis and treatment of TCM on prevention and treatment of CAD to a certain extent; more accurate conclusions need the broader, deeper and large-scale clinical survey.

Keywords

Coronary Artery Disease, Traditional Chinese Medicine, Advantage, Disadvantages, Expert Survey

1. Introduction

Traditional Chinese Medicine (TCM) has a history as long as two thousand years in the prevention and treatment of coronary artery disease (CAD). However, it is necessary to have a better understanding of its role in the current healthcare setting, and identify its advantages and disadvantages, so as to elevate clinical standards and increase its application. It's necessary to grasp the current situation of Traditional Chinese Medicine (TCM) on prevention and treatment for CAD and the possible advantages and disadvantages.

2. Method

A survey in the form of questionnaire was conducted among 60 cardiovascular disease experts who had attended the 2013 annual meeting of CAD in TCM clinical research alliance. The questionnaire requested the experts to provide their opinions on the current situation of TCM in the prevention and treatment of CAD and its advantages and disadvantages. The findings are reported as follows.

3. Results

3.1. Basic Information of the Experts Who Participated in the Survey

60 experts who participated in the investigation were from 22 provinces, municipalities and autonomous regions of China. 45 males and 15 females, aged 55.47 ± 8.12 years old, participated in the survey. Among them were 34 chief physicians, 26 associate chief physicians, 19 doctoral degree mentors, 35 master's degree mentors, with 26.37 ± 5.86 years of work experience. 53 were from TCM hospital, 3 from Western medicine hospital while 4 were from integrated Chinese and Western Medicine hospital. 58 of them come from tertiary hospitals and 2 of them were from secondary hospitals.

3.2. Expert Authority Coefficient

The assigned scores for the basis of judgments by the experts and the familiarity of the issues were pooled and the average coefficient of authority calculated was 0.92 ± 0.06. The high expert authority coefficient indicates that the survey results have high reliability.

4. Results of the Survey

4.1. The Frequency of Disease

The frequency of CAD seen by the experts in the region they belong to are shown in **Table 1**, the frequency is listed in increasing order.

4.2. The Main Subtypes of Disease

The clinical subtypes of CAD in the survey were angina pectoris (AP), arrhythmia, heart failure (HF), myocardial infarction (MI), sudden death, etc. The experts were to grade the frequency of each disease subtype according to their experience. They were to choose if it was unusual, sometimes, common, frequent and constantly and the corresponding scores were 0, 1, 2, 3 and 4. Finally, the scores would be pooled (total score of 240) and average will be calculated. The responses and scores are shown in **Table 2**.

4.3. The Prevention and Treatment of Disease

The investigation on the common methods used for CAD by each experts show that only 3 experts use purely TCM, 2 experts use Western medicine only, while 55 experts use both Chinese traditional and Western medicine. The popularity and effectiveness of the prevention and treatment methods used by experts in CAD were also studied. The methods included in the investigation were TCM decoction, oral proprietary TCM, TCM intravenous preparations, oral western medicine, western medicine intravenous preparations, percutaneous coronary intervention (PCI), coronary artery bypass grafting (CABG) and combination of TCM and western medicine treatment. The popularity was assigned with 4 levels and they were not commonly used, commonly used, more commonly used and strong commonly used. The given scores for the four levels were 0, 1, 2 and 3 correspondingly. The effectiveness was also assigned with 4 levels and they were no effect, effective, more effective and strong effective. The given scores for the four levels were also 0, 1, 2 and 3 correspondingly. Finally, the scores would be summed (total score of 180) and average would be calculated. The responses from the experts and the

Table 1. The frequency of disease.

Level	Unusual	Sometimes	Common	Frequent	Constantly
The number of expert	0	0	10	14	36

Table 2. The inquiry on main subtypes of disease.

Type/Grade	Unusual	Sometimes	Common	Frequent	Constantly	Total Score	Average Score
AP	0	0	18	15	27	189	3.15
Arrhythmia	0	0	26	24	10	164	2.73
HF	0	0	24	23	13	169	2.82
MI	0	10	25	17	8	143	2.38
Sudden death	2	33	19	5	1	55	0.92

scores are shown in **Table 3** and **Table 4**.

4.4. Potential Advantages of TCM

The potential advantages of TCM in comparison to western medicine in the prevention and treatment of CAD are listed in the questionnaire. The clinical advantages were relieving angina pectoris, improving symptoms, enhancing the quality of life, increasing exercise tolerance, improving physiochemical markers, intervening restenosis (RS) after percutaneous coronary intervention (PCI), regulating arrhythmias, improving cardiac function, secondary prevention of myocardial infarction, decreasing endpoint events, etc. The effectiveness advantages were overall conditioning, individual diagnosis, mild effect, safety, low cost, comprehensive benefit, well received by patients, etc. For the above-mentioned advantages, experts were to select from the options of no, possible, general, definite or prominent and the corresponding scores for each option were 0, 1, 2, 3 and 4, at which the scores will be summed (a total of 240 points) and averaged. The result of the investigation is shown in **Table 5**.

4.5. Shortcomings of TCM

There are still shortcomings of TCM in the prevention and treatment of CAD as compared to western medicine, they include plausible curative effect, lack of clinical evidence, slow onset of effect, non-standardized use of medication, decoction is tedious to prepare, unpleasant taste of herbal decoction, toxicity of TCM, narrow variety of TCM proprietary medicine, prominent side effect of Chinese intravenous drugs, high treatment cost, etc. Experts were to choose either yes or no according to their experience and knowledge and results is shown in **Table 6**.

5. Discussion

A person who is very knowledgeable and has great experience in a particular area will be called an expert. The viewpoint of an expert will therefore be a representation of the current level of knowledge in the particular research field. The survey gathers the experience and knowledge of the experts, analyses the results and then makes conclusions corresponding to the objective of the study.

The sixty experts who participated in this survey were from 22 different regions (province/city/municipality) of China. The experts who participated in the investigation were highly professional with high expert authority coefficient. Therefore, this survey result is reliable and scientific and can be a regional representation.

The results demonstrate that CAD, in particular the subtype angina pectoris, is common in most regions of China. Along with the increasing standard of life and advancement in the diagnosis and treatment techniques, heart failure being the end-stage of CAD has also become more common. Arrhythmia and myocardial infarction are the presentations of CAD frequently seen.

More than 91% experts choose to integrate traditional and western medicine for treatment and prevention of CAD. The survey shows that TCM proprietary medicine, traditional herbal decoction and intravenous TCM are

Table 3. The popularity inquiry of prevention and treatment of disease.

Methods/Levels	Not Commonly Used	Commonly Used	More Commonly Used	Strong Commonly Used	Total Scores	Average Scores
TCM decoction	2	5	20	33	144	2.40
Oral proprietary TCM	2	1	22	35	150	2.50
TCM intravenous preparations	2	11	22	25	130	2.17
Oral western medicine	3	2	18	37	149	2.48
Western medicine intravenous preparations	4	11	32	13	114	1.90
PCI	9	15	17	19	106	1.77
CABG	27	16	8	9	59	0.98
Combination of TCM and western medicine	5	2	6	47	155	2.58

Table 4. The effectiveness inquiry of prevention and treatment of disease.

Methods/Levels	No Effect	Effective	More Effective	Strong Effective	Total Scores	Average Scores
TCM decoction	0	7	34	19	132	2.20
Oral proprietary TCM	0	16	37	7	111	1.85
TCM intravenous preparations	0	11	36	13	122	2.03
Oral western medicine	0	2	38	20	138	2.30
Western medicine intravenous preparations	0	5	30	25	140	2.33
PCI	0	3	21	36	153	2.55
CABG	0	4	29	27	143	2.38
Combination of TCM and western medicine	0	1	11	48	167	2.78

widely used in the clinical work, but western medicine injection, coronary artery intervention and coronary artery bypass grafting are more effective than TCM treatment. The mechanism of TCM is unclear and there is a lack of clinical evidence to support the function of the medicine; thus, healthcare providers are less confident with its use.

Moreover, the results of the survey indicate that there are greater approvals with the use of TCM decoction than proprietary medicine and intravenous drugs. This might be due to the narrow variety of proprietary medicine available and the adverse events reported in the use of intravenous drugs.

Clinical advantages of TCM in the prevention of CAD that are listed in the questionnaire include improving symptoms, enhancing quality of life, increasing exercise tolerance, improving cardiac function, relieving angina, secondary prevention of myocardial infarction, etc. These advantages have gained high recognition, and they are consistent with clinical practice and findings [1]-[5]. In addition, individualized treatment, treatment as a whole, safety, well-received by patients, mild effect and comprehensive benefits, etc. were advantages that experts valued. There are still inadequacies in TCM prevention and treatment of CAD, and most experts agree that the shortcomings include troublesome brewing of herbal medicine, unpleasant taste of decoction, minimal clinical evidence, slow onset of effects, non-standardized prescription of medicine, etc. In particular, the hassle in brewing medicine and the unpleasant taste of the decoction were the direct cause to the refusal of treatment by the patients. Currently, efforts have been made to improve traditional Chinese medicine formulations and simplify administration of medicine. The slow onset of effect is in comparison with western medicine; in fact, there are a lot of fast-acting TCM preparations for clinical use. Non-standardized medication and less clinical evidence reflect the current situation of TCM. Standardized medication helps to systematically review the group effect of

Table 5. Investigation of potential advantages in TCM prevention and treatment of CAD.

Advantage/Grade	No	Possible	General	Definite	Prominent	Total Score	Average Score
Relieve angina pectoris	0	0	12	38	10	178	2.97
Improve symptoms	0	1	1	27	31	208	3.47
Enhance the quality of life	0	1	2	32	25	201	3.35
Increase exercise tolerance	1	3	2	34	20	189	3.15
Improve physiochemical indexes	2	3	29	22	4	143	2.38
Intervene restenosis (RS) after PCI	1	10	16	26	7	148	2.47
Regulate arrhythmias	1	3	17	28	11	165	2.75
Improve cardiac function	1	3	7	33	16	180	3.00
Secondary prevention of myocardial infarction	1	3	6	39	11	176	2.93
Decrease endpoints	1	4	20	24	11	160	2.67
Overall conditioning,	0	0	0	20	40	220	3.67
Individual diagnosis	0	0	0	14	46	226	3.77
Mild effect	0	2	5	29	24	195	3.25
Safety	1	2	5	22	30	198	3.30
Low cost	2	1	31	12	14	155	2.58
Comprehensive benefit	0	0	11	29	20	189	3.15
Well received by patients	0	0	6	30	24	198	3.30

Table 6. Shortcomings of TCM.

Insufficiency/Grade	No	Yes	Insufficiency/Grade	No	Yes
Plausible curative effect	30	30	Poor taste of medicinal borth	7	53
Lack of clinical evidence	10	50	Toxicity of TCM	57	3
Slow onset of effects	11	49	Few species of Chinese patent medicine	44	16
Improper use of medication	12	48	Prominent side effect of Chinese injection	42	18
Tedious to prepare decoction	3	57	High treatment cost	40	20

TCM in the prevention of CAD so as to obtain high scientific and authoritative clinical evidence.

Expert opinions and recommendations have been important clinical evidence for local and international guidelines in the treatment of CAD. The results of the survey can reflect the current clinical setting of the treatment and prevention of CAD, which are essential guides and references for clinical use. It should also be noted that the vast majority of the experts involved in the survey are from TCM hospitals, and thus the survey result mainly reflects the basic situation in TCM hospitals. Most experts are from third grade hospitals, so it is unable to accurately reflect the situation in primary hospital. Hence, we should also carry out investigations in western hospitals and primary hospitals in the future, in order to have a complete picture of the clinical diagnosis and treatment of TCM in the prevention of CAD. This will enable us to fully recognize our advantages and disadvantages, make use of the advantages, discover potential advantages, strive to make up for our shortcomings, and make further contributions to the prevention and treatment of the disease.

References

[1]   Mao, J.Y., Bi, Y.F., Zhang, B.L., *et al.* (2010) Study on Clinical Therapeutic Effect of Acute Coronary Syndrome Patients Treated in the Unit Integrated TCM and Western Medicine. *Beijing Journal of Traditional Chinese Medicine*, **29**,

10-13.

[2]   Zhang, M.Z., Liu, Z.Y., Zou, X., *et al.* (2003) Effect of Tongguan Capsule on the Diastolic Function of Left Heart in Patients with Coronary Artery Disease. *Journal of Practical Traditional Chinese Internal Medicine*, **17**, 81-82.

[3]   Zhang, J.H., Shang, H.C., Zhang, B.L., *et al.* (2008) Compound Salvia Droplet Pill, a Traditional Chinese Medicine, for the Treatment of Unstable Angina Pectoris: A Systematic Review. *Medical Science Monitor*, **14**, RA1-RA7.

[4]   Lu, Z., Kou, W., Du, B., *et al.* (2008) Effect of Xuezhikang, an Extract from Red Yeast Chinese Rice, on Coronary Events in a Chinese Population with Previous Myocardial Infarction. *The American Journal of Cardiology*, **101**, 1689-1693. http://dx.doi.org/10.1016/j.amjcard.2008.02.056

[5]   Xu, H.J., Ren, M., Zhang, B.L., *et al.* (2010) Baseline Characteristics of Myocardial Infarction Secondary Prevention Study in Traditional Chinese Medicine (MISPS-TCM). *Heart*, **96**, A119. http://dx.doi.org/10.1136/hrt.2010.208967.383

23

Evaluation of the Safety of Three Phenolic Compounds from *Dipteryx alata* Vogel with Antiophidian Potential

Edson Hideaki Yoshida[1], Miriéle Cristina Ferraz[1], Natália Tribuiani[1],
Renata Vasques da Silva Tavares[1], José Carlos Cogo[2], Márcio Galdino dos Santos[3],
Luiz Madaleno Franco[4], Cháriston André Dal-Belo[5], Rone A. De Grandis[6],
Flávia Aparecida Resende[6], Eliana Aparecida Varanda[6], Pilar Puebla[7],
Arturo San-Feliciano[7], Francisco Carlos Groppo[8], Yoko Oshima-Franco[1*]

[1]Post-Graduate Program in Pharmaceutical Sciences, University of Sorocaba, Sorocaba, Brazil
[2]Serpentarium of the University of Vale do Paraíba, São José dos Campos, Brazil
[3]Post-Graduate Program in Environmental Sciences, Tocantins Federal University, Palmas, Brazil
[4]Methodist University of Piracicaba, Piracicaba, Brazil
[5]Laboratory of Neurobiology and Toxinology, Federal University of Pampa, São Gabriel, Brazil
[6]Department of Biological Sciences, São Paulo State University, Araraquara, Brazil
[7]Department of Pharmaceutical Chemistry, Salamanca University, Salamanca, Spain
[8]Department of Physiological Sciences, University of Campinas, Piracicaba, Brazil
Email: [*]yoko.franco@prof.uniso.br

Abstract

Phenolic compounds from *Dipteryx alata* Vogel were assayed against the *in vitro* neurotoxic effect induced by *Bothrops jararacussu* (Bjssu) venom. Mutagenicity was assessed by the Ames test using *Salmonella typhimurium* strains TA98, TA97a, TA100, and TA102, in experiments with and without metabolic activation. Anti-bothropic activity was obtained by using mouse phrenic nerve-diaphragm (PND) preparation and myographic technique. Control experiments with physiological Tyrode solution were used for keeping the PND preparations alive (n = 4). Concentrations of phenolic compounds were as follow: protocatechuic and vanillic acids (200 µg/mL, n = 4), vanillin (50 µg/mL, n = 4). These compounds were used alone or pre-incubated with the venom (40 µg/mL), 30 min prior the addition to the organ bath (n = 4). Phenolic compounds significantly inhibited the neuromuscular blockade of Bjssu in the following order of potency: vanillic acid > protocatechuic = vanillin. Vanillic acid added 10 min after the Bjssu venom was also able to avoid the venomblockade evolution. The mutagenicity assay indicated that all phytochemicals were unable to increase the number of revertants, demonstrating the absence of mutagenic activity. This study

---

[*]Corresponding author.

demonstrated both the safety and therapeutical potential of the three phenolic compounds as novel complementary anti-bothropic agents.

Keywords

Ames Test, Baru, *Bothrops jararacussu* Venom, Vanillic Acid, Vanillin

---

1. Introduction

Natural phenolic compounds have an aromatic ring bearing one or more hydroxyl or etherified substituents, being known due the ability to complex proteins by hydrogen bonding. Among them, compounds such as protocatechuic (1, PCA) and vanillic (2, VA) acids, both universal among the angiosperms [1]; and the aldehyde vanillin (3, VN) have closely related structures (**Figure 1**), which justify the similarity in their biological activity [2].

Dipteryx alata Vogel (Leguminosae), a native plant from the Brazilian savannah and popularly known as *baru* [3], contains 18 compounds already identified and among them the three phenolic derivatives (PCA, VA, and VN) of biomedical relevance [4].

The biological activity of these compounds has been characterized, and revealed their potential as antioxidants [5], scavengers of active oxygen species and electrophiles [6], blockers of nitration [7], and metal chelators [8]. Despite of their environmental relevance considering the endangered situation of the Brazilian Cerrado biome, a preliminary survey for biological activities justifies the bio-prospection, due to the potential of *baru* as a source for medicinal use, nutritional food, pharmaceutical, and cosmetic compounds. The controlled bio-prospection could allow the valorization of Cerrado's plants, and their sustainable use, contributing to the environment protection.

One of the medicinal interests on *baru* compounds is their use as anti-ophidian medicine. *Bothrops* snakebites, including the *Bothrops jararacussu* snake, are the most relevant snake accidents in Brazil, not only because the number of accidents, but also by the severity of symptoms, which includes high level of pain, inflammation, hemorrhage and myonecrosis. The attributed clinical signs result from proteases/phospholipases/thrombin-like enzymes and peptides present in the venom [9] [10]. Despite of the systemic antigen-antibody action of the antiserum, the local manifestations of *Bothrops* envenomation are only partially avoided [11]. Thus, strategies to minimize the effects at the bite local would corroborate to avoid unwanted sequels, such as a limb amputation.

Nanotechnology, an innovation of the pharmaceutical sciences, can contribute to the development of a supplementary medicine in order to improve serum therapy [12]. Nevertheless, before this step is achieved, the safety assessment is a crucial protocol.

In this study, PCA, VA, and VN from *Dipteryx alata* were assayed in a pre-incubation model of a mouse phrenic nerve-diaphragm (PND) preparation, used to measure the *in vitro* neuromuscular activity of *B. jararacussu* venom [13]. The mutagenic activity of these compounds were assessed by the *Salmonella* microsome assay (Ames test), using *S. typhimurium* test strains TA98, TA97a (to detect frameshift mutations), TA100 (to detect base-pair-substitution mutations) and TA102 (normally used to detect mutagens that cause oxidative damage and base-pair-substitution mutations), in the presence or absence of *in vitro* metabolizing systems [14]-[16]. Results of genetic toxicological tests, combined with an adequate pharmacology profile, have been used to

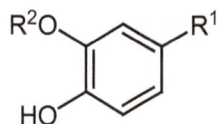

Figure 1. The structures of tested antibothropic phenolics. 1: protocatechuic acid (PCA), 2: vanillic acid (VA), 3: vanillin (VN).

approve clinical trials of novel drug candidates [17].

2. Material and Methods

2.1. Plant Material and Extraction

The barks of an adult *Dipteryx alata* Vogel tree were collected in Pedro Afonso (Tocantins, Brazil), and identified by Institute of Agronomy of Campinas. The voucher specimen was deposited (IAC 50629) at the herbarium of Institute of Agronomy of Campinas. The *D. alata* barks (1.269 kg) were dried at 37°C over 48 h and then powdered, ground in a mill, macerated (200 g, during 5 days) in 2 L of 70% ethanol, being the suspension percolated (under protection against light) at 20 drops/min, resulting in a 20% (m/v) hydroalcoholic extract. Then, the extract was concentrated under reduced pressure and lyophilized, providing a residue of 170 g, reaching 85% of efficiency [18].

2.2. Isolation

Part of the above described residue (50 g) was dissolved in a 80:20 MeOH:H$_2$O mixture, and partitioned successively with the corresponding solvents to give hexane (1.5 g), dichloromethane (CH$_2$Cl$_2$, 18 g), ethyl acetate (EtOAc, 3.7 g) and methanol (MeOH residue, 21 g) fractions. The CH$_2$Cl$_2$ fraction was submitted to a silica-gel flash column chromatography and eluted with hexane-EtOAc (9:1 to EtOAc) to give 12 subfractions. These subfractions were further successively flash-chromatographed in silica gel and purified by Sephadex LH-20 column chromatography, eluted with hexane-CH$_2$Cl$_2$-MeOH-H$_2$O (2:2:1) to yield 18 compounds, among them the phenolic derivatives protocatechuic acid (PCA, 1), vanillic acid (VA, 2) and vanillin (VN, 3) [4].

2.3. Compounds Solubilization

In order to use the phenolic derivatives in the pharmacological assays (see below), they were previously solubilized as follows: PCA (compound 1) in 30 µL of dimethyl sulfoxide (DMSO, Sigma Chemical Co., St. Louis, MO, USA); VA and VN (compounds 2 and 3, respectively) in 15 µL of polyethylene glycol (PEG 400). The concentration of the solubilizing agents did not cause changes on basal response of the neuromuscular preparations, according to Cintra-Francischinelli *et al.* [19].

2.4. Pharmacological Assays

2.4.1. Crude Snake Venom

Bothrops jararacussu venom (Bjssu) was collected from two adult specimens kept in the "Serpentário do Centro de Estudos da Natureza"—*Center for Nature Studies Snake Pit*-CEN. The venom was lyophilized and certified by Professor Dr. José Carlos Cogo from University of Vale do Paraiba, Univap, SP, Brazil.

2.4.2. Animals

Male Swiss white mice (26 - 32 g) were supplied by Anilab (Animais de Laboratório, Paulínia, SP, Brazil). The animals were housed at 25°C ± 3°C on a 12 h light/dark cycle and they had access to food and water *ad libitum*. This study (protocol number A013/CEUA/2011) was approved by the institutional Committee for Ethics in Research of University of Vale do Paraiba, and the experiments were performed following the guidelines of the Brazilian College for Animal Experimentation.

2.4.3. Mouse Phrenic Nerve-Diaphragm Muscle (PND) Preparation

The phrenic nerve-diaphragm [20] was obtained from mice previously anesthetized with halothane (Cristália, Brazil) and killed by exsanguination. The diaphragm was removed and mounted under a tension of 5 g/cm in a 5 mL organ bath containing aerated Tyrode solution (control) with the following composition (mM): NaCl 137; KCl 2.7; CaCl$_2$ 1.8; MgCl$_2$ 0.49; NaH$_2$PO$_4$ 0.42; NaHCO$_3$ 11.9; and glucose 11.1. After equilibration with 95% O$_2$/5% CO$_2$ (v/v), the pH of this solution was 7.0. The PND preparations were indirectly stimulated with supramaximal stimuli (4× threshold, 0.06 Hz, 0.2 ms) delivered from an electrical stimulator (model ESF-15D, Ribeirão Preto, Brazil) directly to the nerve by bipolar electrodes. Isometric twitch tension was recorded with a force displacement transducer (cat. 7003, Ugo Basile, Italy) coupled to a 2-Channel Recorder Gemini physiograph device (cat. 7070, Ugo Basile) via a Basic Preamplifier (cat. 7080, Ugo Basile). The PND myographic recording was performed according to Ferraz et al. [21]. PND was allowed to stabilize for at least 20 min before the experiments.

2.4.4. Experimental Protocols

Control PND preparations (n = 4) were submitted to Tyrode nutritive solution in order to maintain them. Other PND preparations were submitted to the following phenolic derivatives concentrations, which were based in previous studies [21]: PCA and VA (200 µg/mL, n = 4), VN (50 µg/mL, n = 4) and B. jararacussu venom 40 µg/mL (n = 4). New PND preparations were also pre-incubated with the same concentrations of the phenolic derivatives, during 30 min prior to addition into the organ bath. This assay was carried out in order to verify the ability of the phenolic compounds to neutralize the in vitro neurotoxic effect of the Bjssu crude venom (n = 4).

2.5. In Vitro Mutagenicity Assay

Mutagenic activity was tested by the Salmonella/microsome assay, using the S. typhimurium tester strains TA98, TA100, TA102 and TA97a [22], which were kindly provided by B. N. Ames (Berkeley, CA, USA), with and without metabolization by the preincubation method [15]. The strains from frozen cultures were grown overnight for 12 - 14 h, in Oxoid Nutrient Broth No. 2. The S9 fraction, prepared from livers of Sprague-Dawley rats treated with the polychlorinated biphenyl mixture Aroclor 1254 (500 mg/kg), was purchased from Molecular Toxicology Inc. (Boone, NC, USA) and freshly prepared before each test. The metabolic activation system consisted of 4% of S9 fraction, 1% of 0.4 M $MgCl_2$, 1% of 1.65 M KCl, 0.5% of 1 M D-glucose-6-phosphate disodium, 4% of 0.1 M NADP, 50% of 0.2 M phosphate buffer, and 39.5% sterile distilled water [15]. The phenolic compounds of D. alata extract were dissolved in DMSO in order to obtain the nontoxic concentrations. The tested concentrations were selected based on a preliminary toxicity test. In all subsequent assays, the upper limit of the dose range tested was either the highest nontoxic dose or the lowest toxic dose determined in this preliminary assay. Toxicity was apparent either as a reduction in the number of histidine revertants (His+), or as an alteration in the auxotrophic background (i.e., background lawn). The concentrations varied from 0.78 to 6.25 mg/plate for PCA, 0.39 to 3.13 mg/plate for VA and 0.1 to 0.78 mg/plate for VN.

All concentrations of the phenolic compounds to be tested were previously added to 0.5 mL of 0.2 M sodium phosphate buffer (pH 7.4), or to 0.5 mL de 4% S9 mixture, with 0.1 mL of bacterial culture and then incubated at 37°C for 20 min. Next, 2 mL of top agar (0.6% agar, histidine and biotin 0.5 mM each, and 0.5% NaCl) was added, and the mixture was poured on to a plate containing minimal glucose agar (1.5% Bacto-Difco agar and 2% glucose in Vogel-Bonner medium E). The plates were incubated at 37°C for 48 h and the His(+) revertant colonies were counted manually. All experiments were carried out in triplicate. The standard mutagens used as positive controls in experiments without S9 mix were 4-nitro-O-phenylenediamine (10 µg/plate) for TA98 and TA97a, sodium azide (1.25 µg/plate) for TA100 and mitomycin (0.5 µg/plate) for TA102. 2-anthramine (1.25 µg/plate) was used with TA98, TA97a and TA100 and 2-aminofluorene (1.25 µg/plate) with TA102 in the experiments with metabolic activation. DMSO (solvent) was used as a negative control (50 µL/plate).

The mutagenic index (MI) was calculated for each concentration tested, and considered as the average number of revertants per plate obtained by the test compound divided by the average number of revertants per plate in the negative (solvent) control. A sample was considered mutagenic when a dose-response relationship was detected and a two-fold increase in the number of mutants (MI ≥ 2) was observed with at least one concentration [23].

2.6. Statistical Analysis

Each experimental protocol from the pharmacological assays was repeated at least four times and the results are shown as mean ± SEM. The number of experiments (n) is indicated in the legend of each figure. Student's t-test was used for statistical comparison of the data and the confidence level was set as 5% (alpha = 0.05). The results of the mutagenicity tests were analyzed with the Salanal statistical software package (US Environmental Protection Agency, Monitoring Systems Laboratory, Las Vegas, NV, version 1.0, from Research Triangle Institute, RTP, North Carolina, USA), adopting the Bernstein et al. [24] model. The data (revertants/plate) were assessed by analysis of variance (ANOVA), followed by linear regression.

3. Results and Discussion

The deforestation process and associated factors have been studied. Both science and technology have been used to protect human health and environment, and to promote innovative green-business practices [25]. Plants with medicinal properties take important role in the sustainability concept. This concept creates and maintains the condition in which human beings and nature can coexist in a productive harmony, allowing social, economic and other requirements of the present and future generations [26].

The Brazilian biome known as *Cerrado* has been extensively threatened in the last decades. Many species of plants could disappear even before their medicinal properties could be studied [27]. *D. alata* is a very appreciated specimen by the Cerrado population due to its great value for wood-industry, to recover deforested areas, and specially as a food source [28]. In addition, its medicinal properties as antiophidian agent was previously recognized [4] [21] [29].

The antiophidian properties of three natural phenolic compounds PCA (1), VA (2), and VN (3) found in *D. alata* [4], whose structures are shown in **Figure 1**, is showed here for the first time in the literature.

Vanillic acid is an oxidized form of VN and exhibits more free radical scavenging activity than VN [30]. VA has antioxidant, antimicrobial and anti-mutagenic activities and can exhibit a chemopreventive effect in experimentally induced carcinogenesis in rats [31]-[34].

Moreover, VA can scavenge free radical species, having cardioprotective properties, and it could repress fibrogenesis and inflammation in the chronically injured liver [35]-[37]. VN is used as a flavoring agent in food and cosmetics, having well-studied antimicrobial [38] [39], anti-mutagenic, antioxidant, and anti-carcinogenic activities [39]-[41].

Vanillic acid and PCA are commonly derivatives of hydroxybenzoic acid or benzoic acid. According to Anter *et al.* [42], PCA did not exhibit any genotoxic effect. However, it has an antigenotoxic property against the hydrogen-peroxide effects, exhibiting tumoricidal activity, and apoptosis-induction in HL-60 leukemic cells.

Figure 2 shows the pharmacological effect of the phenolic compounds. VN exhibited bigger potency (around 4×) than VA and PCA, since only 50 µg/mL vanillin was used in comparison to the 200 µg/mL of VA and PCA. VN also exhibited a facilitatory effect measured by increased twitches amplitude, at least during 40 min ($p < 0.05$ when compared to the control group).

Probably the facilitatory effect of VN was associated to its reactive electrophilic character. The ideal phytochemical substance for further neutralization assays with Bjssu could be VA, since it showed the better profile, having no significant difference with control (Tyrode solution). It is important to observe that VN and PCA

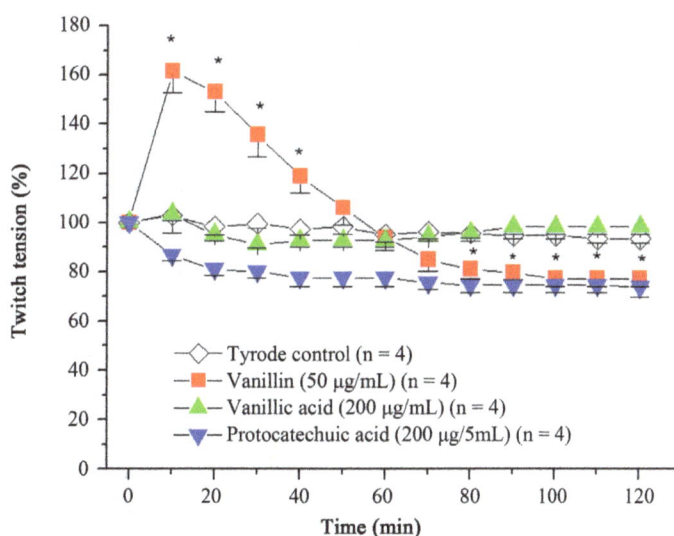

Figure 2. Pharmacological activity evaluation (mouse phrenic nerve-diaphragm preparation, indirect stimuli). The phenolic compounds profile at the selected concentrations and number of experiments (n) are shown in the figure. Each point represents the mean ± SEM. $^* = p < 0.05$ in comparison with the Bjssu venom.

showed significant differences when compared to the control group from 80 min to 120 min.

Figure 3 shows the *in vitro* preincubation with each phytochemical prior the addition of Bjssu venom and the effect of the crude Bjssu venom alone. The *in vitro* irreversible neuromuscular blockade of *B. jararacussu* venom (Bjssu) is well-known [13].

Bothrops jararacussu venom has two basic phospholipase A$_2$ homologues, namely bothropstoxin-I (BthTX-I, a Lys49-PLA2) [43] and bothropstoxin-II (BthTX-II, an Asp49-PLA2) [44] [45]. BthTX-I is considered the main myotoxin from the venom since it is able to reproduce *in vitro* the neurotoxicity and the myonecrosis of the crude venom [43], being this characteristic the main reason of the interest in the myotoxin. BthTX-I has a pre-synaptic nature at 0.35 µM, which is not sufficient to cause muscle fiber depolarization [46]. The Asp49 to Lys49 substitution in the catalytic center (only in the calcium-binding loop) explains the lack of enzymatic action in BthTX-I, due to the loss of ability to bind Ca^{2+} [47].

Chemically, the mechanism of interaction between the snake venom and the plant includes hydrogen-bonds, electrostatic bonds, Vand der Waals forces, hydrophobic bonds, formation of inactive acid-base complexes protein precipitation and covalent bonds [48]-[52]. The tested phenolic compounds protected the PND preparation against the neurotoxic effect of the venom in the following order: VA > PCA = VN.

Acid-base complexation does not explain PCA activity, since PCA did not show the same ability in neutralizing the venom neuromuscular blockade as VA, and the phenolic groups probably have an important role. The chemical difference between VA and PCA is the methylation of the meta-hydroxyl group. This methylation did facilitate the interaction between the *para*-hydroxyl groups with venom's constituents, making VA a better venom-inhibitor than PCA. PCA has both hydroxyl groups bonded intramolecularly. Interestingly, VA was isolated from the active fraction 7 of *D. alata* against Bjssu [29], showing the importance of biomonitoring studies.

Vanillic acid was also evaluated after 10 min of Bjssu venom action (**Figure 4**), in a post-venom model. Even in this condition, VA was able to counteract the venom myotoxic activity, significantly protecting (*p < 0.05) the tissue against the venom damage.

This post-venom model has been commonly used to observe the plant extract potency, in a better mimic model of the ophidian accident than the preincubation model. Hydroalcoholic extracts of leaves from *Casearia gossypiosperma* [53] and *Vellozia flavicans* [54] were validated using the same post-venom model. In all cases, the initial damage induced by the crude Bjssu venom was irreversible, but the damage progression was controlled, conferring an anti-bothropic property to those plants.

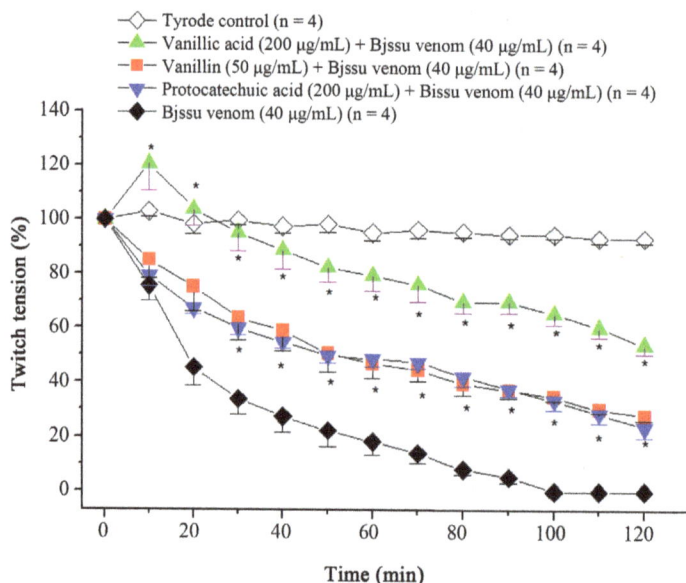

Figure 3. Pharmacological activity evaluation (mouse phrenic nerve-diaphragm preparation, indirect stimuli). Each phenolic compound was pre-incubated prior Bjssu addition. The concentrations and the number of experiments (n) are shown in the figure. Each point represents the mean ± SEM. *= p < 0.05 in comparison with the Bjssu venom.

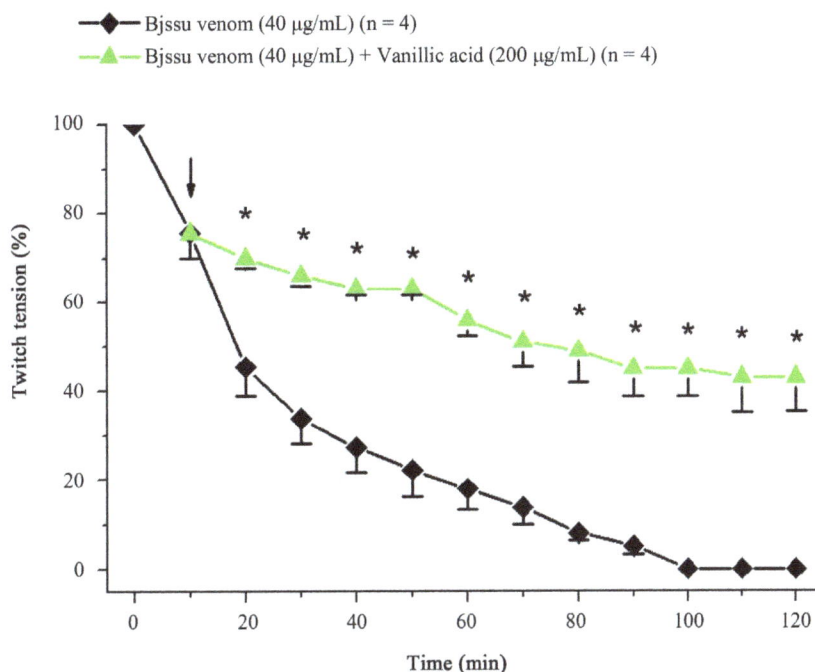

Figure 4. Pharmacological activity evaluation (mouse phrenic nerve-diaphragm preparation, indirect stimuli) of Vanillic acid in a post-venom model. The concentrations and the number of experiments (n) are shown in the figure. Each point represents the mean ± SEM. * = p < 0.05 in comparison with the venom. Arrow: time of Vanillic acid addition.

The balance between the therapeutic and toxicological effects of a compound is a very important measure of its usefulness as a drug. Therefore, the determination of the potential mutagenic effect of any drug under development is mandatory [55]. The Ames assay, which is recommended for testing the mutagenicity of chemical compounds with potential pharmacological application [56] was used in the present study.

In previous studies, Esteves-Pedro *et al.* [18] showed that the *D. alata* Vogel extract had no mutagenic effect by Ames test on the strains tested, in either the presence or absence of metabolic activation. To complement the preliminary results [18] and considering the promising results obtained in the present study, the mutagenic activity of the isolated compounds of *D. alata* Vogel extract was also assessed (**Tables 1-3**). These Tables list the mean number of revertants/plate (M), the standard deviation (SD) and the mutagenic index (MI) after the treatments with VA, PCA and VN respectively, observed in *S. typhimurium* strains TA98, TA100, TA102 and TA97a in the presence (+S9) and absence (−S9) of metabolic activation.

The mutagenicity assays show that none of the phenolic compounds induced any increase in the number of revertant colonies compared to the negative control group, indicating the absence of any mutagenic activity. The absence of mutagenicity against *S. typhimurium* bacterial strains in the Ames assay of these compounds is a positive step towards determining its safe use in medicine. Considering the biological properties of these compounds, a lack of mutagenic effect in the bacterial systems tested is highly relevant.

In addition, the genotoxic and anti-genotoxic effects of VA were determinated on mitomycin C-induced DNA damage in human blood lymphocyte cultures *in vitro* by the cytokinesis-block micronucleus test and the alkaline comet assay. The results showed that VA could prevent oxidative damage to DNA and chromosomes when used at appropriate low doses [57]. VA also induced an inhibitory effect on the mutagenicity of 3-(5-nitro-2-furyl) acrylic acid (5NFAA) and sodium azide [58]. Stagos *et al.* [59] evaluated the mutagenicity of the PCA; and the results showed no mutagenic effect and no significant effect on bleomycin-induced mutagenicity. According to Shaughnessy *et al.* [60], VN is a dietary antimutagen that reduces the spontaneous mutant frequency in *S. typhimurium* strain TA104 (*his*G428, *rfa*, *uvrB*, pKM101) by 50%, when added to assay plates.

Taken together our results, which are also corroborated with data from literature, these phytochemicals are not mutagenic, and they act as antimutagens according to other studies [39] [41] [42] [57] [59]. These results should stimulate new research in order to provide medicines using these safe molecules and nanotechnology to treat

Table 1. Mutagenic activity expressed as the mean and standard deviation of the number of revertants/plate and the mutagenic index (in brackets), for the strains TA98, TA100, TA102, and TA97 of *S. typhimurium* after treatment with phytochemical 4-hydroxy-3-methoxybenzoic (Vanillic acid) isolated from *D. alata* Vogel, with (+S9) and without (−S9) metabolic activation.

Treatments		Number of revertants (M ± SD)/plate and (MI)							
		TA 98		TA 100		TA 102		TA 97a	
	mg/plate	−S9	+S9	−S9	+S9	−S9	+S9	−S9	+S9
Vanillic acid	0.0[a]	28 ± 2	24 ± 2	104 ± 15	95 ± 6	271 ± 18	461 ± 21	125 ± 15	96 ± 10
	0.39	28 ± 5 (1.0)	21 ± 3 (0.9)	113 ± 11 (1.1)	95 ± 11 (1.0)	241 ± 25 (0.9)	518 ± 13 (1.1)	98 ± 13 (0.8)	98 ± 5 (1.0)
	0.78	41 ± 2 (1.5)	18 ± 3 (0.8)	115 ± 15 (1.1)	88 ± 14 (0.9)	237 ± 13 (0.9)	522 ± 16 (1.1)	108 ± 10 (0.9)	108 ± 2 (1.1)
	1.56	31 ± 5 (1.1)	21 ± 2 (0.9)	91 ± 7 (0.9)	89 ± 7 (0.9)	268 ± 10 (1.0)	500 ± 20 (1.1)	113 ± 9 (0.9)	103 ± 13 (1.1)
	2.34	27 ± 2 (1.0)	20 ± 1 (0.8)	96 ± 11 (0.9)	84 ± 7 (0.9)	315 ± 8 (1.2)	487 ± 15 (1.1)	96 ± 3 (0.8)	103 ± 18 (1.1)
	3.13	27 ± 5 (1.0)	21 ± 4 (0.9)	99 ± 8 (0.9)	92 ± 12 (1.0)	293 ± 19 (1.1)	471 ± 13 (1.0)	84 ± 6 (0.7)	97 ± 5 (1.0)
	Ctrol+	2064 ± 87[b]	1213 ± 33[e]	1252 ± 124[c]	1870 ± 69[e]	1173 ± 47[d]	1822 ± 102[f]	1968 ± 77[b]	1850 ± 67[e]

M ± SD = mean and standard deviation; MI = mutagenicity index; [a]Negative control: dimethylsulfoxide (DMSO-50 µL/plate); Ctrol+ = Positive control-[b]4-nitro-*o*-phenylenediamine (NOPD-10.0 µg/plate-TA98, TA97a); [c]sodium azide (1.25 µg/ plate-TA100); [d]mitomycin (0.5 µg/plate-TA102), in the absence of S9 and [e]2-anthramine (1.25 µg/plate-TA 97a, TA98, TA100); [f]2-aminofluorene (10.0 µg/plate-TA102), in the presence of S9.

Table 2. Mutagenic activity expressed as the mean and standard deviation of the number of revertants/plate and the mutagenic index (in brackets), for the strains TA98, TA100, TA102, and TA97 of *S. typhimurium* after treatment with phytochemical 3,4-dihydroxybenzoic acid (Protocatechuic acid) isolated from *D. alata* Vogel, with (+S9) and without (−S9) metabolic activation.

Treatments		Number of revertants (M ± SD)/plate and (MI)							
		TA 98		TA 100		TA 102		TA 97a	
	mg/plate	−S9	+S9	−S9	+S9	−S9	+S9	−S9	+S9
Protocatechuic acid	0.0[a]	28 ± 2	24 ± 2	104 ± 15	95 ± 6	271 ± 18	461 ± 21	125 ± 15	96 ± 10
	0.78	30 ± 7 (1.1)	24 ± 6 (1.0)	113 ± 17 (1.1)	94 ± 11 (1.0)	273 ± 6 (1.0)	502 ± 34 (1.1)	116 ± 10 (0.9)	105 ± 16 (1.1)
	1.56	26 ± 2 (0.9)	22 ± 5 (0.9)	104 ± 3 (1.0)	100 ± 9 (1.0)	261 ± 18 (1.0)	475 ± 51 (1.0)	121 ± 24 (1.0)	101 ± 4 (1.1)
	3.13	24 ± 2 (0.9)	19 ± 4 (0.8)	100 ± 9 (1.0)	96 ± 6 (1.0)	257 ± 6 (0.9)	492 ± 37 (1.1)	124 ± 12 (1.0)	120 ± 2 (1.3)
	4.69	25 ± 2 (0.9)	21 ± 2 (0.9)	94 ± 19 (0.9)	97 ± 7 (1.0)	299 ± 29 (1.1)	498 ± 7 (1.1)	124 ± 4 (1.0)	113 ± 26 (1.2)
	6.25	32 ± 9 (1.1)	17 ± 3 (0.7)	114 ± 10 (1.3)	103 ± 7 (1.1)	372 ± 10 (1.4)	490 ± 21 (1.1)	107 ± 6 (0.9)	120 ± 18 (1.3)
	Ctrol+	2064 ± 87[b]	1213 ± 33[e]	1252 ± 124[c]	1870 ± 69[e]	1173 ± 47[d]	1822 ± 102[f]	1968 ± 77[b]	1850 ± 67[e]

M ± SD = mean and standard deviation; MI = mutagenicity index; [a]Negative control: dimethylsulfoxide (DMSO-50 µL/plate); Ctrol+ = Positive control-[b]4-nitro-*o*-phenylenediamine (NOPD-10.0 µg/plate-TA98, TA97a); [c]sodium azide (1.25 µg/ plate-TA100); [d]mitomycin (0.5 µg/plate-TA102), in the absence of S9 and [e]2-anthramine (1.25 µg/plate-TA 97a, TA98, TA100); [f]2-aminofluorene (10.0 µg/plate-TA102), in the presence of S9.

several pathological conditions, such as snakebite envenoming.

4. Conclusion

Phenolic compounds from *D. alata* significantly protected the neuromuscular preparation against the irreversible neuromuscular blockade-induced by *B. jararacussu* venom, at different levels: VA > PCA = VN, by unclear mechanisms. VA significantly inhibited the venom-blockade evolution in a post-venom model. Moreover, the results indicated the absence of any mutagenic activity by Ames test; it is important to guarantee its safe use in humans.

Table 3. Mutagenic activity expressed as the mean and standard deviation of the number of revertants/plate and the mutagenic index (in brackets), for the strains TA98, TA100, TA102, and TA97 of *S. typhimurium* after treatment with phytochemical 4-hydroxy-3-metoxibenzaldehído (Vanillin) isolated from *D. alata* Vogel, with (+S9) and without (−S9) metabolic activation.

| Treatments | | Number of revertants (M ± SD)/plate and (MI) | | | | | | | |
| | | TA 98 | | TA 100 | | TA 102 | | TA 97a | |
mg/plate		−S9	+S9	−S9	+S9	−S9	+S9	−S9	+S9
	0.0[a]	20 ± 2	30 ± 2	115 ± 7	121 ± 9	313 ± 24	411 ± 17	151 ± 8	143 ± 8
	0.10	20 ± 3 (1.0)	33 ± 3 (1.1)	103 ± 8 (0.9)	142 ± 9 (1.2)	375 ± 15 (1.2)	453 ± 27 (1.1)	171 ± 11 (1.1)	192 ± 6 (1.3)
	0.20	17 ± 1 (0.9)	35 ± 3 (1.2)	111 ± 11 (1.0)	148 ± 11 (1.2)	430 ± 19 (1.4)	496 ± 13 (1.2)	205 ± 22 (1.4)	167 ± 12 (1.2)
Vanillin	0.39	19 ± 3 (0.9)	30 ± 4 (1.0)	110 ± 2 (1.0)	143 ± 10 (1.2)	422 ± 43 (1.4)	503 ± 14 (1.2)	186 ± 12 (1.2)	163 ± 7 (1.1)
	0.59	16 ± 2 (0.8)	37 ± 3 (1.2)	108 ± 6 (0.9)	144 ± 13 (1.2)	367 ± 26 (1.2)	489 ± 27 (1.2)	167 ± 17 (1.1)	167 ± 5 (1.2)
	0.78	20 ± 2 (1.0)	34 ± 6 (1.1)	108 ± 10 (0.9)	116 ± 3 (1.0)	325 ± 41 (1.0)	445 ± 21 (1.1)	173 ± 7 (1.1)	170 ± 13 (1.2)
	Ctrol+	1319 ± 41[b]	1696 ± 41[e]	1708 ± 27[e]	1480 ± 52[e]	1220 ± 24[d]	1825 ± 55[f]	1875 ± 62[b]	1623 ± 48[e]

M ± SD = mean and standard deviation; MI = mutagenicity index; [a]Negative control: dimethylsulfoxide (DMSO-50 μL/plate); Ctrol+ = Positive control-[b]4-nitro-*o*-phenylenediamine (NOPD-10.0 μg/plate-TA98, TA97a); [c]sodium azide (1.25 μg/ plate-TA100); [d]mitomycin (0.5 μg/plate-TA102), in the absence of S9 and [e]2-anthramine (1.25 μg/plate-TA 97a, TA98, TA100); [f]2-aminofluorene (10.0 μg/plate-TA102), in the presence of S9.

Acknowledgements

The authors thank to Roseli B. Torres for the plant identification. This study was supported by FAPESP (04/09705-8; 07/53883-6; 08/50669-6; 08/52643-4; 08/11005-5); Capes/Prosup; Probic/Uniso; and USAL:18KAC9/463AC01.

References

[1] Harborne, J.B. (1998) Phytochemical Methods. A Guide to Modern Techniques of Plant Analysys. 3rd Edition, Chapman & Hall, London.

[2] Lee, S., Monnappa, A.K. and Mitchell, R.J. (2012) Biological Activities of Lignin Hydrolysate-Related Compounds. *Biochemistry and Molecular Biology Reports*, **45**, 265-275.

[3] Lorenzi, H. (1992) Árvores Brasileiras: Manual de Identificação e Cultivo de Plantas Arbóreas Nativas do Brasil. Plantarum, Nova Odessa.

[4] Puebla, P., Oshima-Franco, Y., Franco, L.M., Dos Santos, M.G., Da Silva, R.V., Rubem-Mauro, L. and Feliciano, A.S. (2010) Chemical Constituents of the Bark of *Dipteryx alata* Vogel, an Active Species against *Bothrops jararacussu* Venom. *Molecules*, **15**, 8193-8204. http://dx.doi.org/10.3390/molecules15118193

[5] Kaga, V.E. and Tyurinov, Y.Y. (1998) Recycling and Redox Cycling of Phenolic Antioxidants. *Annals of the New York Academy of Sciences*, **854**, 425-434. http://dx.doi.org/10.1111/j.1749-6632.1998.tb09921.x

[6] Zhou, Y.C. and Zheng, R.L. (1991) Phenolic Compounds and an Analog as Superoxide Anion Scavengers and Antioxidants. *Biochemical Pharmacology*, **42**, 1177-1179. http://dx.doi.org/10.1016/0006-2952(91)90251-Y

[7] Kono, Y., Shibata, H., Kodama, Y. and Sawa, Y. (1995) The Suppression of the N-Nitrosating Reaction by Chlorogenic Acid. *Biochemical Journal*, **312**, 947-953.

[8] Brune, M., Rossander, L. and Hallberg, L. (1989) Iron Absorption and Phenolic Compounds: Importance of Different Phenolic Structures. *European Journal of Clinical Nutrition*, **43**, 547-548.

[9] Jorge, M.T., De Campos, F.P., Martins, F.P., Bousso, A., Cardoso, J.L., Ribeiro, L.A., Fan, H.W., França, F.O., Sano-Martins, I.S., Cardoso, D., Ide Fernandez, C., Fernandes, J.C., Aldred, V.L., Sandoval, M.P., Puorto, G., Theakston, R.D. and Warrell, D.A. (1997) Snake Bites by the Jararacuçu (*Bothrops jararacussu*): Clinicopathological Studies of 29 Proven Cases in São Paulo State, Brazil. *Quarterly Journal of Medicine*, **90**, 323-334. http://dx.doi.org/10.1093/qjmed/90.5.323

[10] Ministério da Saúde (2001) Manual de Diagnóstico e tratamento de acidentes por animais peçonhentos. 2nd Edition, Ministério da Saúde, Brazil.

[11] Warrell, D.A. (1992) The Global Problem of Snaked Bite: Its Prevention and Treatment. In: Gopalakrishnakone, P. and

Tan, C.K., Eds., *Recent Advances in Toxinology Research*, National University of Singapore, Singapore, 121-153.

[12] Dwivedi, R. (2014) Silver Nanoparticles Ecofriendly Green Synthesis by Using Two Medicinal Plant Extract. *International Journal of Bio-Technology and Research*, **3**, 61-68.

[13] Rodrigues-Simioni, L., Borgese, N. and Ceccarelli, B. (1983) The Effects of *Bothrops jararacussu* Venom and Its Components on Frog Nerve-Muscle Preparation. *Neuroscience*, **10**, 475-489. http://dx.doi.org/10.1016/0306-4522(83)90147-1

[14] Ames, B.N., McCann, J. and Yamasaki, E. (1975) Methods for Detecting Carcinogens and Mutagens with the *Salmonella*/Mammalian-Microsome Mutagenicity Test. *Mutation Research*, **31**, 347-364. http://dx.doi.org/10.1016/0165-1161(75)90046-1

[15] Maron, D.M. and Ames, B.N. (1983) Revised Methods for the *Salmonella* Mutagenicity Test. *Mutation Research/Environmental Mutagenesis and Related Subjects*, **113**, 173-215. http://dx.doi.org/10.1016/0165-1161(83)90010-9

[16] Gatehouse, D., Haworth, S., Cebula, T., *et al.* (1994) Recommendations for the Performance of Bacterial Mutation Assays. *Mutation Research/Environmental Mutagenesis and Related Subjects*, **312**, 217-233. http://dx.doi.org/10.1016/0165-1161(94)90037-X

[17] Santos, J.L., Varanda, E.A., Lima, L.M. and Chin, C.M. (2010) Mutagenicity of New Lead Compounds to Treat Sickle Cell Disease Symptoms in a *Salmonella*/Microsome Assay. *International Journal of Molecular Sciences*, **11**, 779-788. http://dx.doi.org/10.3390/ijms11020779

[18] Esteves-Pedro, N.M., Borim, T., Nazato, V.S., Silva, M.G., Gerenutti, M., Oshima-Franco, Y., Lopes, P.S., dos Santos, M.G., Dal Belo, C.A., Primila Cardoso, C.R., Varanda, E.A. and Groppo, F.C. (2012) *In Vitro* and *in Vivo* Safety Evaluation of *Dipteryx alata* Vogel Extract. *BioMed Central Complementary and Alternative Medicine*, **12**, 9. http://dx.doi.org/10.1186/1472-6882-12-9

[19] Cintra-Francischinelli, M., Silva, M.G., Andreo-Filho, N., Cintra, A.C.O., Leite, G.B., da Cruz Höfling, M.A., Rodrigues-Simioni, L. and Oshima-Franco, Y. (2008) Effects of Commonly Used Solubilizing Agents on a Model Nerve-Muscle Synapse. *Latin American Journal of Pharmacy*, **27**, 721-726.

[20] Bülbring, E. (1946) Observation on the Isolated Phrenic Nerve Diaphragm Preparation of the Rat. *British Journal of Pharmacology*, **1**, 38-61.

[21] Ferraz, M.C., Parrilha, L.A.C., Moraes, M.S.D., Amaral Filho, J., Cogo, C.J., dos Santos, M.G., Franco, L.M., Groppo, F.C., Puebla, P., Feliciano, A.S. and Oshima-Franco, Y. (2012) The Effect of Lupane Triterpenoids (*Dipteryx alata* Vogel) in the *in Vitro* Neuromuscular Blockade and Myotoxicity of Two Snake Venoms. *Current Organic Chemistry*, **16**, 2717-2723. http://dx.doi.org/10.2174/138527212804004481

[22] OECD (1997) OECD Guideline for Testing of Chemicals, Bacterial Reverse Mutation Test.

[23] Varella, S.D., Pozetti, G.L., Vilegas, W. and Varanda, E.A. (2004) Mutagenic Activity of Sweepings and Pigments from a Household-Wax Factory Assayed with *Salmonella typhimurium*. *Food and Chemical Toxicology*, **42**, 2029-2035. http://dx.doi.org/10.1016/j.fct.2004.07.019

[24] Bernstein, L., Kaldor, J., McCann, J. and Pike, M.C. (1982) An Empirical Approach to the Statistical Analysis of Mutagenesis Data from the *Salmonella* Test. *Mutation Research/Environmental Mutagenesis and Related Subjects*, **97**, 267-281. http://dx.doi.org/10.1016/0165-1161(82)90026-7

[25] El-Abbas, M.M., Csaplovics, E. and Deafalla, T.H. (2013) Remote Sensing and Spatial Analysis Based Study for Detecting Deforestation and the Associated Drivers. *Proceedings of SPIE* 8893, *Earth Resources and Environmental Remote Sensing/GIS Applications IV*, 88930O, Dresden, 24 October 2013.

[26] US Environmental Protection Agency (EPA). http://www.epa.gov/sustainability/basicinfo.htm

[27] Santos, M.G., Lolis, S.F. and Dal Belo, C.A. (2006) Levantamentos etnobotânicos realizados em duas comunidades de remanescentes de negros da região do Jalapão, Estado do Tocantins. In: Pires, A.L., Cardoso, S. and Oliveira, R., Eds., *Sociabilidade Negras. Comunidades Remanescentes, Escravidão e Cultura*, Daliana, Belo Horizonte, 29-49.

[28] Togashi, M. and Sgarbieri, V.C. (1995) Avaliação nutricional da proteína e do óleo de semente de baru (*Dipteryx alata* Vog.). *Ciência e Tecnologia de Alimentos*, **15**, 66-69.

[29] Nazato, V.S., Rubem-Mauro, L., Vieira, N.A.G., Rocha, D.S., Silva, M.G., Lopes, P.S., Dal-Belo, C.A., Cogo, J.C., Dos Santos, M.G., Da Cruz-Höfling, M.A. and Oshima-Franco, Y. (2010) *In Vitro* Antiophidian Properties of *Dipteryx alata* Vogel Bark Extracts. *Molecules*, **15**, 5956-5970. http://dx.doi.org/10.3390/molecules15095956

[30] Sasaki, Y.F., Ohta, T., Imanishi, H., Watanabe, M., Matsumoto, K., Tomoko Kato, T. and Shirasu, Y. (1990) Suppressing Effects of Vanillin, Cinnamaldehyde, and Anisaldehyde on Chromosome Aberrations Induced by X-Rats in Mice. *Mutation Research Letters*, **243**, 299-302. http://dx.doi.org/10.1016/0165-7992(90)90146-B

[31] Tsuda, H., Uehara, N., Iwahori, Y., Asamoto, M., Ligo, M., Nagao, M., Matsumoto, K., Ito, M. and Hirono, I. (1994) Chemopreventive Effects of β-Carotene, α-Tocopherol and Five Naturally Occurring Antioxidants on Initiation of He-

patocarcinogenesis by 2-Amino-3-methylimidazo[4,5-f] Qumoline in the Rat. *Japanese Journal of Cancer Research*, **85**, 1214-1219. http://dx.doi.org/10.1111/j.1349-7006.1994.tb02932.x

[32] Raja, B. and Mol, S.D. (2010) The Protective Role of Vanillic Acid against Acetaminophen Induced Hepatotoxicity in Rats. *Journal of Pharmacy Research*, **3**, 1480-1484.

[33] Tai, A., Sawano, T., Yazama, F. and Ito, H. (2011) Evaluation of Antioxidant Activity of Vanillin by Using Multiple Antioxidant Assays. *Biochimica et Biophysica Acta*, **1810**, 170-177. http://dx.doi.org/10.1016/j.bbagen.2010.11.004

[34] Tai, A., Sawano, T. and Ito, H. (2012) Antioxidative Properties of Vanillic Acid Esters in Multiple Antioxidant Assays. *Bioscience, Biotechnology, and Biochemistry*, **76**, 314-318. http://dx.doi.org/10.1271/bbb.110700

[35] Prince, P.S.M., Dhanasekar, K. and Rajakumar, S. (2011) Preventive Effects of Vanillic Acid on Lipids, Bax, Bcl-$_2$ and Myocardial Infarct Size on Isoproterenol-Induced Myocardial Infracted Rats: A Biochemical and *in vitro* Study. *Cardiovascular Toxicology*, **11**, 58-66. http://dx.doi.org/10.1007/s12012-010-9098-3

[36] Itoh, A., Isoda, K. and Kondoh, M., Masaya, K., Kiyohito, Y., Masakazu, K. and Makoto, T. (2009) Hepatoprotective Effect of Syringic Acid and Vanillic Acid on Concanavalin A-Induced Liver Injury. *Biological and Pharmaceutical Bulletin*, **32**, 1215-1219. http://dx.doi.org/10.1248/bpb.32.1215

[37] Itoh, A., Isoda, K., Kondoh, M., Masaya, K., Akihiro, W., Kiyohito, Y., Masakazu, K. and Makoto, T. (2010) Hepatoprotective Effect of Syringic and Vanillic Acid on CCl$_4$-Induced Liver Injury. *Biological and Pharmaceutical Bulletin*, **33**, 983-987. http://dx.doi.org/10.1248/bpb.33.983

[38] Santosh Kumar, S., Priyadarsini, K.I. and Sainis, K.B. (2002) Free Radical Scavenging Activity of Vanillin and *o*-Vanillin Using 1,1-diphenyl-2-picrylhydrazyl (DPPH) Radical. *Redox Report*, **7**, 35-40. http://dx.doi.org/10.1179/135100002125000163

[39] Lirdprapamongkol, K., Kramb, J.P., Suthiphongchai, T., Surarit, R., Srisomsap, C., Dannhardt, G. and Svasti, J. (2009) Vanillin Suppresses Metastatic Potential of Human Cancer Cells through PI3K Inhibition and Decreases Angiogenesis *in Vivo*. *Journal of Agricultural and Food Chemistry*, **58**, 3055-3063. http://dx.doi.org/10.1021/jf803366f

[40] Liang, J.-A., Wu, S.-L., Lo, H.-Y., Hsiang, C.-Y. and Ho, T.-Y. (2009) Vanillin Inhibits Matrix Metalloproteinase-9 Expression through Down-Regulation of Nuclear Factor-κB Signaling Pathway in Human Hepatocellular Carcinoma Cells. *Molecular Pharmacology*, **75**, 151-157. http://dx.doi.org/10.1124/mol.108.049502

[41] Tabassum, S., Amir, S., Arjmand, F., Pettinari, C., Marchetti, F., Masciocchi, N., Lupidi, G. and Pettinari, R. (2013) Mixed-Ligand Cu(II)-Vanillin Schiff Base Complexes; Effect of Coligands on Their DNA Binding, DNA Cleavage, SOD Mimetic and Anticancer Activity. *European Journal of Medicinal Chemistry*, **60**, 216-232. http://dx.doi.org/10.1016/j.ejmech.2012.08.019

[42] Anter, J., Romero-Jiménez, M., Fernández-Bedmar, Z., Villatoro-Pulido, M., Analla, M., Alonso-Moraga, A. and Muñoz-Serrano, A. (2011) Antigenotoxicity, Cytotoxicity, and Apoptosis Induction by Apigenin, Bisabolol, and Protocatechuic Acid. *Journal of Medicinal Food*, **14**, 276-283. http://dx.doi.org/10.1089/jmf.2010.0139

[43] Heluany, N.F., Homsi-Brandeburgo, M.I., Giglio, J.R., Prado-Franceschi, J. and Rodrigues-Simioni, L. (1992) Effects Induced by Bothropstoxin, a Component from *Bothrops jararacussu* Snake Venom, on Mouse and Chick Muscle Preparations. *Toxicon*, **30**, 1203-1210. http://dx.doi.org/10.1016/0041-0101(92)90436-9

[44] Gutiérrez, J.M., Núñez, J., Díaz, C., Cintra, A.C., Homsi-Brandeburgo, M.I. and Giglio, J.R. (1991) Skeletal Muscle Degeneration and Regeneration after Injection of Bothropstoxin-II, a Phospholipase A$_2$ Isolated from the Venom of the Snake *Bothrops jararacussu*. *Experimental Molecular Pathology*, **55**, 217-229. http://dx.doi.org/10.1016/0014-4800(91)90002-F

[45] Pereira, M.F., Novello, J.C., Cintra, A.C., Giglio, J.R., Landucci, E.T., Oliveira, B. and Marangoni, S. (1998) The Amino Acid Sequence of Bothropstoxin-II, an Asp-49 Myotoxin from *Bothrops jararacussu* (Jararacucu) Venom with Low Phospholipase A$_2$ Activity. *Journal of Protein Chemistry*, **17**, 381-386.   · http://dx.doi.org/10.1023/A:1022563401413

[46] Oshima-Franco, Y., Leite, G.B., Belo, C.A., Hyslop, S., Prado-Franceschi, J., Cintra, A.C., Giglio, J.R., da Cruz-Höfling, M.A. and Rodrigues-Simioni, L. (2004) The Presynaptic Activity of Bothropstoxin-I, a Myotoxin from *Bothrops jararacussu* Snake Venom. *Basic & Clinical Pharmacology & Toxicology*, **95**, 175-182. http://dx.doi.org/10.1111/j.1742-7843.2004.pto_950405.x

[47] Angulo, Y., Olamendi-Portugal, T., Alape-Girón, A., Hyslop, S., Prado-Franceschi, J., Cintra, A.C., Giglio, J.R., da Cruz-Höfling, M.A. and Rodrigues-Simioni, L. (2002) Structural Characterization and Phylogenetic Relationships of Myotoxin II from Atropoides (*Bothrops*) *nummifer* Snake Venom, a Lys49 Phospholipase A$_2$ Homologue. *The International Journal of Biochemistry & Cell Biology*, **34**, 1268-1278. http://dx.doi.org/10.1016/S1357-2725(02)00060-2

[48] de Oliveira, M., Cavalcante, W.L., Arruda, E.Z., Melo, P.A., Dal-Pai Silva, M. and Gallacci, M. (2003) Antagonism of Myotoxic and Paralyzing Activities of Bothropstoxin-I by Suramin. *Toxicon*, **42**, 373-379. http://dx.doi.org/10.1016/S0041-0101(03)00166-1

[49] Melo, R.F., Farrapo, N.M., Rocha Jr., D.S., Silva, M.G., Cogo, J.C., Dal Belo, C.A., Rodrigues Simioni, L., Groppo, F.C. and Oshima-Franco, Y. (2009) Antiophidian Mechanisms of Medicinal Plants. In: Keller, R.B., Ed., *Flavonoids: Biosynthesis, Biological Effects and Dietary Sources*, Nova Science Publishers, New York, 249-262.

[50] Cotrim, C.A., de Oliveira, S.C., Diz Filho, E.B., Fonseca, F.V., Baldissera Jr., L., Antunes, E., Ximenes, R.M., Monteiro, H.S., Rabello, M.M., Hernandes, M.Z., de Oliveira Toyama, D. and Toyama, M.H. (2011) Quercetin as an Inhibitor of Snake Venom Secretory Phospholipase A2. *Chemico-Biological Interactions*, **189**, 9-16. http://dx.doi.org/10.1016/j.cbi.2010.10.016

[51] Dos Santos, J.I., Cardoso, F.F., Soares, A.M., Dal Pai Silva, M., Gallacci, M. and Fontes, M.R. (2011) Structural and Functional Studies of a Bothropic Myotoxin Complexed to Rosmarinic Acid: New Insights into Lys49-PLA$_2$ Inhibition. *Public Library of Science One*, **6**, e28521.

[52] Li, C.M., Zhang, Y., Yang, J., Zou, B., Dong, X.Q. and Hagerman, A.E. (2013) The Interaction of a Polymeric Persimmon Proanthocyanidin Fraction with Chinese Cobra PLA$_2$ and BSA. *Toxicon*, **67**, 71-79. http://dx.doi.org/10.1016/j.toxicon.2013.03.005

[53] Camargo, T.M., Nazato, V.S., Silva, M.G., Cogo, J.C., Groppo, F.C. and Oshima-Franco, Y. (2010) *Bohrops jararacussu* Venom-Induced Neuromuscular Blockade Inhibited by *Casearia gossypiosperma* Briquet Hydroalcoholic Extract. *The Journal of Venomous Animals and Toxins Including Tropical Diseases*, **16**, 432-441. http://dx.doi.org/10.1590/S1678-91992010000300009

[54] Tribuiani, N., da Silva, A.M., Ferraz, M.C., Silva, M.G., Bentes, A.P., Graziano, T.S., dos Santos, M.G., Cogo, J.C., Varanda, E.A., Groppo, F.C., Cogo, K. and Oshima-Franco, Y. (2014) *Vellozia flavicans* Mart. ex Schult. Hydroalcoholic Extract Inhibits the Neuromuscular Blockade Induced by *Bothrops jararacussu* Venom. *BMC Complementary Alternative Medicine*, **14**, 48. http://dx.doi.org/10.1186/1472-6882-14-48

[55] Resende, F.A., Barbosa, L.C., Tavares, D.C., de Camargo, M.S., de Souza Rezende, K.C., e Silva M.L. and Varanda, E.A. (2012) Mutagenicity and Antimutagenicity of (-)-Hinokinin a Trypanosomicidal Compound Measured by *Salmonella* Microsome and Comet Assays. *BioMed Central Complementary and Alternative Medicine*, **12**, 203. http://dx.doi.org/10.1186/1472-6882-12-203

[56] Müller, R., Kikuchi, Y., Probst, G., Schechtman, L., Shimada, H., Sofuni, T. and Tweats, D. (1999) ICH-Harmonised Guidance on Genotoxicity Testing of Pharmaceuticals: Evolution. *Mutation Research/Reviews in Mutation Research*, **436**, 195-225. http://dx.doi.org/10.1016/S1383-5742(99)00004-6

[57] Erdem, M.G., Cinkilic, N., Vatan, O., Yilmaz, D., Bagdas, D. and Bilaloglu, R. (2012) Genotoxic and Anti-Genotoxic Effects of Vanillic Acid against Mitomycin C-Induced Genomic Damage in Human Lymphocytes *in Vitro*. *Asian Pacific Journal of Cancer Prevention*, **13**, 4993-4998. http://dx.doi.org/10.7314/APJCP.2012.13.10.4993

[58] Birosová, L., Mikulásová, M. and Vaverková, S. (2005) Antimutagenic Effect of Phenolic Acids. *Biomedical Papers*, **149**, 489-491.

[59] Stagos, D., Kouris, S. and Kouretas, D. (2004) Plant Phenolics Protect from Bleomycin-Induced Oxidative Stress and Mutagenicity in *Salmonella typhimurium* TA102. *Anticancer Research*, **24**, 743-745.

[60] Shaughnessy, D.T., Setzer, R.W. and DeMarini, D.M. (2001) The Antimutagenic Effect of Vanillin and Cinnamaldehyde on Spontaneous Mutation in *Salmonella* TA104 Is Due to a Reduction in Mutations at GC but Not AT Sites. *Mutation Research*, **480-481**, 55-69. http://dx.doi.org/10.1016/S0027-5107(01)00169-5

24

Effects of Exogenous Growth Hormone on Growth Hormone-Insulin-Like Growth Factor Axis of Human Gastric Cancer Cell

Daoming Liang*, Yi Zhang, Jiayong Chen, Hua Wang, Tao Huang, Xin Xue

Gastrointestinal Surgery Department, Second Affiliated Hospital of Kunming Medical University, Kunming, China
Email: *daomingliang@sina.cn

Abstract

Aim: To study effects of recombinant human growth hormone (rhGH) on growth hormone-insulin-like growth factor axis (GH-IGFs) of human gastric cancer cell *in vivo* in order to reveal part mechanism of growth effects of rhGH on gastric cancer. Methods: Nude mice were randomly divided into control group, cisplatin (DDP) group, rhGH group and DDP + rhGH group after human gastric cancer xenograft model of node mice was successfully founded and drugs were used for 6 days. We investigated volume of tumor, inhibitory rate of tumor and cell cycle by slide gauge and flow cytometry. In addition, We also respectively investigated insulin-like growth factor-I (IGF-I) and insulin-like growth factor binding protein-3 (IGFBP-3) of blood serum of nude mice, IGF-ImRNA, insulin-like growth factor-I receptor (IGF-IR) mRNA and IGFBP-3 mRNA of xenograft of nude mice by enzyme linked immunosorbent assay (ELISA) and semiquantitative reverse transcriptase-polymerase chain reaction (RT-PCR) on the first day of completing use of drugs later. Results: Tumor grew obviously slowly and tumor inhibitory rate obviously rose in DDP group and DDP + rhGH group compared with control group and rhGH group ($p < 0.05$), but they were not remarkably different between DDP group and DDP + rhGH group or between control group and rhGH group. Cells of gastric cancer xenograft in S phase distinctly diminished in DDP group and DDP + rhGH group compared with control group and rhGH group ($p < 0.05$), but they were not statistically significant between DDP group and DDP + rhGH group or between control group and rhGH group. IGF-I and IGFBP-3 of blood serum of nude mice obviously rose, but ratio of IGF-I and IGFBP-3 obviously lowered in rhGH group and DDP + rhGH group compared with control group and DDP group ($p < 0.05$). Expressions of IGF-I mRNA and IGF-IR mRNA were not obviously different in all groups. But expression of IGFBP-3 mRNA obviously increased in rhGH group, DDP group and DDP + rhGH group compared with control group; meanwhile, expression of IGFBP-3 mRNA also obviously increased in DDP + rhGH group compared with control group, DDP group and rhGH group. Conclu-

---

*Corresponding author.

sion: Our results indicated rhGH in short-time use did not improve proliferation of human gastric cancer cells and its mechanism was possible that rhGH in short-time use raised simultaneously IGF-I and IGFBP-3 of blood serum and increased IGFBP-3 mRNA, but degraded ratio of IGF-I and IGFBP-3 of blood serum in human gastric cancer cells.

Keywords

Human Growth Hormone, Stomach Neoplasm, Insulin-Like Growth Factor, Insulin-Like Growth Factor Binding Protein-3, RT-Polymerase Chain Reaction

1. Introduction

The effect of growth hormone/insulin-like growth factor (GH/IGF) axis on normal cells was very clear; meanwhile, many evidences manifested that GH/IGF axis promoted growth of tumor tissue [1] [2]. Furthermore, epidemiologic survey hinted that GH/IGF axis and long-term use of growth hormone (GH) were tumorigenic possible factors. But other data showed that long-term use of GH could not promote tumorigenesis [3]-[6]. Since 1996, we have always undertaken the clinical research that recombinant human growth hormone (rhGH) was applied in postoperative patients with gastrointestinal malignant tumor for metabolic intervention. We found that rhGH improved patients' rehabilitation, raised patients living quality and did not raise relapse rate and transfer rate of cancer compared with control group [7] [8]. Lots of overseas clinical data showed that hGH did not improve cancer growth and could decrease peroperative complications incidence and death rate in postoperative patients with gastrointestinal malignant tumor [9]-[13]. Our previous empirical study has also demonstrated that rhGH did not accelerate the proliferation of human gastric cancer cell line BGC823 in vitro and in vivo [14] [15]. But mechanism that rhGH did not accelerate the proliferation of human gastric cancer cell was unknown. GH should upgrade the blood level of IGF-I by promoting the transcription and expression of IGF gene. The major effects of IGF were induced by IGF-1R. 1% of IGF was free and effective in vivo, while 99% was combined with insulin-like growth factor binding protein (IGFBP). It showed that IGFBP was important to the regulation of IGF effects in vivo. We analyzed contents of insulin-like growth factor-I (IGF-I), insulin-like growth factor binding protein-3 (IGFBP-3) of blood serum and expression IGF-ImRNA, insulin-like growth factor-I receptor (IGF-IR) mRNA, and IGFBP-3 mRNA of transplantation tumor of nude mice with gastric cancer after rhGH was used in nude mice for short term. Our experiment results would reveal part mechanism of growth effects of rhGH on gastric cancer.

2. Materials and Methods

2.1. Materials

Nu/Nu nude mice were obtained from Beijing Wei Tong Li Hua experimental animal technology limited company and animal certificate number was SCXK (Jing) 2002-003. The mice were 6 wk old, with weights ranging between 15 - 21 g and they were allowed free access to the normal diets and water in specific-pathogen free laboratory in the emphasis natural drugs and pharmacology laboratory of Yunnan province China. The animal experiments were performed according to the European Community guidelines for the care and use of animals, and approved by the Animal Research Ethics Committee, Kunming Medical University. Human gastric cancer cell line MKN45 was supplied by the Cell Bank of Shanghai Cell Biology Institute of Chinese Academy of Sciences. rhGH (Saizen) was supplied by Serono (Switzerland), cisplatin (DDP) by Gejiu Biotechnology and Pharmacology Limited Company. Immunoreagent kit of insulin-like growth factor-I (IGF-I) and insulin-like growth factor binding protein-3 (IGFBP-3) was supplied by Immunodiagnostic Systems Limited, USA and 5× Reverse Transcriptase Buffer, dNTP Mixture, RNase Inhibitor, Oligo (dT) 18 Primer and AMV Reverse Primer all by Takara Biotechnology (Dalian) Limited Company. In addition, enzyme linked immunosorbent assay implement was M262154, USA. PCR implement was supplied by Biometra Company, Germany and its type was UNO-Thermoblock.

2.2. Methods

The cells of human gastric cancer cell line MKN45 were cultured in laboratory and the density of single cell suspension was adjusted to 1×10^7/L for further use. Later, cell suspension (0.2 mL) was inoculated subcutaneously into right gluteal of nude mice.

After long diameter of gastric cancer xenograft was observed to be 1.0 centimeter by measuring its long diameter and short diameter, nude mice were executed and xenograft was divided into lots of mass-their volume were $2 \times 2 \times 2$ mm^3. Then, the mass were respectively inoculated subcutaneously into right gluteal of 30 nude mice and gastric cancer xenograft models of nude mice were founded.

On the fourteenth day of inoculation, nude mice whose xenograft grew well were randomly divided into 4 groups: control group, rhGH group, DDP group and rhGH + DDP group, and 6 in each group. Later, the following drugs were administrated for 6 consecutive days: normal saline (NS) was subcutaneously injected in control group, 0.1 mL/d; rhGH group with rhGH, 2 IU/kg per day; L-OUP group with L-OHP by celiac injection, 1.3 mg/kg per day; and rhGH + L-OHP group with both rhGH and L-OHP of the same dosage as rhGH group and L-OHP group, respectively. The nude rice was killed on the first day of completing administration.

After length and breadth of tumor were measured by slide gauge, volume of tumor was computed before use of drug. On the first day of drugs completing administration, tumor was measured by slide gauge also and volume of tumor and tumor inhibitory rate was computed. In addition, the xenograft was confirmed in pathological observation by HE dyeing. Then, 1 - 1.5 mL eyeballs blood of nude mice was obtained and was centrifuged 3000 rpm/second centrifugal separation of serum 10 min, drawing the upper serum, placed in $-20°C$ refrigerator for enzyme-linked immunosorbent assay (ELISA) detection of IGF-I and IGFBP-3. ELISA detection methods include: coating, dispensing, plus HRP, substrate Yexian add color, to terminate the reaction; results found: on a white background can be a direct observation with the naked eye: the deeper the color reaction hole, the positive degree stronger negative reaction is a colorless or very light, measured by ELISA detector optical density (OD) of each hole.

Calculation formula:

$$\text{Volume of tumor } V = ab^2/2$$

(V: volume of tumor, a: length of tumor, b: breadth of tumor) [16]

$$\text{Tumor growth inhibitory rate } (\%) = \frac{\text{volume in control group} - \text{volume in experiment group}}{\text{volume in control group}} \times 100\%$$

Tissue of tumor was taken and was detected by flow cytometry and by reverse transcriptase-polymerase chain reaction (RT-PCR) after nude mice were killed on the first day of drugs completing administration respectively.

Flow cytometry procedures:

Part of tumor was made into a single-cell suspension for flow cytometry by grinding, centrifugating and washing. After fixed with 70% alcohol, the cells were kept at 4°C overnight, then, dyed with fluorescence. Finally the cell cycle was examined at 488 nm wavelength. Barlogie cell cycle assay was used.

RT-PCR procedures:

1) Extraction of total tissue RNA

1 μg RNA was taken and the first chain of cDNA was synthesized by reverse transcription. Then, according to the instruction of AMV reverse transcriptase, the liquid was shifted in 42°C thermostatic bath and incubated one hour and cooling 2 minutes in ice water in turn after it was lightly stirred and was placed for 10 minutes in room temperature. The last, the reaction product was used for PCR reaction.

2) Primer sequence and reaction condition were shown in **Table 1** and PCR carried out in the volume of 25 μl:

PCR reaction included 94°C denaturing for 3 minutes and lots of cycles which were 94°C denaturing for 30 seconds, annealing for 30 seconds, extending 72°C for 30 seconds and the last extending 72°C for 3 minutes.

3) Electrophoresis after agarose gel electrophoresis, 5 μg/mL ethidium bromide dyeing for 10 minutes and pure water flush, gel was analyzed by Quantity-One software (BIO-RAD, Hercules, CA) and was image analyzed.

2.3. Statistical Analysis

Statistics were computed using the statistics program SPSS 13.0 software (SPSS Inc., Chicago, Ill., USA) for

Table 1. Primer sequence and reaction conditions of RT-PCR.

	Primer sequence	Annealing temperature (°C)	Product (bp)
IGF-1	ATTTCAACAAGCCCACAG TCCCTCTACTTGCGTTCT	56	219
IGF-1R	CCTACAACATCACCGACCCG CCACGACCCATTCCCAGA	58	464
IGFBP-3	CCCTCTACTTGCTCGATTC ACGTGCCTACCCACCTTC	54	240
GAPDH	GGAGCCAAACGGGTCATCATCTC GAGGGGCCATCCACAGTCTTCT	62	233

Windows. Data are presented as mean ± SEM and differences among experimental groups were analyzed by one-way analysis of variance or rank test. Statistical significance was set at $p < 0.05$.

3. Results

3.1. Pathomorphology of Xenograft by HE Dyeing

We observed pathomorphology of xenograft in optical microscope by HE dyeing and we found that the tumor cells of xenograft were round, amount, big nucleus, more pathological division, multiple nucleoli, tumor cells arranging in disorder, plentiful blood sinusoid (**Figure 1**). So we thought that gastric cancer xenograft models of nude mice were successfully founded.

3.2. Volume of Tumor and Tumor Inhibitory Rate

Tumor grew obviously slowly and tumor inhibitory rate obviously rose in DDP group and DDP + rhGH group compared with control group and rhGH group ($p < 0.05$); but they were not remarkably different between DDP group and DDP + rhGH group or between control group and rhGH group (**Table 2**).

3.3. ELISA Detection

As shown in **Table 3**, IGF-I and IGFBP-3 of blood serum of nude mice obviously stepped up in rhGH group or DDP + rhGH group compared with Control group or DDP group but ratio of IGF-I and IGFBP-3 obviously lowered and there was significant difference among them.

3.4. Cell Cycle

Cells of gastric cancer xenograft in S phase distinctly diminished in DDP group and DDP + rhGH group compared with control group and rhGH group ($p < 0.05$); but there was not statistically significant between DDP group and DDP + rhGH group or between control group and rhGH group (**Table 4**, **Figure 2**).

3.5. RT-PCR Detection

Relative abundance of mRNA was accounted in accordance with glyceraldehyde phosphate dehydrogenase (GAPDH) strap which optical density value was set for 1.000. Expression of IGF-ImRNA IGF-IR and mRNA has no statistical difference among all groups, but expression of IGFBP-3 mRNA obviously raised in DDP group, rhGH group and DDP + rhGH group compared with control group and it also obviously raised in DDP + rhGH group compared with other groups ($p < 0.05$) (**Table 5**, **Figure 3**).

4. Discussions

In our experiment, we successfully founded gastric cancer xenograft models of nude mice and cancer models were confirmed by HE dying. Then, after we detected volume of tumor, tumor growth inhibitory rate and cell cycle, we thought that the short term usage of rhGH would not accelerate the growth of human gastric cancer cells and it was in accord with our earlier studies and other data [14] [15] [17]. The results lay the foundation for next study.

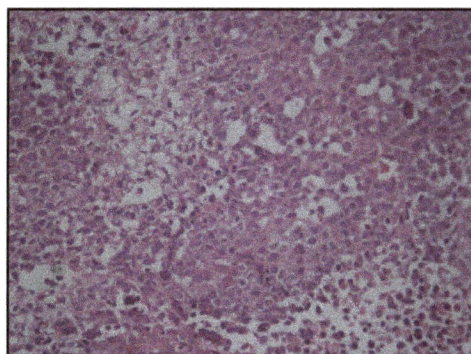

Figure 1. Pathomorphology of xenograft in control group by HE dyeing (×40). There were big nucleus, more pathological division, multiple nucleoli, tumor cells arranging in disorder.

Table 2. Volume of tumor and tumor inhibitory rate of gastric cancer before and after use of drug.

Groups	Volume of tumor before use of drug (cm^3)	Volume of tumor after use of drug (cm^3)	Tumor inhibitory rate (%)
Control Group	0.56 ± 0.35	1.54 ± 0.96	0
DDP Group	0.55 ± 0.27	$0.60 \pm 0.22^*$	60.75^*
rhGH Group	0.58 ± 0.36	1.57 ± 0.93	-0.21
DDP + rhGH Group	0.40 ± 0.22	$0.45 \pm 0.24^*$	70.76^*

$^*p < 0.05$, control group or rhGH group vs DDP group or DDP + rhGH group.

Table 3. IGF-I, IGFBP-3 and IGF-I/IGFBP-3 of blood serum of nude mice by ELISA ($\bar{x} \pm s$).

Groups	IGF-I (ng/mL)	IGFBP-3 (ng/mL)	IGF-I/IGFBP-3
Control Group	1727.3 ± 69.2	565.0 ± 106.3	3.20 ± 0.94
DDP Group	1735.3 ± 80.2	627.5 ± 176.4	2.84 ± 0.84
rhGH Group	$1916.1 \pm 93.7^*$	$1194.2 \pm 245.9^*$	$1.65 \pm 0.28^*$
DDP + rhGH Group	$1909.5 \pm 118.7^*$	$1181.7 \pm 342.8^*$	$1.71 \pm 0.42^*$

$^*p < 0.05$, rhGH group or DDP + rhGH group vs control group or DDP group.

Table 4. Cell cycle of gastric cancer after use of drug.

Groups	G0-G1 phase	S phase	G2-M phase
Control Group	66.80 ± 4.95	11.13 ± 5.33	20.03 ± 2.72
DDP Group	71.33 ± 6.23	$5.27 \pm 3.21^*$	23.37 ± 3.65
rhGH Group	66.03 ± 5.59	12.68 ± 4.41	21.28 ± 4.11
DDP + rhGH Group	69.87 ± 8.51	$5.72 \pm 2.41^*$	24.42 ± 10.65

$^*p < 0.05$, control group or rhGH group vs DDP group or DDP + rhGH group.

Table 5. Expression of IGF-I, IGF-IR and IGFBP-3mRNA in tumor by RT-PCR.

Groups	IGF-ImRNA	IGF-IR mRNA	IGFBP-3 mRNA
Control Group	0.675 ± 0.221	0.646 ± 0.282	$0.021 \pm 0.001^{\#}$
DDP Group	0.724 ± 0.224	0.681 ± 0.203	$0.283 \pm 0.103^{*\#}$
rhGH Group	0.566 ± 0.184	0.495 ± 0.212	$0.215 \pm 0.087^{*\#}$
DDP + rhGH Group	0.618 ± 0.243	0.652 ± 0.193	$0.534 \pm 0.189^*$

$^*p < 0.05$, DDP group, rhGH group or DDP + rhGH group vs control group; $^{\#}p < 0.05$, control group, DDP group or rhGH group vs DDP + rhGH group.

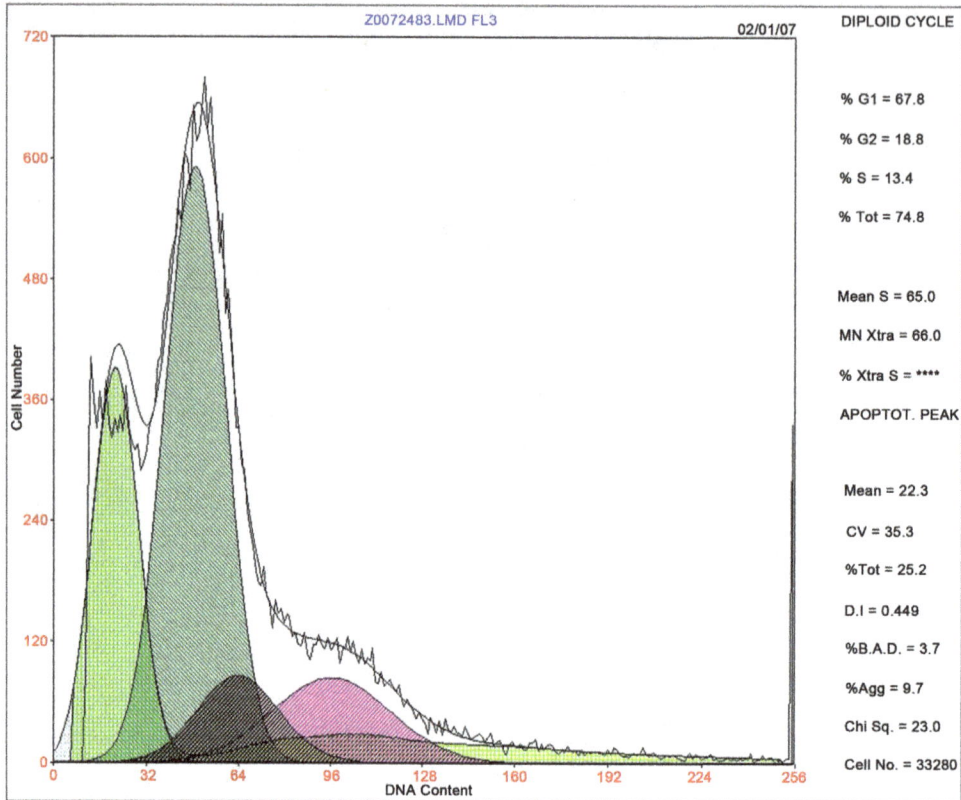

(a)

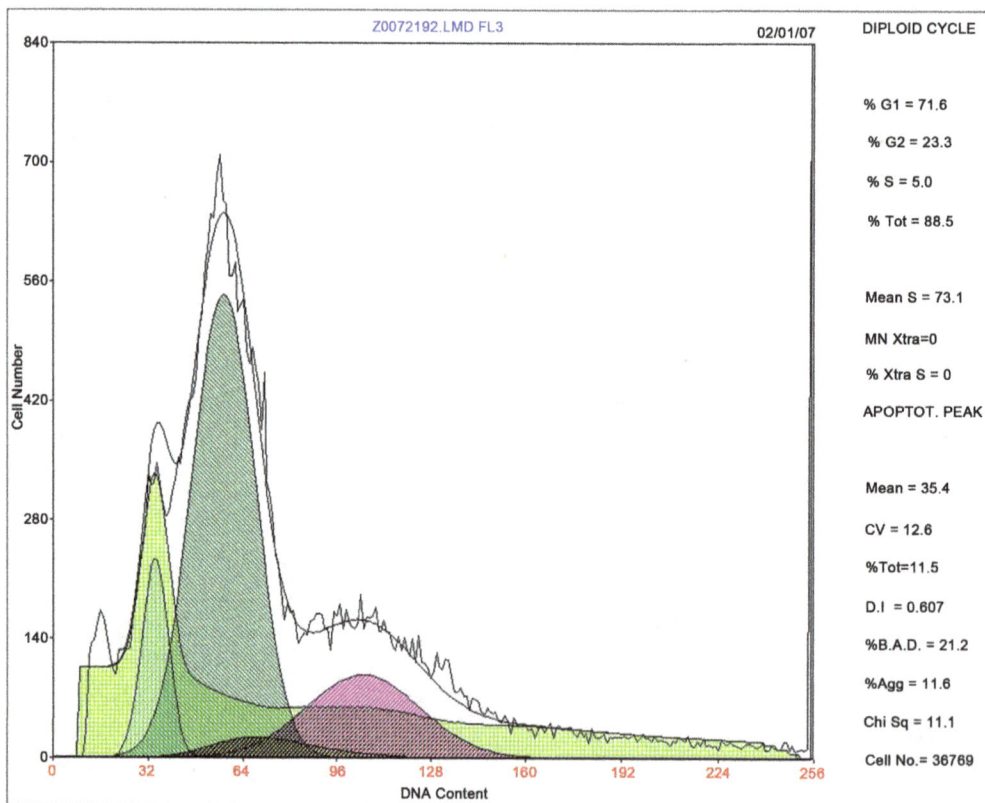

(b)

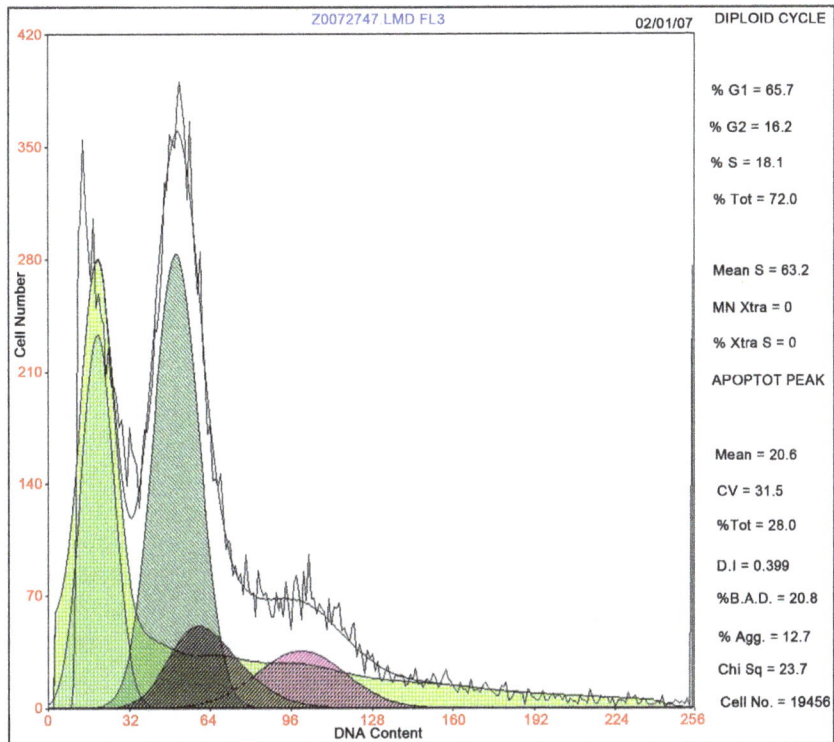

(c)

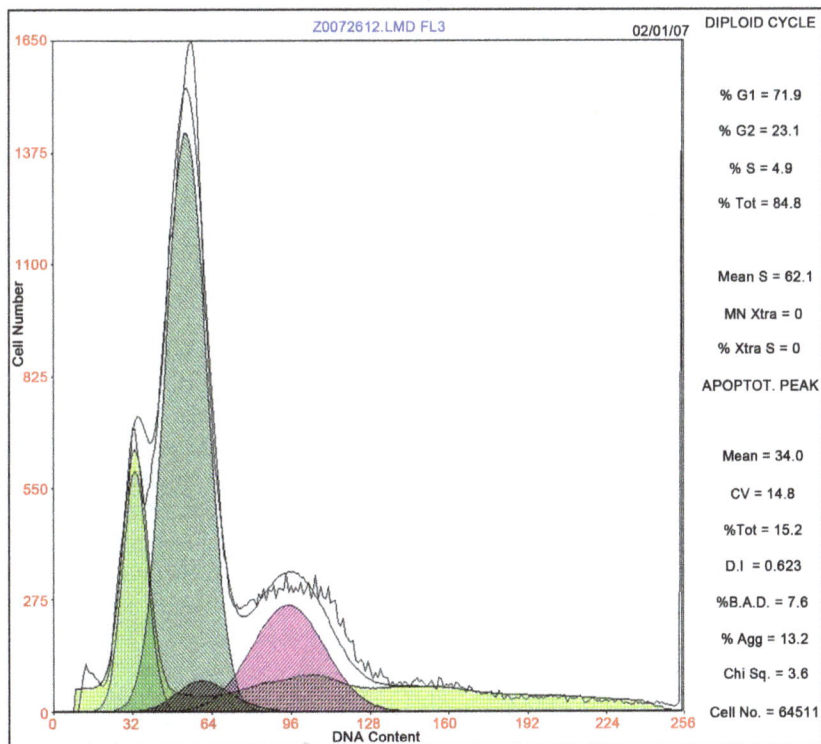

(d)

Figure 2. Scanogram of cell cycle of gastric cancer cells after use of drug by flow cytometry: (a) control group; (b) DDP group; (c) rhGH group; (d) DDP + rhGH group green stands for G0-G1 phase gray stands for S phase; pink stands for G2-M cells in S phase distinctly diminished in DDP group and DDP + rhGH group compared with control group and rhGH group ($p < 0.05$).

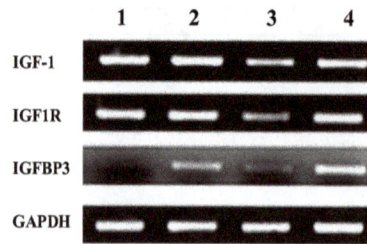

Figure 3. Expression of IGF-I, IGF-IR and IGFBP-3mRNA in tumor by RT-PCR. 1: control group, 2: DDP group, 3: rhGH group, 4: DDP + rhGH group. Expression of IGFBP-3 mRNA obviously raised in DDP group, rhGH group and DDP + rhGH group compared with control group and it obviously raised in DDP + rhGH group compared with other groups ($p < 0.05$).

The growth hormone-insulin-like growth factor axis (GH-IGFs) contains GH, IGFs, IGFR, IGFBP, and IGFBP protease. IGF-1, one of the IGFs, was effective on cell caryocinesia and metabolism. GH could stimulate liver to produce and release IGF, and there was positive correlation between the GH level and the released IGF level. Growth hormone played on its metabolic effects in directly or indirectly by IGF-I [18] [19]. Simultaneously, IGF-I mediated multiple roles of growth hormone promoting growth and synthesis [20]. Furthermore, both growth hormone and IGF-I have roles of saving lean body tissue and maintaining anabolic effect of protein synthesis [21]-[24].

The GH-IGFs acted as a strong promoter not only on cell proliferation in normal tissue but also on tumor formation, development and transference. In many prospective researches, the investigated people were distributed into different 4 groups by their IGF-I levels, and the tumor such as prostatic carcinoma, lung cancer, rectal cancer and breast cancer occurred double or triple times in the highest IGF-I level group than in the lowest IGF-I level group [25] [26]. IGF-I was detected in almost every normal tissue type, it was positive on cell proliferation and differenciation. IGF-1 was also a strong motigen in tumor tissues, and it was regarded as a messenger of GH which was related with several tumor occurrence [27]. Research has shown IGF-I to stimulate the proliferation of pancreatic [28], colon [29], and breast [30] adenocarcinoma cell lines, with blockade of the IGF-1R leading to a downregulation in growth [28] [31] [32]. Studies about breast [33] and colon cancer [34] have demonstrated higher IGF-I levels to be associated with increased risk of adenocarcinoma development. But in recent researches, it was suggested that GH should act differently in tumor tissues according to the IGF-I gene polymorphism and the tumor tissue type [35]-[37]. In addition, Shitara *et al.* found that genetic polymorphisms of IGF-I may have a substantial effect on recurrence for gastric cancer patients who have undergone curative gastrectomy [38]. Felice *et al.* thought GH action in the T47D cells was independent of changes in IGF-I and IGF-I receptor (IGF-IR) expression and IGF-IR signaling, suggesting that GH can exert direct effects on breast cancer cells [39].

IGFBP included IGFBP-1, 2, 3, 4, 5, 6 and them were separated and were identified, and IGFBP-3 was regarded as the major binding protein. In some special cases, IGFBP-3 could increase the activities of IGF-I by its self-degradation. The dual regulating mechanisms were controlled by IGFBP protease and GH *et al*. Because IGFBP was more effective than IGF-1R on binding with IGF-I, it should decrease the activity of IGF-I by the way of competitive inhibition. Besides, IGFBP should suppress cell growth directly. In tumor tissue, the level of IGF-I and IGFBP was effective on tumor occurrence, development, and prognosis, as well as the ratio between IGF-I and IGFBP. It was reported in a research of tumor-bearing mice that the tumor grew little when the mice had ingested the compound protein of IGF-I and IGFBP-3 while the protein production and nutritional status of the mice were improved apparently [40]. It was believed in part of researchers that the proper usage of GH should be related to the treatment periods and the doses of GH as well as the blood level of IGF-1 and IGFBP-3 [41]. It was reported that IGF-1 and IGF-1/IGFBP-3 molar ratio might increase the risk of cancer by increasing mammographic density [42]. In our experiment, the short term treatment of exogenous human growth hormone had increased not only the blood level of IGF-I and IGFBP-3 but also the mRNA expression of IGFBP-3 gene in tumor tissue, but had decreased the rate of IGF-I/IGFBP-3 in the mean time. The increased blood level of IGF-I and IGFBP-3 was also reported in the research of applying rhGH to the dystrophic patients who had been treated with total parenteral nutrition [43].

In the experiment, the short term treatment of exogenous human growth hormone had increased not only the blood level of IGF-I and IGFBP-3 but also the mRNA expression of IGFBP-3 gene in tumor tissue. In the mean time, the short term treatment of which rhGH had decreased the rate of IGF-I/IGFBP-3, especially when the treatment was associated with chemical therapy. In our earlier and before researches, it showed that the short term usage of rhGH would not accelerate the growth of human gastric cancer cells [13] [14]. Considering the results of both research, it should be suggested that the short term usage of rhGH would decrease the rate of IGF-I/IGFBP-3 in blood and would increase the protein level of IGFBP-3 in blood and gastric cancer tissue both, and the increased IGFBP-3 would bind with IGF-I as well as competitively inhibited the combination between IGF-I and its receptors, so it was one of mechanism of that the short term usage of rhGH would not accelerate the growth of human gastric cancer cells.

5. Conclusions

RhGH in short-time use did not improve proliferation of human gastric cancer cells and its mechanism was possible that rhGH in short-time use raised simultaneously IGF-I and IGFBP-3 of blood serum and increased IGFBP-3 mRNA, but degraded ratio of IGF-I and IGFBP-3 of blood serum in human gastric cancer cells.

Finally, we didn't do some long-term experiments about the research for death of nude mice in DDP group, and this also is the defect of our experiment.

Acknowledgements

We are grateful to anonymous reviewers for their valuable suggestions and comments. This work was supported by research grants from Natural Science Foundation of China (No. 81060114).

Conflict of Interest

The authors state no conflict of interest.

Foundation

Supported by the Natural Science Foundation of China, No. 81060114.

References

[1]   Smith, G.D., Gunnell, D. and Holly, J. (2000) Cancer and Insulin-Like Growth Factor-I. A Potential Mechanism Linking the Environment with Cancer Risk. *BMJ*, **321**, 847-848. http://dx.doi.org/10.1136/bmj.321.7265.847

[2]   Samani, A.A., Yakar, S., LeRoith, D. and Brodt, P. (2007) The Role of the IGF System in Cancer Growth and Metastasis: Overview and Recent Insights. *Endocrine Reviews*, **28**, 20-47. http://dx.doi.org/10.1210/er.2006-0001

[3]   Bogarin, R. and Steinbok, P. (2009) Growth Hormone Treatment and Risk of Recurrence or Progression of Brain Tumors in Children: A Review. *Child's Nervous System*, **25**, 273-279. http://dx.doi.org/10.1007/s00381-008-0790-6

[4]   Losa, M., Gatti, E., Rossini, A. and Lanzi, R. (2008) Replacement Therapy with Growth Hormone and Pituitary Tumor Recurrence: The Relevance of the Problem. *Journal of Endocrinological Investigation*, **31**, 75-78.

[5]   Arnold, J.R., Arnold, D.F., Marland, A., Karavitaki, N. and Wass, J.A. (2009) GH Replacement in Patients with Non-Functioning Pituitary Adenoma (NFA) Treated Solely by Surgery Is Not Associated with Increased Risk of Tumor Recurrence. *Clinical Endocrinology*, **70**, 435-438. http://dx.doi.org/10.1111/j.1365-2265.2008.03391.x

[6]   Rohrer, T.R., Langer, T., Grabenbauer, G.G., Buchfelder, M., Glowatzki, M. and Dörr, H.G. (2010) Growth Hormone Therapy and the Risk of Tumor Recurrence after Brain Tumor Treatment in Children. *Journal of Pediatric Endocrinology and Metabolism*, **23**, 935-942. http://dx.doi.org/10.1515/jpem.2010.150

[7]   Chen, J.Y., Zhang, J., Tan, J., Gan, P., Sun, M. and Chen, X.Z. (1999) Evaluation of Human Growth Hormone on Gastric and Gastric Cancer Patients after Surgery. *Chinese Journal of Base and Clinics in General Surgery*, **6**, 365-367.

[8]   Chen, J.Y., Gan, P., Xu, P.Y., Zhang, J., Tan, J. and Sun, M. (2000) Effects of Growth Hormone on Protein Catabolism and Immunologic Function of Postoperative Old Age Patients with Digestive Tract Tumor. *Chinese Journal of Gerontology*, **20**, 162-163.

[9]   Harrison, L.E., Blumberg, D., Berman, R., Ng, B., Hochwald, S., Brennan, M.F. and Burt, M. (1996) Effect of Human Growth Hormone on Human Pancreatic Carcinoma Growth, Protein and Cell Cycle Kinetic. *Journal of Surgical Research*, **61**, 317-322. http://dx.doi.org/10.1006/jsre.1996.0123

[10] Tacke, J., Bolder, U., Herrmann, A., Berger, G. and Jauch, K.W. (2000) Long-Term Risk of Gastrointestinal Tumor Recurrence after Postoperative Treatment with Recombinant Human Growth Hormone. *JPEN*, **24**, 140-144.

http://dx.doi.org/10.1177/0148607100024003140

[11] Bartlett, D.L.T., Stein, P., Torosian, M.H., Philadelphia, P.A. and Camden, N.J. (1995) Effect of Growth Hormone and Protein Intake on Tumor Growth and Host Cachexia. *Surgery*, **117**, 260-267. http://dx.doi.org/10.1016/S0039-6060(05)80199-0

[12] Beentjes, J.A., van Gorkom, B.A., Sluiter, W.J., de Vries, E.G., Kleibeuker, J.H. and Dullaart, R.P. (2000) One Year Growth Hormone Replacement Therapy Does Not Alter Colonic Epithelial Cell Proliferation in Growth Hormone Deficient Adults. *Clinical Endocrinology*, **52**, 457-462. http://dx.doi.org/10.1046/j.1365-2265.2000.00993.x

[13] Blethen, S.L., Allen, D.B., Graves, D., August, G., Moshang, T. and Rosenfeld, R. (1996) Safety of Recombinant Deoxyribonucleic Acid-Derived Growth Hormone: The National Cooperative Growth Study Experience. *Journal of Clinical Endocrinology and Metabolism*, **81**, 1704-1710.

[14] Chen, J.Y., Liang, D.M., Gan, P., Zhang, Y. and Lin, J. (2004) *In Vitro* Effects of Recombinant Human Growth Hormone on Growth of Human Gastric Cancer Cell Line BGC823 Cells. *World Journal of Gastroenterology*, **10**, 1132-1136.

[15] Liang, D.M., Chen, J.Y., Zhang, Y., Gan, P., Lin, J. and Chen, A.B. (2006) Effects of Recombinant Human Growth Hormone on Growth of a Human Gastric Carcinoma Xenograft Model in Nude Mice. *World Journal of Gastroenterology*, **12**, 3810-3813.

[16] Osieka, R., Houchens, D.P., Goldin, A. and Johnson, R.K. (1977) Chemotherapy of Human Colon Cancer Xenografts in Athymic Nude Mice. *Cancer*, **40**, 2640-2650.

[17] Lin, Y., Li, S., Cao, P., Cheng, L., Quan, M. and Jiang, S. (2011) The Effects of Recombinant Human GH on Promoting Tumor Growth Depend on the Expression of GH Receptor *in Vivo*. *Journal of Endocrinology*, **211**, 249-256. http://dx.doi.org/10.1530/JOE-11-0100

[18] Heemskerk, V.H., Daemen, M.A. and Buurman, W.A. (1999) Insulin-Like Growth Factor-I (IGF-I) and Growth Hormone (GH) in Immunity and Inflammation. *Cytokine & Growth Factor Reviews*, **10**, 5-14.

[19] Berneis, K. and Keller, U. (1996) Metabolic Actions of Growth Hormone: Direct and Indirect. *Baillière's Clinical Endocrinology and Metabolism*, **10**, 337-352. http://dx.doi.org/10.1016/S0950-351X(96)80470-8

[20] LeRoith, D. and Yakar, S. (2007) Mechanisms of Disease: Metabolic Effects of Growth Hormone and Insulin-Like Growth Factor I. *Nature Clinical Practice. Endocrinology & Metabolism*, **3**, 302-310.

[21] Hayes, V.Y., Urban, R.J., Jiang, J., Marcell, T.J., Helgeson, K. and Mauras, N. (2001) Recombinant Human Growth Hormone and Recombinant Human Insulin-Like Growth Factor I Diminish the Catabolic Effects of Hypogonadism in Man: Metabolic and Molecular Effects. *Journal of Clinical Endocrinology & Metabolism*, **86**, 2211-2219.

[22] Mauras, N. and Haymond, M.W. (2005) Are the Metabolic Effects of GH and IGF-I Separable? *Growth Hormone & IGF Research*, **15**, 19-27.

[23] Mauras, N., Martinez, V., Rini, A. and Guevara-Aguirre, J. (2000) Recombinant Human Insulin-Like Growth Factor Has Significant Anabolic Effects in Adults with Growth Hormone Receptor Deficiency: Studies on Protein, Glucose, and Lipid Metabolism. *Journal of Clinical Endocrinology & Metabolism*, **85**, 3036-3042.

[24] Shimoda, N., Tashiro, T., Yamamori, H., Takagi, K., Nakajima, N. and Ito, I. (1997) Effects of Growth Hormone and Insulin-Like Growth Factor I on Protein Metabolism, Gut Morphology, and Cell-Mediated Immunity in Burned Rats. *Nutrition*, **13**, 540-516.

[25] Shaneyfelt, T., Husein, R., Bubley, G. and Mantzoros, C.S. (2000) Hormonal Predictors of Prostate Cancer: A Meta-Analysis. *Journal of Clinical Oncology*, **18**, 847-853.

[26] Toniolo, P., Bruning, P.F., Akhmedkhanov, A., Bonfrer, J.M., Koenig, K.L., Lukanova, A., Shore, R.E. and Zeleniuch-Jacquotte, A. (2000) Serum Insulin-Like Growth Factor-I and Breast Cancer. *International Journal of Cancer*, **88**, 828-832. http://dx.doi.org/10.1002/1097-0215(20001201)88:5<828::AID-IJC22>3.0.CO;2-8

[27] Ibrahim, Y.H. and Yee, D. (2004) Insulin-Like Growth Factor-I and Cancer Risk. *Growth Hormone & IGF Research*, **14**, 261-269. http://dx.doi.org/10.1016/j.ghir.2004.01.005

[28] Tomizawa, M., Shinozaki, F., Sugiyama, T., Yamamoto, S., Sueishi, M. and Yoshida, T. (2010) Insulin-Like Growth Factor-I Receptor in Proliferation and Motility of Pancreatic Cancer. *World Journal of Gastroenterology*, **16**, 1854-1858. http://dx.doi.org/10.3748/wjg.v16.i15.1854

[29] Koenuma, M., Yamori, T. and Tsuruo, T. (1989) Insulin and Insulin-Like Growth Factor I Stimulate Proliferation of Metastatic Variants of Colon Carcinoma 26. *Cancer Science*, **80**, 51-58. http://dx.doi.org/10.1111/j.1349-7006.1989.tb02244.x

[30] Lippman, M.E. (1985) Growth Regulation of Human Breast Cancer. *Clinical Research*, **33**, 375-382.

[31] Li, S.L., Liang, S.J., Guo, N., Wu, A.M. and Fujita-Yamaguchi, Y. (2000) Single-Chain Antibodies against Human Insulin-Like Growth Factor I Receptor: Expression, Purification, and Effect on Tumor Growth. *Cancer Immunology*,

Immunotherapy, **49**, 243-252. http://dx.doi.org/10.1007/s002620000115

[32] Reinmuth, N., Liu, W., Fan, F., Jung, Y.D., Ahmad, S.A., Stoeltzing, O., Bucana, C.D., Radinsky, R. and Ellis, L.M. (2002) Blockade of Insulin-Like Growth Factor I Receptor Function Inhibits Growth and Angiogenesis of Colon Cancer. *Clinical Cancer Research*, **8**, 3259-3569.

[33] Key, T.J., Appleby, G.N., Reeves, G.K. and Roddam, A.W. (2010) Insulin-Like Growth Factor I (IGF1), IGF Binding Protein 3 (IGFBP3), and Breast Cancer Risk: Pooled Individual Data Analysis of 17 Prospective Studies. *Lancet Oncology*, **11**, 530-542. http://dx.doi.org/10.1016/S1470-2045(10)70095-4

[34] Ma, J., Pollak, M.N., Giovannucci, E., Chan, J.M., Tao, Y., Hennekens, C.H. and Stampfer, M.J. (1999) Prospective Study of Colorectal Cancer Risk in Men and Plasma Levels of Insulin-Like Growth Factor (IGF)-I and IGF-Binding Protein-3. *Journal of the National Cancer Institute*, **91**, 620-625. http://dx.doi.org/10.1093/jnci/91.7.620

[35] Cleveland, R.J., Gammon, M.D., Edmiston, S.N., Teitelbaum, S.L., Britton, J.A., Terry, M.B., Eng, S.M., Neugut, A.I., Santella, R.M. and Conway, K. (2006) IGF1 CA Repeat Polymorphisms, Lifestyle Factors and Breast Cancer Risk in the Long Island Breast Cancer Study Project. *Carcinogenesis*, **27**, 758-765. http://dx.doi.org/10.1093/carcin/bgi294

[36] Zecevic, M., Amos, C.I., Gu, X., Campos, I.M., Jones, J.S., Lynch, P.M., Rodriguez-Bigas, M.A. and Frazier, M.L. (2006) IGF1 Gene Polymorphism and Risk for Hereditary Nonpolyposis Colorectal Cancer. *Journal of the National Cancer Institute*, **98**, 139-143. http://dx.doi.org/10.1093/jnci/djj016

[37] McGrath, M., Lee, I.M., Buring, J. and De Vivo, I. (2011) Common Genetic Variation within IGFI, IGFII, IGFBP-1, and IGFBP-3 and Endometrial Cancer Risk. *Gynecologic Oncology*, **120**, 174-178. http://dx.doi.org/10.1016/j.ygyno.2010.10.012

[38] Shitara, K., Ito, S., Misawa, K., Ito, Y., Ito, H., Hosono, S., Watanabe, M., Tajima, K., Tanaka, H., Muro, K. and Matsuo, K. (2012) Genetic Polymorphism of IGF-I Predicts Recurrence in Patients with Gastric Cancer Who Have Undergone Curative Gastrectomy. *Annals of Oncology*, **23**, 659-664. http://dx.doi.org/10.1093/annonc/mdr293

[39] Felice, D.L., El-Shennawy, L., Zhao, S., Lantvit, D.L., Shen, Q., Unterman, T.G., Swanson, S.M. and Frasor, J. (2013) Growth Hormone Potentiates 17β-Estradiol-Dependent Breast Cancer Cell Proliferation Independently of IGF-I Receptor Signaling. *Endocrinology*, **154**, 3219-3227. http://dx.doi.org/10.1210/en.2012-2208

[40] Wang, W., Iresjö, B.M., Karlsson, L. and Svanberg, E. (2000) Provision of rhIGF-I/IGFBP-3 Complex Attenuated Development of Cancer Cachexia in an Experimental Tumor Model. *Clinical Nutrition*, **19**, 127-132. http://dx.doi.org/10.1054/clnu.1999.0090

[41] Cohen, P., Clemmons, D.R. and Rosenfeld, R.G. (2000) Does the GH-IGF Axis Play a Role in Cancer Pathogenesis? *Growth Hormone & IGF Research*, **10**, 297-305. http://dx.doi.org/10.1054/ghir.2000.0171

[42] Izzo, L., Meggiorini, M.L., Nofroni, I., Pala, A., De Felice, C., Meloni, P., Simari, T., Izzo, S., Pugliese, F., Impara, L., Merlini, G., Di Cello, P., Cipolla, V., Forcione, A.R., Paliotta, A., Domenici, L. and Bolognese, A. (2012) Insulin-Like Growth Factor-I (IGF-1), IGF-Binding Protein-3 (IGFBP-3) and Mammographic Features. *Il Giornale di Chirurgia*, **33**, 153-162.

[43] Justová, V., Lacinová, Z., Melenovský, V., Marek, J., Holly, J.M. and Hass, T. (2001) The Changes of IGF Binding Proteins after rhGH Administration to Patients Totally Dependent on Parenteral Nutrition. *Growth Hormone & IGF Research*, **11**, 407-415. http://dx.doi.org/10.1054/ghir.2001.0257

Permissions

All chapters in this book were first published in CM, by Scientific Research Publishing; hereby published with permission under the Creative Commons Attribution License or equivalent. Every chapter published in this book has been scrutinized by our experts. Their significance has been extensively debated. The topics covered herein carry significant findings which will fuel the growth of the discipline. They may even be implemented as practical applications or may be referred to as a beginning point for another development.

The contributors of this book come from diverse backgrounds, making this book a truly international effort. This book will bring forth new frontiers with its revolutionizing research information and detailed analysis of the nascent developments around the world.

We would like to thank all the contributing authors for lending their expertise to make the book truly unique. They have played a crucial role in the development of this book. Without their invaluable contributions this book wouldn't have been possible. They have made vital efforts to compile up to date information on the varied aspects of this subject to make this book a valuable addition to the collection of many professionals and students.

This book was conceptualized with the vision of imparting up-to-date information and advanced data in this field. To ensure the same, a matchless editorial board was set up. Every individual on the board went through rigorous rounds of assessment to prove their worth. After which they invested a large part of their time researching and compiling the most relevant data for our readers.

The editorial board has been involved in producing this book since its inception. They have spent rigorous hours researching and exploring the diverse topics which have resulted in the successful publishing of this book. They have passed on their knowledge of decades through this book. To expedite this challenging task, the publisher supported the team at every step. A small team of assistant editors was also appointed to further simplify the editing procedure and attain best results for the readers.

Apart from the editorial board, the designing team has also invested a significant amount of their time in understanding the subject and creating the most relevant covers. They scrutinized every image to scout for the most suitable representation of the subject and create an appropriate cover for the book.

The publishing team has been an ardent support to the editorial, designing and production team. Their endless efforts to recruit the best for this project, has resulted in the accomplishment of this book. They are a veteran in the field of academics and their pool of knowledge is as vast as their experience in printing. Their expertise and guidance has proved useful at every step. Their uncompromising quality standards have made this book an exceptional effort. Their encouragement from time to time has been an inspiration for everyone.

The publisher and the editorial board hope that this book will prove to be a valuable piece of knowledge for researchers, students, practitioners and scholars across the globe.

List of Contributors

Pou Kuan Leong, Hoi Yan Leung, Hoi Shan Wong, Ji Hang Chen, Wing Man Chan and Kam Ming Ko
Division of Life Science, Hong Kong University of Science and Technology, Hong Kong, China

Chung Wah Ma and Yi Ting Yang
Infinitus (China) Company Ltd., Guangzhou, China

Yongxing Yan, Lizhen Liang, Yonghui Shen and Yanjing Cao
Department of Neurology, The Third People's Hospital of Hangzhou, Hangzhou, China

Tao Xie
Department of Neurology, University of Chicago Medicine, Chicago, USA

Allah Nawaz, Saira Bano, Zeeshan Ahmed Sheikh, Khan Usmanghani and Aqib Zahoor
Research and Development Department, Herbion Pakistan (Pvt.) Limited, Karachi, Pakistan

Allah Nawaz
First Department of Internal Medicine, Faculty of Medicine, Graduate School of Medical & Pharmaceutical Sciences, University of Toyama, Toyama, Japan

Khan Usmanghani
Jinnah University for Women, Karachi, Pakisntan

Iqbal Ahmad
Baqai Institute of Pharmaceutical Sciences, Baqai Medical University, Karachi, Pakistan

Syed Faisal Zaidi
Department of Basic Medical Sciences, College of Medicine, King Saud bin Abdulaziz University of Health Sciences, Jeddah, KSA

Irshad Ahmad
Department of Pharmacy, The Islamia University of Bahawalpur, Bahawalpur, Pakistan
Clinical Pharmacy and Health Care, Jinnah University for Women, Karachi, Pakistan

Dalin Song, Tongliang Han and Hua Zhang
Department of Geriatric Cardiology, Geriatric Institute, Qingdao Municipal Hospital, Qingdao, China

Yongjun Mao, Mengfen Hu and Dalin Song
Qingdao University, Qingdao, China

Tao Tian
Department of Geriatric Cardiology, Linyi People's Hospital, Linyi, China

Bingwen Lu and Xingwei Wu
Ophthalmology Department, Shanghai First People's Hospital, Shanghai, China

Chunqing Li and Haochang Du
Nephrology Department of Wuxi No. 3 Hospital, Wuxi, China

Wei Sun and Chunqing Li
Discipline of Chinese and Western Integrative Medicine, Nanjing University of Chinese Medicine, Nanjing, China

Dong Zhou, Jihong Chen, Lu Zhang, Jiade Shao and Wei Sun
Nephrology Department of Jiangsu Province Hospital of Traditional Chinese Medicine, Nanjing, China

Liang Zhang, Changming Li and Shangju Xie
Research Institute of Orthopedics, Zhejiang Chinese Medical University, Hangzhou, China

Renfu Quan
Department of Orthopedics, Xiaoshan Traditional Chinese Medical Hospital, Hangzhou, China

Pei Yang, Xiwen Li, Hong Zhou and Hui Yao
Institute of Medicinal Plant Development, Chinese Academy of Medical Sciences and Peking Union Medical College, Beijing, China

Wei Sun and Xiwen Li
Institute of Chinese Materia Medica, China Academy of Chinese Medical Sciences, Beijing, China

Yitao Wang and Hao Hu
State Key Laboratory of Quality Research in Chinese Medicine, Institute of Chinese Medical Sciences, University of Macau, Macau, China

Hui Zhang
Development Center of Traditional Chinese Medicine and Bioengineering, Changchun University of Chinese Medicine, Changchun, China

Bingwen Lu and Xingwei Wu
Ophthalmology Department, Shanghai First People's Hospital, Shanghai, China

Hui Zhang, Xiangeng Zhang, Xiaoli Liang, Jin Gao, Qin Liu and Hongyan Wang
The School of Nursing, Chengdu University of TCM, Chengdu, China

Han Lai
The School of Foreign Language, Chengdu University of TCM, Chengdu, China

Sheeraz Siddiqui and Khan Usmanghani
Faculty of Eastern Medicine, Hamdard University, Karachi, Pakistan

Khan Usmanghani, Aqib Zahoor, Zeeshan Ahmed Sheikh and Saleha Suleman Khan
Research and Development Department, Herbion Pakistan (Pvt.) Limited, Karachi, Pakistan

Adrián Ángel Inchauspe
School of Medical Sciences, National University of La Plata, Buenos Aires, Argentina

Peng Wang and Zefeng Zhang
Department of Pediartic Orthopaedic, Nantong Rich Hospital Affiliated to Yangzhou University, Yangzhou, China

Peng Wang and Zefeng Zhang
Jiangsu ZhouKe Medical Instrument Technological Co., Ltd., Nantong, China

Tiebao Gu
Department of Pain, Nantong Convalescence Hospital Affiliated to Nantong University, Nantong, China

Huiqun Wu
Medical College Affiliated to Nantong University, Nantong, China

Dafeng Ji
Digital Medical Center, Fudan University, Shanghai, China

Hoishan Wong, Jihang Chen, Poukuan Leong, Hoiyan Leung, Wingman Chan and Kamming Ko
Division of Life Science, Hong Kong University of Science and Technology, Hong Kong, China

Shiyu Zou, Jiangping Li and Chungwah Ma
Infinitus (China) Company Ltd., Guangzhou, China

Lei Li, Clara W. C. Chan and Kwai Ching Lo
School of Chinese Medicine, The University of Hong Kong, Hong Kong, China

Oroma B. Nwanodi and Melanie M. Tidman
Department of Interdisciplinary Health Studies, A. T. Still University Arizona School of Health Sciences, Mesa, USA

Guohua Lin, Xushan Cha and Qian Li
The First Affiliated Hospital of Guangzhou University of Traditional Chinese Medicine, Guangzhou, China

Yunkuan Yang
Chengdu University of Traditional Chinese Medicine, Chengdu, China

Hongxing Zhang
Wuhan NO.1 Hospital, Wuhan, China

Lixia Li and Chuyun Chen
Guangzhou Hospital of Traditional Chinese Medicine, Guangzhou, China

Yue Liu
The Second Hospital of Traditional Chinese Medicine of Guangdong Province, Guangzhou, China

Chung Wah Ma and Shi Yu Zou
Infinitus (China) Company Ltd., Guangzhou, China

Pou Kuan Leong, Hoi Yan Leung, Wing Man Chan, Ji Hang Chen, Hoi Shan Wong and Kam Ming Ko
Division of Life Science, The Hong Kong University of Science & Technology, Hong Kong SAR, China

Simao Xu, Weichun Liu and Minhua Li
Department of Physical Education, Guangxi Normal University, Guilin, China

Bo Shuai, Yanping Yang, Lin Shen and Hui Ke
Department of Integrated Traditional Chinese and Western Medicine, Union Hospital, Tongji Medical College, Huazhong University of Science and Technology, Wuhan, China

Aref Abu-Rabia
Ben-Gurion University of the Negev, Beersheba, Israel

Ying-Fei Bi, Jing-Yuan Mao, Xian-Liang Wang, Zhi-Qiang Zhao, Bin Li and Ya-Zhu Hou
Cardiovascular Department, First Teaching Hospital of Tianjin University of Chinese Medicine, Tianjin, China

Edson Hideaki Yoshida, Miriéle Cristina Ferraz, Natália Tribuiani, Renata Vasques da Silva Tavares and Yoko Oshima-Franco
Post-Graduate Program in Pharmaceutical Sciences, University of Sorocaba, Sorocaba, Brazil

José Carlos Cogo
Serpentarium of the University of Vale do Paraíba, São José dos Campos, Brazil

Márcio Galdino dos Santos
Post-Graduate Program in Environmental Sciences, Tocantins Federal University, Palmas, Brazil

Luiz Madaleno Franco
Methodist University of Piracicaba, Piracicaba, Brazil

Cháriston André Dal-Belo
Laboratory of Neurobiology and Toxinology, Federal University of Pampa, São Gabriel, Brazil

Rone A. De Grandis, Flávia Aparecida Resende and Eliana Aparecida Varanda
Department of Biological Sciences, São Paulo State University, Araraquara, Brazil

Arturo San-Feliciano and Pilar Puebla
Department of Pharmaceutical Chemistry, Salamanca University, Salamanca, Spain

Francisco Carlos Groppo
Department of Physiological Sciences, University of Campinas, Piracicaba, Brazil

Daoming Liang, Yi Zhang, Jiayong Chen, Hua Wang, Tao Huang and Xin Xue
Gastrointestinal Surgery Department, Second Affiliated Hospital of Kunming Medical University, Kunming, China